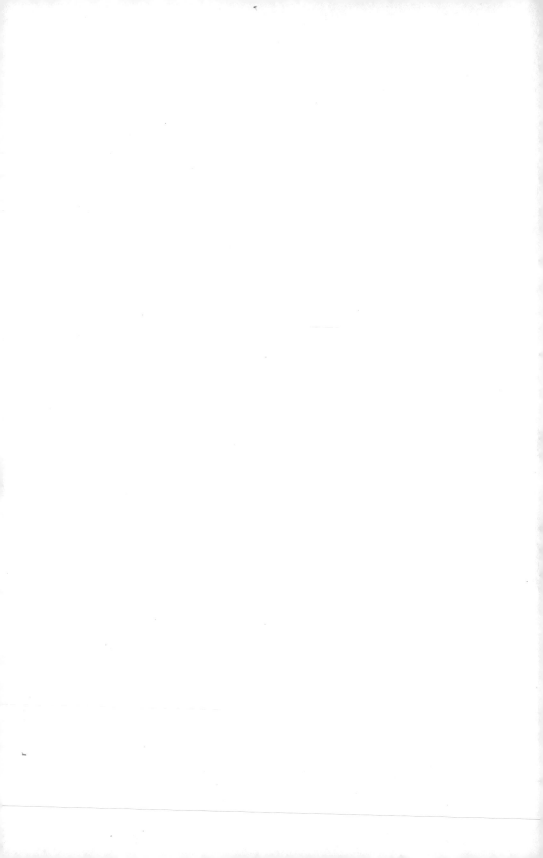

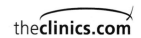

# CHILD AND ADOLESCENT PSYCHIATRIC CLINICS OF NORTH AMERICA

## Training

GUEST EDITOR
Christopher K. Varley, MD

CONSULTING EDITOR
Andrés Martin, MD, MPH

January 2007 • Volume 16 • Number 1

**SAUNDERS**

An Imprint of Elsevier, Inc.
PHILADELPHIA   LONDON   TORONTO   MONTREAL   SYDNEY   TOKYO

**W.B. SAUNDERS COMPANY**
*A Division of Elsevier Inc.*

Elsevier Inc. • 1600 John F. Kennedy Boulevard • Suite 1800 • Philadelphia, Pennsylvania 19103-2899

http://www.childpsych.theclinics.com

| | |
|---|---|
| **CHILD AND ADOLESCENT PSYCHIATRIC CLINICS** | **Volume 16, Number 1** |
| **OF NORTH AMERICA** | **ISSN 1056–4993** |
| **January 2007** | **ISBN-13: 978-1-4160-4283-9** |
| Editor: Sarah E. Barth | **ISBN-10: 1-4160-4283-0** |

*Reprints*: For copies of 100 or more, of articles in this publication, please contact the Commercial Reprints Department, Elsevier Inc., 360 Park Avenue South, New York, New York 10010-1710. Tel. (212) 633-3813; Fax: (212) 462-1935; email: reprints@elsevier.com.

The ideas and opinions expressed in *Child and Adolescent Psychiatric Clinics of North America* do not necessarily reflect those of the Publisher. The Publisher does not assume any responsibility for any injury and/or damage to persons or property arising out of or related to any use of the material contained in this periodical. The reader is advised to check the appropriate medical literature and the product information currently provided by the manufacturer of each drug to be administered to verify the dosage, the method and duration of administration, or contraindications. It is the responsibility of the treating physician or other health care professional, relying on independent experience and knowledge of the patient, to determine drug dosages and the best treatment for the patient. Mention of any product in this issue should not be construed as endorsement by the contributors, editors, or the Publisher of the product or manufacturers' claims.

*Child and Adolescent Psychiatric Clinics of North America* (ISSN 1056-4993) is published quarterly by Elsevier Inc., 360 Park Avenue South, New York, NY 10010-1710. Months of issue are January, April, July, and October. Business and Editorial Offices: 1600 John F. Kennedy Boulevard, Suite 1800, Philadelphia, PA 19103-2899. Customer Service Offices: 6277 Sea Harbor Drive, Orlando, FL 32887-4800. Periodicals postage paid at New York, NY and additional mailing offices. Subscription prices are $200.00 per year (US individuals), $302.00 per year (US institutions), $103.00 per year (US students), $227.00 per year (Canadian individuals), $356.00 per year (Canadian institutions), $124.00 per year (Canadian students), $200.00 per year (international individuals), $356.00 per year (international institutions), and $124.00 per year (international students). International air speed delivery is included in all *Clinics* subscription prices. All prices are subject to change without notice. **POSTMASTER:** Send address changes to *Child and Adolescent Psychiatric Clinics of North America*, Elsevier Periodicals Customer Service, 6277 Sea Harbor Drive, Orlando, FL 32887-4800. **Customer Service: 1-800-654-2452 (US). From outside of the US, call 1-407-345-4000.**

*Child and Adolescent Psychiatric Clinics of North America* is covered in *Index Medicus, ISI, SSCI, Research Alert, Social Search, Current Contents,* and *EMBASE/Excerpta Medica*.

Printed in the United States of America.

# CONSULTING EDITOR

**ANDRÉS MARTIN, MD, MPH,** Associate Professor of Child Psychiatry and Psychiatry and Director of Medical Studies, Yale Child Study Center, Yale University School of Medicine; and Medical Director, Children's Psychiatric Inpatient Service, Yale–New Haven Children's Hospital, New Haven, Connecticut

# GUEST EDITOR

**CHRISTOPHER K. VARLEY, MD,** Professor, Division of Child and Adolescent Psychiatry, Department of Psychiatry and Behavioral Sciences, University of Washington School of Medicine, Seattle, Washington

# CONTRIBUTORS

**THOMAS F. ANDERS, MD,** Distinguished Professor Emeritus, Department of Psychiatry and Behavioral Sciences, University of California Davis M.I.N.D. Institute, Sacramento, California

**RICHARD BELITSKY, MD,** Dean for Medical Education, Yale University School of Medicine, New Haven, Connecticut

**DEBORAH A. BILDER, MD,** Assistant Professor, Department of Psychiatry, University of Utah School of Medicine, Salt Lake City, Utah

**EUGENE BERESIN, MD,** Associate Professor of Psychiatry, Harvard Medical School; Director of Child and Adolescent Psychiatry Residency Training, Massachusetts General Hospital and McLean Hospital, Boston, Massachusetts

**MICHAEL BLOCH, MD,** Yale Child Study Center, New Haven, Connecticut

**ALLAN K. CHRISMAN, MD,** Assistant Clinical Professor, Department of Psychiatry and Behavioral Sciences, Duke University Medical Center; Program Training Director, Duke University Hospital Child & Adolescent Psychiatry Residency Training Program, Duke Child & Family Study Center, Durham, North Carolina

**JENNIFER S. COLVIN, MD,** Child and Adolescent Psychiatry Resident, Duke University Hospital Child and Adolescent Psychiatry Residency Training Program, Department of Psychiatry and Behavioral Sciences, Duke Child & Family Study Center, Durham, North Carolina

**MATTHEW R. DeJOHN, MD,** Child and Adolescent Psychiatry Resident, Duke University Hospital Child and Adolescent Psychiatry Residency Training Program, Department of Psychiatry and Behavioral Sciences, Duke Child & Family Study Center, Durham, North Carolina

**ARDEN D. DINGLE, MD,** Associate Professor, Department of Psychiatry and Behavioral Sciences; Training Director, Child and Adolescent Psychiatry, Emory University School of Medicine, Atlanta, Georgia

**MARTIN J. DRELL, MD,** Carl P. Adatto Professor of Community Psychiatry; Head of Infant, Child, and Adolescent Psychiatry, Louisiana State University Health Sciences Center; and Clinical Director, New Orleans Adolescent Hospital and Community System of Care, New Orleans, Louisiana

**MICHAEL EBERT, MD,** Department of Psychiatry, Yale University School of Medicine, New Haven, Connecticut

**FLORENCE F. EDDINS-FOLENSBEE, MD,** Department of Psychiatry and Behavioral Sciences, Child and Adolescent Psychiatry, Baylor College of Medicine, Houston, Texas

**HARRY T. ENDERLIN, MD,** Chief, Child and Adolescent Psychiatry Resident, Duke University Hospital Child and Adolescent Psychiatry Residency Training Program, Department of Psychiatry and Behavioral Sciences, Duke Family & Child Study Center, Durham, North Carolina

**ROWLAND W. FOLENSBEE, PhD,** Clinical Associate Professor of Psychiatry and Behavioral Sciences, Baylor College of Medicine, Houston, Texas

**GERI FOX, MD, MHPE,** Professor of Clinical Psychiatry, Director of Psychiatry Undergraduate Medical Education, Director of Graduate Medical Education Programming, and Special Assistant to the Senior Associate Dean of Educational Affairs, University of Illinois at Chicago, Chicago, Illinois

**DOUGLAS D. GRAY, MD,** Associate Professor, Department of Psychiatry, University of Utah School of Medicine, Salt Lake City, Utah

**GRAEME HANSON, MD,** Clinical Professor, Departments of Psychiatry and Pediatrics, University of California, San Francisco, San Francisco, California

**ANDREW HARPER, MD,** Associate Professor, Department of Psychiatry and Behavioral Sciences, Assistant Dean, University of Texas Medical School at Houston; and Medical Director, Harris County Psychiatric Center, Houston, Texas

**ELLEN HEYNEMAN, MD,** Professor, Director of Child and Adolescent Psychiatry Residency Training, Department of Psychiatry, University of California, San Diego, San Diego, California

**SHASHANK V. JOSHI, MD,** Assistant Professor, Psychiatry and Pediatrics, and Director of Child and Adolescent Psychiatry Residency Training, Division of Child and Adolescent Psychiatry and Child Development, Stanford University School of Medicine, Stanford, California

**DEBRA A. KATZ, MD,** Associate Professor of Psychiatry and Neurology; Residency Training Director for Psychiatry, Child and Adolescent Psychiatry and Triple Board (Pediatrics/Psychiatry/Child and Adolescent Psychiatry) Programs, Department of Psychiatry, University of Kentucky College of Medicine, Lexington, Kentucky

**WUNJUNG KIM, MD, MPH,** Visiting Professor, Director of Child Psychiatry Inpatient Education, Department of Psychiatry, Medical University of Ohio at Toledo, Ohio

**KERRY LEE LANDRY, MD,** Child and Adolescent Psychiatry Resident, Duke University Hospital Child and Adolescent Psychiatry Residency Training Program, Department of Psychiatry and Behavioral Sciences, Duke Child & Family Study Center, Durham, North Carolina

**JAMES F. LECKMAN, MD,** Neilson Harris Professor of Child Psychiatry, Psychology and Pediatrics, and Director of Research, Yale Child Study Center, New Haven, Connecticut

**HENRIETTA L. LEONARD, MD,** Professor, Department of Psychiatry and Human Behavior, Bradley Hasbro Research Center, Providence, Rhode Island

**ANDRÉS MARTIN, MD, MPH,** Associate Professor of Child Psychiatry and Psychiatry and Director of Medical Studies, Yale Child Study Center, Yale University School of Medicine; and Medical Director, Children's Psychiatric Inpatient Service, Yale–New Haven Children's Hospital, New Haven, Connecticut

**KYLE PRUETT, MD,** Clinical Professor of Child Psychiatry and Nursing, Yale Child Study Center, New Haven, Connecticut

**SONJA L. RANDLE, MD,** Director of Child and Adolescent Outpatient Services, Assistant Professor, Department of Psychiatry and Behavioral Sciences, University of Texas Medical School at Houston, Houston, Texas

**CYNTHIA W. SANTOS, MD,** Director of Child and Adolescent Psychiatry Residency Training; and Associate Professor, Department of Psychiatry and Behavioral Sciences, University of Texas Medical School at Houston, Houston, Texas

**ANN E. SAUNDERS, MD,** Associate Professor, Chief, Division of Child and Adolescent Psychiatry, Department of Psychiatry and Behavioral Sciences, University of Texas Medical School at Houston, Houston, Texas

**SANDRA B. SEXSON, MD,** Professor and Chief, Division of Child, Adolescent and Family Psychiatry, Department of Psychiatry and Health Behavior; and Director of Training in Child and Adolescent Psychiatry, Medical College of Georgia, Augusta, Georgia

**SAUNDRA STOCK, MD,** Associate Professor, Director of Child and Adolescent Psychiatry Residency Training, Department of Psychiatry and Behavioral Medicine, University of South Florida, Tampa, Florida

**MICHAEL G. STORCK, MD,** Assistant Professor of Psychiatry and Behavioral Sciences, Division of Child and Adolescent Psychiatry, University of Washington School of Medicine, Seattle, Washington

**VENETA STOYANOVA, MD,** Resident in Child and Adolescent Psychiatry, Oregon Health and Science University, Portland, Oregon

**DOROTHY STUBBE, MD,** Associate Professor and Director of Residency Training, Yale Child Study Center, Yale University School of Medicine, New Haven, Connecticut

**MARGO THIENEMANN, MD,** Assistant Professor, Psychiatry and Behavioral Sciences, and Director, Anxiety Disorders Clinic, Division of Child and Adolescent Psychiatry and Child Development, Stanford University School of Medicine, Stanford, California

**ANN VANDER STOEP, PhD,** Associate Professor of Psychiatry and Behavioral Sciences, Division of Child and Adolescent Psychiatry, University of Washington School of Medicine, Seattle, Washington

**NANCY C. WINTERS, MD,** Associate Professor of Psychiatry, Director of Training in Child and Adolescent Psychiatry, Oregon Health and Science University, Portland, Oregon

*Cover Artwork Courtesy of Socorro Rivera G., Mexico City, Mexico*

# CONTENTS

This article provides a summary of the history of the development
of the subspecialty of child and adolescent psychiatry and the con-
comitant development of training in the field. The historical perspective provides a context for the discussion of an overview of
child and adolescent psychiatry training in the twenty-first century.
Four challenges are identified: recruitment, funding, curriculum,
and assessment and remediation, each of which is discussed in
some depth. The article concludes with a perspective that focuses
efforts in training more on basic core competencies rather than
the rapidly expanding and changing medical knowledge and specific clinical interventions relevant to the field.

In this article we propose developmentally informed remedies to
the challenges that face research training. The initiatives described
in it have been implemented to various degrees at our institution,
and several are already being replicated or expanded through strategic partnerships across the country. We are fortunate to work in
an environment in which child and adolescent psychiatry is visible
and well represented, but we are aware that many of the settings in
which education and recruitment needs are most pressing may not
have the range of our resources. We view our different programs as

seamlessly interconnected with one another but present them as separate entities to facilitate the incorporation of different components into local realities.

## Recruitment
WunJung Kim

Child and adolescent psychiatry has long been recognized as a shortage specialty by various national studies. The workforce has never increased to the extent that meets society's demand, however. The workforce crisis has continued with declining funding for residency, declining clinical revenues, and declining recruitment of trainees. This article reviews the historical trend of recruitment, recruitment dynamics (training programs and trainees), workforce models, and future direction. It concludes with hope and excitement in the field for recruitment, including the American Academy of Child and Adolescent Psychiatry's 10-year recruitment initiative that has been generating the support of medical/psychiatric educators, governmental agencies, and the public at large to improve the profession's recruitment efforts to provide access to quality care and needed services to the nation's children and adolescents and their families.

## Triple Board Training and New "Portals" into Child Psychiatry Training
Douglas D. Gray, Deborah A. Bilder, Henrietta L. Leonard, and Thomas F. Anders

Originally an experiment in medical education, the triple board program has established itself as a permanent and successful training program. It offers a viable 5-year alternative to the traditional 7 to 8 years of residency training required for board eligibility in pediatrics, general psychiatry, and child and adolescent psychiatry. One primary objective of the creation of this program was to address the workforce shortage of child psychiatrists by recruiting medical students who may have otherwise pursued general pediatrics. The second objective was to bridge the gap between child psychiatry and pediatrics by training physicians proficient in the culture, language, and content of both specialty fields. Although the shortage crisis continues, both objectives were met. The success of the triple board experiment has facilitated further consideration and support for the development of other novel training portals into child psychiatry.

## Teaching Development in Undergraduate and Graduate Medical Education
Geri Fox, Debra A. Katz, Florence F. Eddins-Folensbee, and Rowland W. Folensbee

Faculty members from three different institutions, each with long-standing experience teaching development, present strategies for teaching normal development in undergraduate and graduate medical education. This article provides an overview of licensing body requirements, teaching methodology, audiovisual and textbook resources, goals and objectives (knowledge, skills, and attitudes), and sample curricula for teaching human development to medical students, general psychiatry residents, and child and adolescent psychiatry residents. The challenges of teaching development to various groups of trainees with different required course lengths and expected levels of competency using lifespan and topical approaches are reviewed.

Psychopathology is one of the core aspects of a curriculum in child and adolescent psychiatry. Because there is no best-evidence method described for teaching this topic, an approach must be developed in each program that meets the standards set out by the Residency Review Committee and fully prepares its graduates to be competent child and adolescent psychiatrists. Methods used for teaching psychopathology may vary widely among programs and should be based on a sound educational rationale and adult learning principles that emphasize life-long, self-directed learning. This article describes an overall approach to curriculum design and expands on the use of problem-based learning as an educational method for teaching psychopathology in a child and adolescent psychiatry residency program.

This article reviews the various definitions of case formulation, differences between diagnosis and case formulation, how case formulation for the child patient differs from the adult patient, and case formulation in the context of residency training, including challenges for residents transitioning from adult psychiatry. It presents a suggested structure for constructing a biopsychosocial formulation that can be applied in a training setting. Several specialized types of psychotherapy formulation are reviewed in more detail. The article concludes with a case example of a child psychiatry resident's case formulation before and after discussion in supervision.

In this article, the authors seek to instill a readiness and enthusiasm for appreciating the manyfaceted influences in the lives and struggles of developing children and their families. A framework for clinical investigation is proposed that draws from ecologic, ethno-graphic and attributional perspectives and therein augments and extends contemporary notions of culturally competent care. This framework can be used to help illuminate the clinically-relevant geography of the child's world such as 1) health care and social welfare zones, 2) child activity zones, and 3) cultural and religious spheres of influence. Training tools and strategies are offered for building insightful, respectful and convivial co-investigator part-nerships with patients and their families.

Pediatric psychopharmacology is taught at the Duke University Hospital Child and Adolescent Psychiatry Residency Training Pro-gram within the context of an evidence-based medicine model. The basic goal of the course is to develop competence in the psycho-pharmacologic management of psychiatric problems of children and adolescents as part of a biopsychosocial/developmental model of care. Associated with this overarching goal is the demonstration of specific attitudes, knowledge, and skills. This article discusses the educational model with examples and each of these goals in depth.

Currently our field is actively involved in developing new ways to characterize and treat children and adolescents with psychiatric disorders and in evaluating the effects of our therapies. We also are beginning to examine the effectiveness of our teaching meth-ods. This article presents evidence for, ideas about, and a philoso-phy to guide individuals who are privileged to train child psychiatrists in psychotherapies. Specifically, it discusses the issues of the evidence base for diagnosis and for nonspecific and specific active elements of child psychotherapy. Evidence for methods of training is presented. The article addresses the need for supervising psychiatrists to keep abreast of developments in teaching methods so that we can best train competent, curious, and compassionate child psychiatrists.

This article documents the diminution over the past 25 years in the focus on training in psychodynamic psychotherapy in psychiatry residencies. The author contends that the diminution is currently at the point that it endangers the "holding environment" necessary for the acquisition of this valuable skill. The article also outlines societal factors that contribute to this situation and societal responses that might be taken to counteract a decline in the practice of psychodynamic psychotherapy by psychiatrists.

## FORTHCOMING ISSUES

## RECENT ISSUES

ELSEVIER
SAUNDERS

Child Adolesc Psychiatric Clin N Am
16 (2007) xiii–xv

CHILD AND
ADOLESCENT
PSYCHIATRIC CLINICS
OF NORTH AMERICA

Foreword

# Pipeline Promise

The future ain't what it used to be.

— *Yogi Berra*

Training in child and adolescent psychiatry has traditionally been cast in an apprenticeship mold, one in which the "see one, do one, teach one" formula has been a guiding and accepted ethos. It has revolved around the three core elements of didactic instruction, clinical immersion, and individual supervision. Its major aim has been to place practitioners into the workforce who are capable of providing sorely needed services, while remaining attuned to larger systems issues necessary for the smooth collaboration with schools and other stakeholders. Over the past few decades this approach has delivered on these goals and produced the nearly 10,000 specialists currently active in America. Furthermore, it has trained countless others who have since returned to their countries of origin to adapt the specialty to local needs. By setting uniform standards for education and board certification, training programs have played a critical role in sculpting the specialty and the professional identity of those dedicated to it.

Important and welcome as these accomplishments are, a self-critical and honest appraisal suggests that we have not been as successful as we should have been. Specifically, we continue to face limitations in recruitment and retention, and our workforce is much smaller than current and projected needs would demand. Perhaps most concerning when looking ahead, we may have lagged in adapting to changes in biomedical research as aggressively as we could have. It seems imperative that we do so now if we are to make major inroads in the understanding and treatment of the major mental disorders of childhood.

The challenges that we face in recruitment are largely shared with general psychiatry training, our "parent" or "feeder" specialty. Fortunately for all, the choice of psychiatry as a specialty has steadily crept up among recently graduating cohorts, and child and adolescent training has become increasingly popular and sought after. Shifting attitudes around mental illness and a gradual erosion in biased perceptions of psychiatry have brought the discipline closer to the medical mainstream, and excitement around applying new technologies to understanding and treating psychopathology

1056-4993/07/$ - see front matter © 2006 Elsevier Inc. All rights reserved.
doi:10.1016/j.chc.2006.09.007                                    *childpsych.theclinics.com*

have attracted more talented students into our fold. While we can feel optimistic about these trends, they remain modest and far from a sufficient solution.

The "casualties" that we have routinely come to see in those graduates who drift away from child and adolescent work toward more general psychiatric practice may have less to do with market pressures or clinical demands than with the late development of an "add-on" identity as a professional dedicated to working with youth. The unique challenges attendant to working with children and families can understandably lead some recent graduates to shift back to the more familiar and secure grounding of treating adults: a regression, so to speak, to earlier developmental stages. The risk may be most pronounced for trainees involved in research. In fact, a resident contemplating investigation may simply forego the additional 2 years of child and adolescent training to delve straight into the lab, thus leaving the ranks of developmental psychopathology with one fewer potential physician-investigator.

There will always be an inevitable lag between research advances and their application to clinical practice. It may well be that the most efficient remedy for this inescapable reality is in the education of a new cadre of practitioners proficient in self-directed learning, conversant in research and methodology, and above all, flexible in the face of a rapidly changing scientific landscape. The child psychiatry that will be practiced a few years hence will have even less to do with the one we practice today than this one has with that of our forebears a few decades ago. Just as we marvel today at the evocative clinical descriptions of Winnicott and other seminal founders, and hard pressed as we are to imagine their child psychiatry practiced without psychotropics, our trainees may all too soon look back from their genomic maps, brain images, and electronic medical records to the quaint old days of 2007. We should relish the opportunity to be one-upped: to look forward to our myths being debunked and our limitations overcome by our students. We should not cower under the threat of our obsolescence: we should embrace our past and our present selves, but remain committed to a brighter future.

This issue of the *Clinics* distills the best of today's child and adolescent psychiatry training. It includes novel approaches to teaching specific skills, to monitoring progress and to remedying deficiencies. It provides roadmaps not only for the way we train today, but for how we may come to adapt education in the years to come. I am grateful to Chris Varley for organizing this issue and for bringing together its exceptional cast of contributing authors.

Like them, we should all take pleasure in recognizing ourselves in our trainees. But we should perhaps be even more excited and hopeful when seeing in them something new and hitherto unknown, something difficult to understand and incorporate into our practice and professional sense of self. Trainees should push the limits and boundaries of our comfort zones.

Training should not only reflect and keep up with advances in our field—it should help define and propel them.

We must shift our emphasis away from shepherding our trainees from one requirement or rotation safely onto the next. If we are to deliver on the latent promise of our discipline, we must train a new generation capable of redefining it. Our educational mission should be less about guiding and monitoring our pilgrims' progress than about aggressively promoting our pipeline's promise.

Andrés Martin, MD, MPH
*Yale Child Study Center*
*Yale University School of Medicine*
*230 South Frontage Road*
*New Haven, CT 06520-7900, USA*

*E-mail address:* andres.martin@yale.edu

ELSEVIER
SAUNDERS

Child Adolesc Psychiatric Clin N Am
16 (2007) xvii–xviii

CHILD AND
ADOLESCENT
PSYCHIATRIC CLINICS
OF NORTH AMERICA

# Preface

This issue of the *Child and Adolescent Psychiatric Clinics of North America* is devoted to child and adolescent psychiatry training. An overarching goal of training is to promote development in our residents of an orientation to life-long learning, with the capacity to recognize, evaluate, and then integrate new information regarding the field as it emerges, with an understanding that there are significant additions to our knowledge base every year. Teaching a commitment to the provision of quality care, provided in the context of complex systems of care and multiple other providers, is another important dimension of training, helping residents fully appreciate that all of the work that we do is imbedded in a developmental framework.

The authors who contributed to this issue are affiliated with important training programs from across the country, and many are—or have been—training directors of child and adolescent psychiatry residencies. We are fortunate to have several residents contributing to this project. Several articles are devoted specifically to recruitment, competencies, and evidenced-based medicine; however, readers will find these themes recurring within the context of numerous other articles. Training new child and adolescent psychiatrists is the life blood of our discipline, and the authors are passionate about this generative process. Entry of young people into our field invigorates the discipline and is essential to meet the pressing national mental health care needs for children and adolescents.

This issue begins with an overview by Sandra Sexson. Four sections then follow. The first section begins with consideration of entry into our field. Creative efforts at Yale Child Study Center to encourage medical students to enter into child and adolescent psychiatry are described in the article by Andrés Martin and colleagues. An article by Dr. WunJung Kim on recruitment follows. The American Academy of Child and Adolescent Psychiatry (AACAP) initiative to expand portals of entry into child and adolescent psychiatry training is described by Doug Gray and colleagues, with a focus on the triple board initiative.

The issue shifts in the second section to key foundational areas of training. This section begins with an article by Geri Fox and colleagues on teaching growth and development, which includes a description of a unique video

1056-4993/07/$ - see front matter © 2006 Elsevier Inc. All rights reserved.
doi:10.1016/j.chc.2006.09.006
*childpsych.theclinics.com*

series created by Dr. Fox. The next article reviews a key seminar for residents on psychopathology, and is written by Cynthia Santos and colleagues, who have developed a case-based curriculum.

An article follows on teaching formulation in the modern era by Nancy Winters and Graeme Hanson, along with a child and adolescent psychiatry resident, Veneta Stoyanova, recognizing that each child has an individual narrative history that is informed by diagnosis and by the child's unique history.

Teaching the critical social and societal contexts in which children live is next described in an article by Michael Storck and Ann Vander Stoep. These important systems include the ecology surrounding a child, issues on family, cultural, and ethnic identity, poverty, abuse, and racism. Specific systems that affect children are also discussed, including schools, the legal system, and foster care. Dr. Storck chairs the AACAP Work Group on Native American Children.

The third section discusses the teaching of specific treatment modalities, beginning with an article on teaching evidence-based psychopharmacology by Allan Chrisman and residents from his program at Duke, Drs. Enderlin, Landry, Colvin, and DeJohn.

Next is an article on evidence-based psychotherapy by Margo Thieneman and Shashank Joshi, followed by an article on psychodynamic psychotherapy in the modern era by Martin Drell.

The last section addresses the requirements we have to ensure that residents are fully and adequately trained. Arden Dingle and Eugene Beresin describe the current ACGME competencies. Finally, Dorothy Stubbe and colleagues review the process of monitoring resident progress and intervening when a resident has performance problems.

This issue attempts to recognize the best of the old and the new in training, with historical foundations in areas such as formulation discussed in the article by Winters and Hanson and psychodynamic psychotherapy discussed in the article by Drell. The articles venture into the modern era of evidence-based teaching, clarify training goals and objectives, and measure outcome in our trainees to ensure that at the end of their training they learn what we believe is essential and that they become competent and safe practitioners, providing the highest quality of care to children and adolescents. Proper training also should orient residents to a life-long commitment to continuing education. New pedagogical strategies are described, as are new methods for establishing that our teaching goals are met and our residents are competent.

Christopher K. Varley, MD
*Children's Hospital and Regional Medical Center*
*4800 Sand Point Way, NE*
*Mailstop W3636*
*Seattle, WA 98105, USA*

*E-mail address:* cvarley@u.washington.edu

ELSEVIER
SAUNDERS

Child Adolesc Psychiatric Clin N Am
16 (2007) 1–16

CHILD AND
ADOLESCENT
PSYCHIATRIC CLINICS
OF NORTH AMERICA

# Overview of Training
# in the Twenty-First Century

## Sandra B. Sexson, MD

*Division of Child, Adolescent and Family Psychiatry, Department of Psychiatry and Health Behavior, Medical College of Georgia, 1515 Pope Avenue, Augusta, GA 30912-3800, USA*

Training and education in child and adolescent psychiatry in the United States has developed in the modern era to prepare physicians to specialize "in the diagnosis and, if indicated, the treatment of disorders of thinking, feeling or behavior affecting children, adolescents and their families" [1]. At the beginning of the twenty-first century, even the most conservative recent estimates suggest that there are far too few child and adolescent psychiatrists to meet the needs of America's children and their families [2,3]. During the first decade of this century, training in child and adolescent psychiatry faces several challenges: (1) Recruitment: who will be trained and how we can increase the numbers of child and adolescent psychiatrists to meet the needs of America's children and families. (2) Funding: how training will be funded in the context of excessive medical student loans and decreasing funding sources. (3) Curriculum: what the core competencies are for the child and adolescent psychiatrist in an age of rapidly changing science and societal demands for physicians who are not only knowledgeable and skillful but also altruistic and dutiful [4]. (4) Evaluation: how the core competencies in child and adolescent psychiatry can best be assessed and how the field addresses the inevitable need for remediation. Within the context of these challenges, psychiatric educators may have as the primary educational objective that of training our resident physicians to adopt the concept of educating themselves throughout their professional lives to prepare future child and adolescent psychiatrists for a professional life of "lifelong learning," providing them with the skills to evaluate and, when appropriate, embrace not only modern manualized therapy, not just the most recent psychopharmacologic agent, but the next one on the horizon and the next and the next.

*E-mail address:* ssexson@mail.mcg.edu

## The historical perspective

### *Development of child and adolescent psychiatry*

Understanding training of child and adolescent psychiatrists in the modern era must begin with the understanding that the field of child and adolescent psychiatry is essentially a twentieth century development (Table 1). In the United States, child and adolescent psychiatry developed in response to the establishment of juvenile courts, the first in Illinois in 1899 [3]. Just a decade later, in 1909, a neurologist, William Healy, developed a program in Chicago to provide consultation to the juvenile court regarding psychological issues related to juvenile detainees [5]. This Juvenile Psychopathic Institute in Chicago was the first organized child psychiatry service in the United States. A few years later in 1917, frustrated by providing evaluations only, Healy and psychologist Augusta Brunner moved to Boston to set up the Judge Baker Foundation, which would provide assessment and treatment to juvenile court detainees [5]. Out of these early efforts the child guidance movement developed in the 1920s. In 1930, Adolph Meyer appointed Leo Kanner to work on integration of psychiatry and pediatrics, and Kanner called himself a child psychiatrist. Five years later he published the first textbook of child and adolescent psychiatry. Shortly thereafter more formalized training for pediatricians in child psychiatry was begun, initiating training for persons who wanted to evaluate and treat children with mental health disorders. The next decade saw the establishment of the American Academy of Child Psychiatry, which later became the American Academy of Child and Adolescent Psychiatry (1986), and the recognition of the American Board of Medical Specialties (ABMS) through the American Board of Psychiatry and Neurology (ABPN) of child psychiatry as a subspecialty of psychiatry. The field of child psychiatry was established [5,6]. Much has happened since then, some of which is chronicled in the history of training.

### *Development of training in child and adolescent psychiatry*

Like all other fields of medicine, child and adolescent psychiatry training evolved in the mid-twentieth century in an apprentice-based model, which, in many ways, continues into the twenty-first century, where working with and being supervised by experienced clinicians remains the mainstay of child psychiatric residency education. Schowalter [3] described the formal development of training in child and adolescent psychiatry, noting its roots in the early development of child psychiatry in the juvenile justice system and its evolution into the child guidance movement (Table 2). Once it became clear that psychiatrists working with children and families needed specific training beyond general psychiatry training, efforts began to formalize areas of expertise required for child and adolescent psychiatrists. In 1944, the Commonwealth Fund, a supporter of the child guidance clinic movement,

Table 1
Historical timeline for the development of child and adolescent psychiatry in America

| Date | Origins | Leader/movement/outcome |
| --- | --- | --- |
| 1909 | Juvenile justice system | Neurologist William Healy established Juvenile Psychopathic Institute in Chicago to advise courts on psychology of juvenile detainees |
| 1917 | Juvenile justice system | Healy and psychologist Augusta Brunner set up Judge Baker Foundation in Boston for assessment and treatment of juvenile detainees |
| 1921 | Chicago and Boston clinics | Child guidance clinic model, which included psychiatrist, psychologist, and social worker in treatment of children and families, rapidly expanded during 1920s |
| 1923–24 | Organized efforts to treat childhood psychiatric disorders convened by Karl Menninger | American Orthopsychiatric Association with Healy as first president—annual meetings, a journal—began to separate child psychiatry from the treatment of adults |
| 1930 | Johns Hopkins Hospital | Adolph Meyer appointed Leo Kanner to integrate psychiatry and pediatrics, and Kanner called himself a child psychiatrist |
| 1935 | Johns Hopkins Hospital | Kanner published first textbook of child psychiatry |
| 1937 | Commonwealth Fund | Supported training for pediatricians in psychiatry |
| 1945–47 | American Association of Psychiatric Clinics for Children | Set up training guidelines in child psychiatry but no accreditation |
| 1953 | Medical school academia | American Academy of Child Psychiatry was formed—very selective |
| 1959 | ABPN | Established child psychiatry as specialty |
| 1986 | AACP | Became American Academy of Child and Adolescent Psychiatry (AACAP) |

*Data from* Musto DF. History of child psychiatry. In: Lewis M, editor. Child and adolescent psychiatry: a comprehensive textbook. 3$^{rd}$ edition. Philadelphia: Lippincott Williams & Wilkins; 2002. p. 1446–9; and Schowalter JE. History of child and adolescent psychiatry in the United States. Psychiatric Times 2003;20(9).

Table 2
History of training and certification in child and adolescent psychiatry in the United States

| Date | Origin/organization | Outcome |
|------|---------------------|---------|
| 1944 | Child guidance clinics in collaboration with Commonwealth Fund | Established areas of expertise for psychiatrists who treated children with focus on development, working with children and parents, serving as administrative leaders of clinics, and working in the community |
| 1946 | Mental Health Act of 1946 | Funded training in child psychiatry |
| 1946 | American Association of Psychiatric Clinics for Children formed | Set up rigorous standard for approving clinics to train child psychiatrists |
| 1953 | American Academy of Child Psychiatry | Set up elite organization for psychiatric leaders and educators, which took over training accreditation from a more medical perspective |
| 1959 | ABPN | First subspecialty examination for certification in child psychiatry |
| 1960 | ACGME through psychiatry RRC | Essentials for child psychiatry |
| 1985 | ABPN and ABP | Innovative 5-year triple board pilot project to provide training in pediatrics, psychiatry and child and adolescent psychiatry |
| 1986 | AACP | Expanded name to American Academy of Child and Adolescent Psychiatry and ABPN and ACGME agreed shortly thereafter |
| 1992 | ABPN and ABP | Triple Board pathway approved nationally |
| 2000 | Psychiatry RRC | Established most recent update of the essentials for child and adolescent psychiatry training |

*Data from* Musto DF. History of child psychiatry. In: Lewis M, editor. Child and adolescent psychiatry: a comprehensive textbook. 3rd ed. Philadelphia: LWW; 2002. p. 1446–9; and Schowalter JE. History of child and adolescent psychiatry in the United States. Psychiatric Times 2003;20(9).

convened a group that defined the specific areas of expertise required for child psychiatrists. These first requirements identified skills common to our modern requirements (ie, a focus on growth and development of the child), which included an understanding of the psychodynamic contributions to development, an integration of work with parents and the community, and an emphasis on the child psychiatrist as the administrative leader of the treatment team [3]. Training programs were organized in several child guidance clinics. The Mental Health Act of 1946, with its funding for training in child psychiatry, bolstered the field, and the organization of the child guidance clinics, the American Association of Psychiatric Clinics for Children, set up a meticulous process that only approved approximately 50% of the training programs that applied [3]. By 1953, child psychiatry as a field had developed sufficiently to foster its own organization, the American Academy of Child Psychiatry, which initially was primarily an organization of child psychiatric educators and outstanding leaders in the field. This new organization immediately took on the responsibility of accrediting training programs, a process that moved the field into a more medically based specialty [3].

With the formalization of training in child psychiatry, recognition of child psychiatry as a subspecialty in medicine became important for the further development of the field. The controversies surrounding which field, psychiatry or pediatrics, was the most appropriate specialty group with which child psychiatry should ally continue to be debated. Leading child psychiatrists were surveyed, however, and psychiatry was chosen as the parent specialty. Still the American Board of Pediatrics negotiated a pediatrician member to the Committee on Certification in Child Psychiatry, a position that continues into the present [3]. Child psychiatrists were first certified by the ABPN in 1959. Once the subspecialty was established, the ACGME through the Residency Review Committee in Psychiatry developed standards for training in child psychiatry in 1960. These requirements, first published in the "Essentials of Approved Residencies" [7] in 1960 defined core competencies for training in child psychiatry that are not that different from the modern ACGME requirements for the specialty. These first requirements [7] focused on medical leadership by experienced child psychiatrists, diversity of patients across age, gender, socioeconomic status, and diagnosis, developmental issues from preschool through adolescence, and clinical experiences in various settings that provided opportunities for evaluation and treatment of children and their families and collaborative work with social work and psychology. Consultative work across many venues was highlighted. Supervision, no less than 2 hours weekly, was considered the cornerstone of the training process, although interdisciplinary conferences and didactic sessions were also required. These requirements, although shorter, differently formatted, and somewhat less specific, mirrored the current 2-year requirements in their basic content and aimed at preparing child psychiatry resident physicians for myriad professional activities that they might pursue as child psychiatrists.

The most recent major innovation in child psychiatry came with the 1985 collaborative project between the ABP and ABPN, the 5-year triple board pilot, which provided training in pediatrics, general psychiatry, and child and adolescent psychiatry in a somewhat abbreviated time frame. After 7 years of careful monitoring by the ABPN, this pilot program was approved in 1992 as a combined residency available to approved applicants nationwide [3]. ACGME accreditation for these programs is not yet available.

## Challenges for training in the twenty-first century

### Recruitment

For decades child and adolescent psychiatry has been perceived as a shortage area in American medicine, indeed, throughout the world [2,3,8–10]. Despite many efforts over the years to increase recruitment into child and adolescent psychiatry, the number of resident physicians per year has remained relatively stable, with a small decrease over the last two decades, and the number of accredited training programs has decreased. This subject is reviewed in detail by Dr. Kim elsewhere in this issue. There is little, if any, controversy over the undersupply of child and adolescent psychiatrists needed to meet the mental health needs of America's children, however. In 2001, the American Academy of Child and Adolescent Psychiatry designated recruitment into child and adolescent psychiatry as its top priority for the next 10 years. Obstacles to recruitment into child and adolescent psychiatry are myriad and include such issues as minimal exposure to medical students during medical school, increasing debt associated with medical school (average for child and adolescent psychiatry residents approaches $40,000) [11], long training sequence without concomitant opportunities for increased remuneration, and limited portals of entry (currently only through general psychiatry and through the modified program referred to as the "triple board") into training. Recognition of these limitations, particularly the portal of entry concerns, has sparked heated debate among leaders in child and adolescent psychiatry regarding such proposals as opening entry into child and adolescent psychiatry from fields (eg, pediatrics or even perhaps family medicine) other than general psychiatry, decreasing the amount of general psychiatry training, and abbreviated training models that would facilitate training in child and adolescent psychiatry in less than the current minimum of 5 years. It is likely that at least some of these proposals may be evaluated as pilot projects over the next decade. Proposals for shortened training during a time of burgeoning scientific knowledge in the field and rapid advances in treatment modalities present a major conundrum. The field is somewhat divided, on the one hand, trying to convince itself that shorter training periods and less general psychiatry training might entice more physicians to pursue training in child and adolescent psychiatry while recognizing, on the other hand, the pitfalls of abbreviated training, which are not likely to increase dramatically the numbers of child and adolescent psychiatrists and are likely to diminish the status of the field by diluting the training and potentially leading to a less competent workforce in the face of increased clinical demands. Whatever the outcome of this controversy, it is important that any proposed changes be evaluated carefully and any changes adequately and objectively assessed over time before general implementation.

Although there is a defined need for more child and adolescent psychiatrists, it is most important to ensure that persons designated as child and adolescent psychiatrists are highly competent to care for our nation's children, adolescents, and families. Within our current context of training, efforts at recruitment should include (1) the identification of outstanding candidates early (undergraduate, medical school, and general psychiatry residencies) and the focused nurturing of the interests of these future child and adolescent psychiatrists, (2) the improvement of the visibility of child and adolescent psychiatrists in medical student and general psychiatry arenas through research and clinical endeavors, (3) the provision of easy entry into child and adolescent psychiatry by expanding the currently available portals to facilitate entry at any level of training from post-graduate year-1 onward and increasing the numbers of truly integrated training sequences that integrate general and child psychiatry and even research in the field from the beginning, and (4) national, regional, and local efforts to improve the image and visibility of the field in public advocacy efforts that work to decrease stigma, promote parity for payment for child mental health services, and showcase our rapidly expanding science. In the meantime, it is also imperative that other obstacles to recruitment, including funding for training and improved reimbursement for clinical services provided by child and adolescent psychiatrists, be addressed aggressively. (See section I of this issue for complete discussions of issues around recruitment and entry into child and adolescent psychiatry.)

*Funding*

Funding for training in child and adolescent psychiatry continues to be a challenge for training in the twenty-first century. During the latter part of the twentieth century several factors impacted funding for child and adolescent psychiatry training negatively [2]. The National Institute of Mental Health discontinued funding for child and adolescent psychiatry training. Progress in the field resulted in deinstitutionalization of many patients, which led to a decrease in state funds for supporting training. Managed care also impacted clinical revenues and decreased funding available from such sources as faculty practice plans, private clinical practices, and psychiatric hospitals. More and more faculty are required to generate their own salaries through clinical revenues, a requirement that eliminates faculty-generated funds for training and decreases the availability of faculty for teaching endeavors. Finally, in efforts to promote primary care and decrease federal funding for training, direct graduate medical education funding has been decreased and a cap has been placed on graduate medical education positions, which has resulted in restraints on expansion of positions in child and adolescent psychiatry even when there are adequate training facilities and interested applicants. Having lost many of the traditional funding sources for training, training slots have become more and more tied to service obligations. Funding training through service obligations complicates training. If funding is limited to time served on a service, who pays for the time all residents must spend "off service" in didactics, continuity experiences, and supervision? How does a training program fund required experiences for which there is no funding source for the experience in a system in which all the funding is tied to some service?

The twenty-first century challenges the field to develop national initiatives for graduate medical education funding, especially for highly needed specialties such as child and adolescent psychiatry. The American Academy of Child and Adolescent Psychiatry and the field at large are working diligently to develop federal initiatives that loosen caps on graduate medical education positions, seek funding for specialized training, promote loan forgiveness programs for individuals who seek training in child and adolescent psychiatry, and work toward better reimbursement for child and adolescent psychiatric services. Another potential solution is the development of faculty/resident clinics to improve reimbursement of resident and faculty time. In some areas, training programs have succeeded in credentialing residents to provide services on managed care panels. This avenue may be one to pursue more aggressively in child and adolescent psychiatry because most child and adolescent psychiatry residents have achieved the level of the potential for first board certification at least by the beginning of their second year. Training programs also must look for local liaisons to provide training venues with a capability of providing funding. New opportunities must be identified to expand funding sources for child and adolescent psychiatry training. Finally, departments of psychiatry must foster faculty development programs that value teaching as a faculty effort and develop programs to reward teaching from promotion and salary perspectives. Modern training challenges will continue to require a focus on funding resources.

*Curriculum*

Curricular challenges are synonymous with training and education in any field because no effective curriculum can be static but always must be evolving. Almost 20 years ago Cohen and Dulcan [12] maintained that training in child and adolescent psychiatry must be couched in those same overarching concepts outlined in the first ACGME requirements, focusing on developmental approaches to prevention, diagnosis, treatment, and consultation. The requirements for training in child and adolescent psychiatry currently being developed by the Psychiatry Residency Review Committee continue to reflect this basic approach. Cohen and Dulcan also highlighted the necessity for programs to ensure that resident physicians learn, read, and evaluate the literature and maintain the flexibility to incorporate, as appropriate, advances into existing clinical regimens. The challenge still remains the same. Training curricula must adapt constantly to the changing face of child and adolescent psychiatry practice, incorporating new innovations while adhering to basic tenets that survive over time, tenets that ensure a developmental approach to understanding mental health issues of infants, children, and adolescents and their families. Training directors must resist capitulation to external and internal factors that potentially impact negatively on the developmental biologic, psychological, and social approach to child and adolescent psychiatry (eg, biologic reductionism and influences of managed care and other restrictions on funding) [13]. Although teaching evidence-based medicine is a lofty goal, much—if not most—of the routine work of medicine is not evidence based and must be learned where the resident physician meets the patient on a day-to-day basis through work with the patient and supervision from experienced practitioners [14]. Curricular development must focus on the core concepts that provide the foundation for our specialty and promote the development within each resident physician of a commitment to lifelong learning. The field of child and adolescent psychiatry, indeed all of medicine, is constantly changing. As Leach stipulates, "...science demonstrates that yesterday's dogma is no longer true," that science continues to approximate the truth but never quite reaches the truth. On the other hand, the art of medicine—in our case, the skills of understanding the developmental process, establishing a working relationship with our patients and our families, taking a good history, and thoughtfully putting together a formulation that helps us understand our patients deeply—is more enduring and continues to stand the test of time [14].

Specific articles in sections II and III address many issues relevant to the basic core of the specialty. A survey published in 2002 of practicing child and adolescent psychiatrists who had graduated between 1996 and 1998 suggested that they perceived their training as appropriate for their practice [15]. They identified cognitive behavioral therapy, work with complex psychopharmacology, children with complicated developmental disabilities, and areas of administration and leadership as areas in which they felt the need for more training. Many psychiatrists identified pediatric consultation and inpatient management as areas with too strong an emphasis. They identified as key their clinical experiences and their work with mentors and supervisors, reiterating the crucial influence of hands-on experiences supervised by experienced clinicians. Clearly, curricular challenges are integrally related to effective teachers and experienced clinicians who serve in didactic and clinical areas of the education and training process.

The challenge regarding curricular development has been raised to a higher level in the past decade with overt societal concerns that physicians are not prepared to meet the health care needs of America's citizens. In response to this perception, the Association of American Medical Colleges and the ACGME have developed strategies to ensure that physicians are competent, not only in knowledge and skill areas but also in attitudes that reflect altruism and duty to patients above all else [4]. The ACGME has defined core competencies for all medical specialties (described in detail elsewhere in this issue by Dingle and Beresin). All training programs will be required to define, implement, and evaluate all of these competencies [16]. Two of these competencies—medical knowledge (clinical science) and patient care—are currently recognized as specialty specific. These specialty-specific competencies involve the basic underpinnings and the changing face of child and adolescent psychiatry practice. The current tendency, one which is likely to continue over the next years, is to look at the other four competencies as generic, across specialties. The ACGME common requirements are likely to include language to which all specialties must adhere in the competencies of interpersonal skills and communication, practice-based learning and improvement, professionalism and ethical behavior, and systems-based care. The specialty may add requirements in these areas, but all specialties will be held to ACGME-defined competencies in these areas.

Training programs must work within the context of the competencies to continue to define the competencies that are necessary for a fully trained child and adolescent psychiatrist. These competencies must be chosen carefully to ensure that resident physicians have the basic skills on which practicing child and adolescent psychiatrists can continue their learning process throughout their practice lives, while adapting to the inevitable continued changes in the face of practice. The challenge is to define what the basic expertise is and ensure that all resident physicians achieve that level of competence, to offer a broad range of exposure to different experiences, and to help resident physicians embrace the competency of continued practice-based learning and improvement. The following efforts are necessary to emphasize the importance of ongoing self-directed learning to prepare the resident physician in child and adolescent psychiatry for the inevitable task of adapting to a constantly changing practice environment: more standardized journal clubs [17], focus on critical incident learning, modified morbidity and mortality conferences [14,18], focus on effective self-directed learning skills to increase intrinsic learning motivation [19], and development of portfolios to highlight the expertise of any particular resident and potentially identify areas of weakness. Instilling curiosity and the commitment to life-long learning, a major component of maintenance of certification, ensures that learning will continue after training so that child and adolescent psychiatrists will remain up-to-date in their approaches to the evaluation and treatment of their patients.

If truly "core" competencies can be defined, perhaps the field will recognize that many of these core skills can be taught in a multitude of settings, allowing training programs to use their strong venues to teach several competencies and avoid the prevalent situation in which programs must use less-than-adequate experiences because of prescribed settings for training. An example might be the teaching of consultative skills. Child and adolescent psychiatry resident physicians must have specific experiences in pediatric, school, community, and forensic consultation. Many programs find themselves struggling to provide one or maybe even two of these experiences. They must put together a rotation that may not meet their educational standards, something that also may be underfunded. If core consultative skills for child and adolescent psychiatrists can be defined, then it is likely that these skills can be taught in a particular setting and easily transferred, with minimal didactic input into other settings. This definition of competencies, not rotations, offers the opportunity for training programs to demonstrate the expertise of their resident physicians, not focus simply on the various experiences that they offer.

*Evaluation and remediation*

Although child and adolescent psychiatry training in the twenty-first century faces the various challenges outlined previously, most of the challenges have been evolving over the last one or two decades. Appropriately, the final two articles in this issue are devoted to the issues of evaluation and remediation in depth. The challenge of evaluation and, when indicated, remediation, is likely to be the most intense challenge in the coming years. The ACGME outcomes project is moving past the development of the core competencies to the implementation of these competencies, including the organized and increasingly objective evaluation of these competencies. Program directors and faculty will be held accountable for the performance of their resident physicians during training through internal resident performance data and externally through standardized in-training examinations and ABMS performance [20]. No longer will it be adequate for program directors and faculty to ascertain in writing a level of competence appropriate for a graduating resident; they will be required to demonstrate the measures used to validate that assertion. The American Board of Psychiatry and Neurology also is working with the field, considering the potential assessment during training of a psychiatry resident physician's ability to establish a relationship with a patient, conduct an interview that accesses adequate history and review of symptoms, and develop an organized and integrated presentation of these findings using a biologic, psychological, and social model. Demonstrating such competency during residency would be considered a credential necessary to sit for the ABPN examination and—ultimately—for certification in the specialty. Although specific discussions concerning the application of this model to child and adolescent psychiatry certification are preliminary and will evolve only should general psychiatry be able to resolve this issue, such consideration may occur in the not-so-distant future. Although methodology to standardize such a process across training programs has not been developed, the advantages for child and adolescent psychiatry are particularly exciting, because such a process conceivably could allow for assessment of the interview, the child and adolescent psychiatric evaluation, and integration of findings across the entire developmental spectrum, not just with adolescents, as is currently possible during the oral examination. It is also possible that resident physicians would not depend on just one assessment of these core child and adolescent psychiatric skills but possibly could have opportunities to demonstrate their competency on several occasions with a varied patient population. Such a program, however, must be well grounded in some framework of objectivity across training programs. Failing resident physicians appropriately in any of their experiences is not an established competence of most training programs at this time.

Remediation is a challenge that many programs undertake occasionally but for which no consensus has been reached. Graduate medical education remains an area in education in which many resident physicians pass through in a defined period of time, regardless of their performance, unless something egregious happens. Program directors are at a loss as how to fund remediation if it cannot be done within the context of the time frame and clinical experiences within a residency. Over the past decade, graduate medical education programs have become more aware of the dual responsibilities of program directors and faculty, the obligation to residents to help them succeed and the obligation to society to be sure that the graduated residents can practice their specialty in a safe and competent manner [21]. ACGME requirements for training in child and adolescent psychiatry require a statement from the program director in the final evaluation that attests to such competency. When program directors talk among themselves, however, it is apparent that there is a concern regarding adequate formal documentation of resident physician inadequacies. Faculty seem to be willing to talk to the program director but unwilling at times to talk to the resident or formally document their concerns about resident performance. The conundrum remains that faculty members believe that identifying incompetencies is a responsibility of the training program, that faculty seem confident that they can recognize incompetence, but that the faculty admittedly refrain from failing residents for which they have concerns [22].

Dudek and colleagues [22] have summarized their findings regarding reasons faculty seem to be unwilling to fail residents, including concerns about the onerous and ill-defined task of documenting supportable evidence of inadequate performance, concerns about the support they will receive should the resident pursue an appeal process, and the concern that remediation either would be their own responsibility or that there would be no good remediation process available to the resident. It is likely that most program directors would not be surprised with these findings. The twenty-first century challenge is to work together to deal with these resistances to adequate performance evaluations through institutional support for defining a resident's performance unsatisfactory as opposed to the all-too-common situation in which the evaluating faculty feels like they are unsupported and undermined. Dudek and colleagues [22] also suggest that program directors with the residency education committee must take on the task of remediation and make it clear to clinical supervisors that they are not responsible for developing and implementing the plan. A critical challenge to child and adolescent training programs in the twenty-first century is enabling faculty supervisors to express their true evaluations of the resident physicians by addressing the cultural and administrative issues within a training program that discourage consistent reports of poor clinical performance.

Working with resident physicians to help them evaluate their own performance successfully is another challenge that programs may face in the next decade. Critical incident learning, the development of portfolios for self-assessment and not just as a method to demonstrate best performances, provides foci to improve residency training that are being discussed actively at the ACGME across specialty training programs. Skills that allow resident physicians to evaluate themselves critically and effectively may be based on the same abilities that foster competence in their work, however [23]. Kruger and Dunning [23] suggest that making a correct judgment uses the same abilities that allow someone to recognize a correct judgment. They suggest "the incompetent will tend to grossly overestimate their skills and abilities." They also note that individuals who function lower than their peers are not effective in recognizing the competency in their peers. Finally, their work suggests that helping the incompetent to be better at self-assessment requires acquisition of more competence within their field. Given this theoretical and somewhat demonstrated framework, as program directors we may find self-assessment a good tool for our more competent resident physicians but a part of remediation for those who are less competent. Optimizing the resident physician's ability to accurately assess his or her performance should be a goal of training, because it is the basis on which self-directed life-long learning can be effective. How to do this is a challenge for the next decade. Self-assessment is a product of repeated and focused practice, a process that must be integrated into our training programs through more focused self-reflection, accurate and consistent feedback, organized approaches to learning from critical incidents, and potentially through specifically created portfolios that require guided portfolio entries to evaluate identified experiences and skills or the lack thereof [14,24].

The challenge of evaluation and remediation represents the major challenge for child and adolescent psychiatry training in the twenty-first century. If academic medicine is to survive, training programs with the program director and the faculty must assume more responsibility for the outcomes of their efforts—outcomes that may be measured by actual patient outcomes, by resident physician performance on in-training evaluations, and by graduate physician's performance on ABMS examinations. Not only must program directors and faculty maintain a commitment to the trainees but also they must prioritize a responsibility to the profession and to society to ensure that individuals who graduate from our training programs are competent to practice child and adolescent psychiatry.

## Summary

Child and adolescent psychiatry training in the early decades of the twenty-first century is faced with many challenges that are replete with exciting opportunities. Recruitment challenges may stimulate us to develop innovative training sequences and evaluate carefully alternative portals to entry into child and adolescent training while increasing visibility of the profession at all levels of secondary, undergraduate, and graduate education. Funding challenges require close collaboration between local programs, community mental health services, and ultimately advocacy efforts through state and national organizations. From a curriculum perspective, training programs are challenged to incorporate the ACGME core competencies across all educational endeavors while identifying core clinical and cognitive skills necessary for the preparation of child and adolescent psychiatrists who progress through the twenty-first century and incorporate the newest, most evidence-based interventions while ensuring that the physicians retain the commitment to duty and altruism. Finally, training programs must develop methods of evaluation that enable faculty and program directors to effectively ascertain that resident physicians acquire the core competencies necessary to provide child and adolescent psychiatric services to their patients and families. Integral to the evaluation process is a commitment to remediation when indicated, and, whenever necessary, to guiding those determined to lack the capability to function competently as a child and adolescent psychiatrist to other fields of medicine.

This modern era is truly a time of exciting advances in our field, changes that often seem to make medical knowledge, and even some clinical interventions, almost immediately obsolete. In view of our rapidly changing field, program directors and faculty may need to ensure that basic medical knowledge and clinical skills are attained. It may be even more important to focus on the underpinnings of our physician responsibilities, that is, emphasizing in our training programs those core competencies of interpersonal skills and communication, practice-based learning and improvement, professionalism, and ethical behavior. If a resident physician is able to communicate with patients and families, assessment and interventions will be facilitated. If training effectively can teach its resident physicians to embrace practice-based learning, effectively evaluate the literature and incorporate appropriate findings into an ongoing practice improvement plan, surely as practicing child and adolescent psychiatrists, they will stay up-to-date, constantly updating their medical knowledge and clinical skills. Finally, addressing issues of professionalism and ethical behavior throughout training may have the greatest impact on the competency of future child and adolescent psychiatrists. Recent research demonstrates that unprofessional behavior, particularly lack of reliability and responsibility, lack of motivation, initiative, and inability to adapt to and improve identified weaknesses, predicts future disciplinary problems during practice [25]. Behaviors that predict later problems must be recognized and addressed across faculty and resident physicians. Fostering the development of complete physicians across all these competencies is truly the goal of child and adolescent psychiatry training in the twenty-first century.

## References

[1] American Academy of Child and Adolescent Psychiatry. The child and adolescent psychiatrist. Washington, DC: American Academy of Child and Adolescent Psychiatry; 2001.

[2] Kim WJ. Child and adolescent psychiatry workforce: a critical shortage and national challenge. Acad Psychiatry 2003;27(4):277–82.

[3] Schowalter J. Recruitment, training, and certification in child and adolescent psychiatry in the United States. In: Lewis M, editor. Child and adolescent psychiatry: a comprehensive textbook. 3rd edition. Philadelphia: Lippincott Williams & Wilkins; 2002. p. 1429–33.

[4] Sexson S, Zima B, Beresin E, et al. Sample core competencies in child and adolescent psychiatry training: a starting point. Acad Psychiatry 2001;25(4):201–13.

[5] Musto D. History of child psychiatry. In: Lewis M, editor. Child and adolescent psychiatry: a comprehensive textbook. 3rd edition. Philadelphia: Lippincott Williams & Wilkins; 2002. p. 1446–9.

[6] Schowalter J. A history of child and adolescent psychiatry in the United States. 2003. Available at: www.psychiatrictimes.com/p030943.html. Accessed June 13, 2006.

[7] ACGME. Child psychiatry: essentials of approved residencies. Chicago (IL): ACGME; 1960. p. 378–80.

[8] Belfer M. Child and adolescent mental health around the world: challenges for progress. JIACAM 2006;1(1):1–7.

[9] Kanapaux W. Child psychiatry faces workforce shortage. 2004. Available at: www.psychiatrictimes.com/p040301a.html. Accessed June 13, 2006.

[10] Thomas CR. The continuing shortage of child and adolescent psychiatrists. J Am Acad Child Adolesc Psychiatry 2006;45(9):1023–31.

[11] Stubbe DETW. A survey of early-career child and adolescent psychiatrists: professional activities and perceptions. J Am Acad Child Adolesc Psychiatry 2002;42(2):123–30.

[12] Cohen RLDM. Conclusions and next steps. In: Cohen RL, editor. Basic handbook of training in child and adolescent psychiatry. Springfield (IL): Charles C. Thomas; 1987. p. 475–9.

[13] Okasha A. The future of medical education and teaching: a psychiatric perspective. Am J Psychiatry 1997;154(6):77–85.

[14] Leach D. Using assessment for improvement: it begins with experience. ACGME Bulletin 2006;4–5.

[15] Stubbe D. Preparation for practice: child and adolescent psychiatry graduates' assessment of training experiences. J Am Acad Child Adolesc Psychiatry 2002;41(2):131–9.

[16] ACGME. Outcome project. ACGME General Competencies 2000. Version 1.3. Available at: www.acgme.org/outcome. Accessed June 13, 2006.

[17] Lee A. Journal club: a tool to teach, assess and improve resident competence in practice-based learning and improvement. ACGME Bulletin 2006;20–2.

[18] Rosenfield J. Morbidity and mortality conference: a practice based learning tool for the performance improvement of residents and residency programs. ACGME Bulletin 2006;23–5.

[19] Mann K. Motivation in medical education: how theory can inform our practice. Acad Med 1999;74(3):237–9.

[20] Derstine P. Improvement through the application of the competencies: turning the challenge into opportunity. ACGME Bulletin 2006;1.

[21] Schartel S. Planning for remediation. ACGME 2006;43–5.

[22] Dudek N, Regehr G. Reluctance to fail poorly performing residents: explanations and potential solutions. ACGME Bulletin 2006;45–8.

[23] Kruger JDD. Unskilled and unaware of it: how difficulties in recognizing one's own incompetence lead to inflated self-assessments. J Pers Soc Psychol 1999;77(6):1121–34.

[24] Clay A. Fostering self-assessment and self-directed learning in the intensive care unit. ACGME Bulletin 2006;36–8.

[25] Teherani A. How can we improve the assessment of professionalism behaviors in graduate medical education? ACGME Bulletin 2006;5–7.

Child Adolesc Psychiatric Clin N Am
16 (2007) 17–43

CHILD AND
ADOLESCENT
PSYCHIATRIC CLINICS
OF NORTH AMERICA

ELSEVIER
SAUNDERS

# From Too Little Too Late to Early and Often: Child Psychiatry Education During Medical School (and Before and After)

Andrés Martin, MD, MPH*, Michael Bloch, MD,
Kyle Pruett, MD, Dorothy Stubbe, MD,
Richard Belitsky, MD, Michael Ebert, MD,
James F. Leckman, MD

*Yale Child Study Center, 230 South Frontage Road, New Haven, CT 06520-7900, USA*

"…we need to make a serious investment in training a new generation of real experts in the science and art of psychopathology. Otherwise, we high-tech scientists may wake up in 10 years and discover that we face a silent spring. Applying technology without the companionship of wise clinicians with specific expertise in psychopathology will be a lonely, sterile, and perhaps fruitless enterprise."
—Nancy C. Andreasen [1]

## Too little too late: the status quo

The shortage of specialists in child and adolescent psychiatry necessary to meet current and projected clinical demands has been recognized for more than a decade. In the United States, the American Academy of Child and Adolescent Psychiatry (AACAP) Task Force on Work Force Needs has examined some of the reasons underlying this state of affairs and proposed viable solutions to remedy it. Some of the reasons identified include inadequate support for child and adolescent psychiatry in academic institutions, limited graduate medical education funding, lower clinical revenues under

This article is supported in part by the Klingenstein Third Generation Foundation, the John and Patricia Klingenstein Fund, and an anonymous associate of the Yale Child Study Center.
* Corresponding author.
*E-mail address:* andres.martin@yale.edu (A. Martin).

doi:10.1016/j.chc.2006.07.005
*childpsych.theclinics.com*

a managed care environment, and a devalued image of the profession. By the group's conservative estimates, even if funding and recruitment were to remain stable at the current levels, there would be 4312 fewer child and adolescent psychiatrists by the year 2020 than needed to maintain the (already suboptimal) 1995 use levels [2]. The AACAP went as far as declaring in 2001 that recruitment into child and adolescent psychiatry would be its top priority for the next decade. Reflecting this commitment, two related articles in this issue of the *Clinics* by key leaders within the AACAP address innovative ways to enhance recruitment [3] and to create innovative portals of entry [4] into the profession.

Many of the efforts to enhance recruitment to date have focused on improving graduate medical education in the specialty. Paradigmatic of this approach was the creation in 1986 of Triple Board Residency Programs by the American Board of Psychiatry and Neurology. Similarly, curriculum requirement changes have been proposed to the Residency Review Committee (RRC) that are aimed at facilitating entry into the subspecialty. Welcome as these and other efforts have been in the United States and abroad, it has become clear that our recruitment efforts should start much earlier. If we are to recruit not only a greater number but also the best possible quality of physicians into our field, we must make concerted efforts to attract them into it early in their medical education.

In addition to the clinical shortage, the number of specialists involved in academic activities and research in pediatric mental health remains limited. The percentage of United States physicians engaged in patient-oriented research has declined steadily, from 4.2% in 1984 to 1.8% in 1999 [5,6]. Various reasons have been posited for this decline, including an increasing portion of students with a large academic debt, an increase in the amount of time required to prepare for a research career, and the perception by physicians that they may not be competitive with PhDs [7–11].

For psychiatry in general and for child and adolescent psychiatry in particular, the decreasing number of physician-scientists is especially problematic. Viewed in the light of challenges such as the public health costs of mental illness and addiction and opportunities to use scientific advances to improve prevention, early intervention, and treatment of psychiatric disorders, the need for psychiatrist-researchers is particularly urgent. In addition to the common concerns about personal economic disincentives and long duration of training, medical students and psychiatry residents face limitations in the availability of appropriate research education and training programs.

In 2001, the National Institute of Mental Health (NIMH), then under the leadership of Steven Hyman, asked the Institute of Medicine to convene an expert committee to study research training during psychiatric residency. The committee concluded that more intensive and better residency-based training is needed to solidify the research career interests of junior psychiatrists. After careful examination of the charge, the committee outlined several specific recommendations and identified obstacles to research training. The recommendations are summarized in the 2003 report "Research Training in Psychiatry Residency: Strategies for Reform" [12]. The report was highly critical of the currently available programs to enhance research training opportunities during psychiatric residencies.

In this article we propose developmentally informed remedies to these challenges. All of the initiatives described in it have been implemented to various degrees at our institution, and several are already being replicated or expanded through strategic partnerships across the country. We are fortunate to work in an environment in which child and adolescent psychiatry is visible and well represented, but we are aware that many of the settings in which education and recruitment needs are most pressing may not have the range of our resources. With this in mind, we encourage readers to see the programs described as models that may be implemented in whole or in parts or adapted freely, depending on local needs and resources. We view our different programs as seamlessly interconnected with one other but present them as separate entities to facilitate the incorporation of different components into local realities.

One final caveat is our exclusive focus throughout this article on child and adolescent psychiatry. Although this choice has been a deliberate one, we believe that several of these initiatives may be relevant to other disciplines involved in pediatric mental health (developmental behavior pediatrics, psychology, social work, nursing, and special education come readily to mind). We are realists and are aware that many, if not most, of the targeted medical students are not likely to pursue careers in child and adolescent psychiatry. Despite this, we believe that other positive outcomes can be expected, such as increasing the relevant knowledge base among future practitioners in other disciplines, attuning them to the mental health needs of their patients, their families, and the population at large, and providing clinical research skills generalizable to other areas of inquiry. Finally, the process is one way of providing a welcome alternative to negative socialization experiences that are generally based on outdated views of our discipline which historically have hurt our recruitment efforts and public perception [13].

### Early and often: proposed developmentally informed remedies

The initiatives that we describe are developmentally informed because they are specifically tailored for different phases of training. We begin by presenting programmatic efforts during medical school. In addition to describing them by year of training, we have divided them broadly into curricular (required) and extracurricular (optional) categories. Table 1 summarizes the different venues that we have used to increase exposure to child and adolescent psychiatry within the medical school experience at Yale. The curricular and extracurricular sections are followed by a third one that

Table 1
Opportunities for child psychiatry involvement in medical education

| Medical school year | Curricular | Extracurricular |
|---|---|---|
| **Preclinical** | | |
| *First* | Child and adolescent development in the practice of medicine<br>Interview skills: school-aged children | Mentorship program initial year: clinical exposure, mentor assigned, monthly seminars<br>Summer research projects, including funded opportunities (eg, AACAP's Jean Spurlock award) |
| *Second* | Child and adolescent psychopathology within psychiatry preclinical module<br>Interview skills: standardized patients (eg, breaking difficult news) | Mentorship program ongoing involvement or leadership year (recruit first-year students, organize seminar series) |
| **Clinical** | | |
| *Third* | Core psychiatry clerkship: child and adolescent inpatient, outpatient, emergency department, and consultation-liaison placements<br>Child and adolescent psychopathology within psychiatry clinical module<br>Interface with pediatric clerkship (eg, pediatric palliative care seminar) | Mentorship program ongoing involvement or broader leadership year (interface with AACAP and mentorship national network)<br>Attendance at AACAP annual meeting<br>Research projects or writing opportunities<br>Psych cinema or other venues for media interface and informal gatherings |
| *Fourth (± Fifth)* | Elective rotations (including at other institutions)<br>Completion (and possible publication) of thesis work | Explore postgraduate training options in child and adolescent psychiatry, including in traditional, triple board, or integrated programs |

describes undergraduate and postgraduate initiatives to maximize recruitment, particularly that of clinician-scientists dedicated to pediatric mental health research.

*Curricular initiatives*

There currently is no uniform list of learning objectives for national medical school accreditation; instead, the individual objectives are left up to the individual schools. The Liaison Committee on Medical Education of the American Medical Association provides broad educational objectives and general requirements but does not provide specific or subject-based learning objectives (http://www.lcme.org/functions2005oct.pdf). Instead, the objectives listed for the United States Medical Licensing Examination (USMLE) board come closest to providing a nationally accepted standard. In light of this, familiarity with USMLE requirements is instrumental to the development of any curricular initiative in medical school, particularly because medical students are often keenly aware of the USMLE requirements.

Box 1 presents content areas relevant to child and adolescent psychiatry, divided according to preclinical and clinical years (Steps 1 and 2, respectively).

At the Yale University School of Medicine we have been able to encompass all of these content areas through initiatives that are spread out across the first 3 years of the curriculum. These offerings are available to all students, regardless of their eventual career interests. We believe in the critical importance of educating future medical professionals in child psychiatry even if they do not pursue careers in the field. Giving future physicians a better understanding of developmental and pediatric mental health principles and an appreciation and understanding of what child psychiatrists actually do is a worthwhile effort unto itself. Interested students also can have a more self-directed experience in their fourth year, either through elective rotations (including at other institutions) or through participation in research, often conducive to the Yale medical school thesis requirement described below.

*First year*

The initial class-wide introduction to child and adolescent psychiatry comes in the spring semester of the first year, through "Child and Adolescent Development in the Practice of Medicine" (CAD), a course that has been in existence for more than two decades. CAD explicitly deals with normal development and specifically emphasizes its social, cognitive, and emotional aspects. It seeks to heighten student awareness of how different phases of development intersect with the clinical practice of medicine. Students learn about different schools of thought on development and about cognitive, language, motor, social, sexual, and interpersonal milestones, from birth through senescence. The course recognizes that it can be challenging for rookie medical students to understand the importance of these normative processes in a clinical vacuum and addresses this challenge by putting normal processes within the context of what happens when they become derailed. With this in mind, the course is constructed as a complement of traditional lectures delivered in the first hour and clinical applications of that developmental phase in the second hour. The schedule for the16-hour course for the 2006 academic year is presented in Table 2.

The specifics of this schedule are not likely to be easily generalizable to other medical schools, because it has been crafted partially around our own colleagues' areas of expertise (eg, prenatal cocaine exposure [14,15], novel gene-finding techniques [16], and disorders that involve disrupted signaling pathways [17]). We choose to include the schedule as a specific example of our approach and to highlight some of the underlying themes guiding it. We believe that in contrast to the specifics of the curriculum, the following general principles can be generalizable and inform adaptations to local ecologies and faculty areas of expertise.

*Early exposure.* When it occurs at all, exposure to child and adolescent psychiatry typically takes place in medical school during the clinical years.

**Box 1. Content areas relevant to child and adolescent psychiatry covered in the United States Medical Licensure Examination (USMLE)**

*Step 1: Basic sciences: gender, ethnic, and behavioral considerations that affect disease treatment and prevention, including psychosocial, cultural, occupational, and environmental*

- Progression through the life cycle, including birth through senescence
  Cognitive, language, motor skills, and social and interpersonal development
  Sexual development (eg, puberty, menopause)
  Influence of developmental stage on physician-patient interview
- Psychological and social factors that influence patient behavior
  Personality traits or coping style, including coping mechanisms
  Psychodynamic and behavioral factors, related past experience
  Family and cultural factors, including socioeconomic status, ethnicity, and gender
  Adaptive and maladaptive behavioral responses to stress and illness (eg, drug-seeking behavior, sleep deprivation)
  Interactions between the patient and the physician or the health care system (eg, transference)
  Patient adherence, including general and adolescent
- Patient interviewing, consultation, and interactions with the family
  Establishing and maintaining rapport
  Data gathering
  Approaches to patient education
  Enticing patients to make lifestyle changes
  Communicating bad news
  Difficult interviews (eg, anxious or angry patients)
  Multicultural ethnic characteristics
- Medical ethics, jurisprudence, and professional behavior
  Consent and informed consent to treatment
  Physician-patient relationships (eg, ethical conduct, confidentiality)
  Death and dying
  Birth-related issues
  Issues related to patient participation in research
  Interactions with other health professionals (eg, referral)
  Sexuality and the profession; other boundary issues

Ethics of managed care
Organization and cost of health care delivery

*Step 2: Clinical sciences: mental disorders*
- Health and health maintenance
Early identification and intervention (eg, suicide potential, depression, alcohol/substance abuse, family involvement in schizophrenia)
- Mechanisms of disease
Biologic markers of mental disorders and mental retardation syndromes
Intended/unintended effects of therapeutic interventions, including effects of drugs on neurotransmitters
- Diagnosis
Mental disorders usually first diagnosed in infancy, childhood, or adolescence (eg, mental retardation, communication disorders, pervasive developmental disorders, attention deficit hyperactivity disorder, disruptive disorders, tic disorders, elimination disorders)
Substance-related disorders (eg, alcohol and other substances)
Schizophrenia and other psychotic disorders
Mood disorders (eg, bipolar disorders, major unipolar depressive disorders, dysthymic disorder, mood disorder caused by a general medical condition, medication-induced mood disorder)
Anxiety disorders (eg, panic disorder, phobia, obsessive-compulsive disorder, posttraumatic stress disorder, generalized anxiety disorder, acute stress disorder, separation anxiety disorder, anxiety caused by a general medical condition, substance-induced anxiety disorder)
Somatoform disorders (eg, factitious disorder, somatization disorder, pain disorder, conversion disorder, hypochondriasis)
Other disorders/conditions (eg, sexual and gender identity disorders, personality disorders, child, spouse, elder abuse, eating disorders, adjustment disorders, dissociative disorders, psychological factors that affect medical conditions)
- Principles of management (with emphasis on topics covered in section on diagnosis)
Pharmacotherapy only
Management decision (treatment/diagnosis steps)
Treatment only

*Adapted from* the USMLE website: http://www.usmle.org/.

Table 2
Child and adolescent development in the practice of medicine course schedule for 2006

| Session | Lecture | Clinical correlation (and select references) |
|---|---|---|
| 1 | Introduction to the course: development across the life cycle; overview of major stages and approaches; relevance to the practice of medicine | Autism and its early detection [43,44,46] |
| 2 | Pregnancy, infancy, and toddlerhood | Research on early-life strains: in utero cocaine exposure and puerperal depression as paradigms [14,15] |
| 3 | Preschool and school age | Daycare, divorce, adoption [47] |
| 4 | Adolescence and beyond | Genetics of neurodevelopmental and childhood psychiatric disorders: obsessive-compulsive disorder [16,48] |
| 5 | Molecular mechanisms underlying learning and memory | Fragile X, Prader Willi, and disorders involving disrupted signaling pathways (eg, neurofibromatosis) [17] |
| 6 | Putting clinical cases together: formulation and integration: attention, mood, and somatoform disorders | Trauma across the life cycle [49] |
| 7 | Psychosocial aspects of chronic and terminal illness | Death and dying in childhood; pediatric palliative care [50] |
| 8 | *Kid Flicks:* a video-based review of course highlights and omissions | *Kid Flicks,* Part 2 [20] |
| Optional | Small group patient interviews | |

We believe that this timing is too late for any substantial change in knowledge, socialization, or career trajectory changes to occur. The most important principle that we espouse throughout all of our initiatives is that of reversing this trend by exposing students to our field as early as possible. To this end, we are fortunate to have the curriculum-sanctioned platform of CAD and encourage others to seek out spots in their preclinical curricula in which similar exposure may take place in a systematic and routine fashion, even if not through as lengthy, organized, or full-fledged a course.

*Differentiation from, and collaboration with, general psychiatry and pediatrics.* Faculty members from general psychiatry and pediatrics are more likely to have regular contact with students during their preclinical years. It behooves child and adolescent psychiatry faculty committed to education reform to establish bridges and working relationships with these colleagues and to contribute to a shared teaching mission. Our colleagues in these disciplines are likely to be welcoming and encouraging of our participation, but unless we let ourselves be known as available and interested, we may not be asked to participate. An assertive yet collegial approach is one way of increasing the visibility of our field within the preclinical years. As a specific case in point, session 7 of the CAD curriculum (chronic and terminal illness, death and pediatric palliative care) deals with issues that could as easily 'belong' to pediatrics.

*Balancing normal and derailed development.* Despite the intuitive appeal to do so, our early efforts to teach normal development in the preclinical years and leave pathology to the clinical years did not meet with much success. Students often complained about normal development being self-evident at best and irrelevant to their future as physicians at worst. More importantly, however, these comments, which may well have been outliers, provided a general sense that normal development and psychopathology were not organically connected, which left our preclinical and clinical efforts dislocated from each other. With this feedback and experience in mind, we have moved to introducing clinical applications and correlations from the outset. This approach has had the additional and welcome effect of engaging students with the patient contact that they are so intrigued about and impatient for. As an example, social referencing and stranger anxiety are abstract concepts that can be hard to grasp. However, by presenting them in the context of children with autism who have not reached these milestones normally, the terms and their critical importance become more apparent and relevant.

*Balancing the 'hard' and 'soft' sides of child psychiatry.* We are well aware of how common preconceived notions or misinformation about psychiatry in general—and child and adolescent psychiatry in particular—continue to be, even among as sophisticated and educated a group of students. Given this reality, we see an ambassadorial mission as integral to CAD and other early exposures to our field. One of the most ingrained and recalcitrant misconceptions deals with the soft, nonmedical, or unscientific nature of the field. We explicitly exploit these prejudicial views by presenting some of the more advanced and cutting edge areas of our research portfolio as part of the lecture series (see the clinical correlation references in Table 2). By doing so we not only have helped dispel myths and inform students about ongoing areas of research but also usually ended up recruiting students into these efforts along the way. Concretely, many of the students who produced theses with us were initially recruited during their exposure to child psychiatry in CAD. Conversely, students immersed in the book- and lab-heavy preclinical years have come to deeply appreciate the softer and clinically textured parts of the course—sections that rely on exposing them to clinical encounters across the lifespan and different interview styles, techniques, and ways of coherently organizing clinical data.

*Live interviews, formulation, and integration.* As an optional offering of the course, students are invited to the inpatient unit to attend patient interviews as small groups of four or five. We have opted for this approach over earlier efforts to conduct live interviews in front of the entire class. The latter approach was logistically complex, and children's and families' responses were often hard to predict or adapt to. By contrast, the self-selected small groups allow for a more intimate and clinically intensive experience, give students a legitimate sense of being in a real clinical situation, and allow for the application, in real time, of another core aspect of the course, namely its emphasis on clinical formulation and integration. Two of the last sessions in the course (6 and 8) are devoted to providing students with ways of approaching clinical complexity in an organized fashion. We do so by briefly reviewing different approaches to formulation, such as the biopsychosocial model [18], the 4 Ps (*P*redisposing, *P*recipitating, *P*erpetuating and *P*rotective factors), or the Four Perspectives model (diagnosis, dimension, behavior, and life story [19]). We first embed these different approaches within a medical, nonpsychiatric example (eg, lung cancer) and only then follow with specific examples of psychopathology. We also focus as much on formulation as on integration—on the ability to capture the big picture or gestalt of a patient [20]. In addition to teaching specific information and skills in child and adolescent psychiatry, we believe that these sessions are useful and well received because they are generalizable to other clinical areas and because they help students bind their natural anxiety around dealing with clinical complexity and uncertainty. As we explain in the course notes for the relevant session:

> Synthesizing complex and at times contradictory information into a cohesive whole that makes sense is one of the challenges of everyday clinical medical practice. Doing so takes knowledge, skill, time, and practice. The purpose of these clinical correlations is to introduce students to this way of thinking, and to make them familiar with some ways of approaching the task in a *systematic* fashion. The goal today will not be to make the 'right' diagnosis or treatment plan: we are well aware that these are knowledge blocks that will come later. Rather, the emphasis will be on honing observation skills, and in the context of the available information and an explicit reference framework, facilitate clinical thinking and the connecting of some of the dots seen thus far, in both this course and others. The term *formulation* has a specific psychiatric connotation, but can be applied (as we hope you will agree) across a wide range of disorders and clinical conditions.

*The role of digital video and desktop editing.* Videotaped materials are not particularly new tools in teaching development and psychopathology; they have been recognized and put to good use by others [21]. More recent and pertinent perhaps is the ease and widespread availability of desktop editing. Like others, we have come to rely heavily on this tool and find it to be engaging for students and didactically effective [22]. One common model that we use is digitally recording an interview or play session with a child after obtaining the appropriate consents. A medical student (typically a third-year student in his or her clinical rotation) is present for the interview with a senior clinician and actively helps conduct it. After the session, the medical student takes the camera and tape, reviews it, and is given the task of 'playing movie director' (ie, editing the material from its 20 or 50 minutes down to a manageable clip of 3–5 minutes). Students are encouraged to find the story that they find compelling within the tape, suggest section titles, reorder segments if helpful to facilitate flow and coherence, and generally use their imagination in the process. Some students edit the tapes themselves; for students who are more skittish around computers, they may provide the timing and order for the clips, with the desktop editing done by the faculty member. The key issue is the active involvement of students in creating the clips: from conducting the interview, to editing the tape, to presenting it to the team. Assuming that the separate assent and consent forms have been secured from the child and family, these clips can be used for educational purposes in other teaching settings. We have come to rely heavily on these video clips for teaching in the CAD (and other) courses. We currently have an extensive enough library to devote the final 2 hours of the course to a "Kid Flicks" series, which is an opportunity to review course highlights (and omissions) through the well-received medium of video.

*Second year*

Unlike the first year, there is no time specifically set aside for a course centrally taught by child psychiatry in the second year. Instead, we have sought out opportunities within courses taught by general psychiatry, pediatrics, or relevant to the practice of medicine more generally, in which our skill set and particular expertise could be put to good use. Some of the openings have been natural ones. For example, we teach three classes on child-specific psychopathology within the "Mechanisms of Disease" module dedicated to psychiatry (attention deficit hyperactivity disorder and learning disabilities, Tourette's syndrome and pediatric obsessive-compulsive disorder, and pervasive developmental disorders). By contrast, other opportunities have been created rather than found. For example, we have partnered with pediatrics in teaching an interview skills module for school-aged children and with internal medicine in coaching students through workshops on breaking difficult news using standardized (actor) adult patients. In both instances, even if the subject matter or the age in question doesn't fall neatly within our realm, our approach adds unique features and has been valued by students. It allows for ongoing exposure to child psychiatry and child psychiatrists rather than for a more isolated and discontinuous experience. Issues relevant to medical students in which the child psychiatry perspective has been especially welcome include greater familiarity with developmental principles, the appreciation and management of boundaries in medicine, or the challenges of balancing privacy and confidentiality while remaining legitimate and real in the clinical setting—what has been aptly dubbed the "HIPAA versus Hippocrates" tension [23].

*Third year*

During their first clinical year, students are immersed in the different hospital wards. Their core psychiatry clerkship is 6 weeks long and incorporates a diverse range of teaching placements, among which child psychiatry understandably represents a minority. In past years students often faced the difficult choice of having to opt for an adult or a child placement, which gave pause even to students potentially interested in pursuing child psychiatry. ("How could I graduate from medical school not having seen an adult with schizophrenia or alcoholism?") Fortunately, changes in the medical school curriculum made effective in July 2005 have restructured the core clerkship into two 3-week-long blocks, one on acute psychiatry (ie, inpatient or emergency room settings), the other on the interface with medicine (ie, consultation liaison). This curricular reorganization has included the input of child psychiatry faculty and allows students to have clinical rotations in adult and child psychiatry settings. It has not made them have to decide between meeting educational objectives and pursuing particular interests. It should be noted that the core rotation also includes continuous (6-week) components: a traditional lecture series and assignments to write-up and interview tutors. Fellows in training have been particularly engaged and effective as write-up or interview tutors, which allows for further exposure to practicing child and adolescent psychiatrists and helps trainees hone their own teaching and mentorship skills.

*Fourth year*

Although not all students pursue either of the options described in this section with a child and adolescent psychiatry focus, they are included under curricular initiatives because all students at Yale have time allotted to elective rotations and all must complete a thesis to graduate.

*Elective rotations.* The fourth year has no formal child psychiatry component, although interested students and students considering a possible career in the field often do a month-long elective rotation. In addition to the local placements that they may (or not) have rotated through in their third year psychiatry clerkships, students can pursue these elective rotations elsewhere. In essence, we have developed an informal, although thriving, exchange program. Our students have performed rotations nationally and internationally (the intramural program at NIMH has been a particularly good fit for our students, and we routinely host eight to ten exchange students per year, half of them typically from abroad).

*The medical school thesis requirement at Yale: a historical tradition and a conducive environment.* Yale University School of Medicine has an extraordinary record of producing academic physician scientists and leaders. We believe that this track record partly results from the 166-year-old tradition of each Yale medical student completing an MD thesis based on original research before graduation, a tradition that is widely supported by our faculty and students and coordinated by the Office of Student Research. The Yale curriculum provides an ideal milieu for encouraging research training by students because the curriculum differs in important ways from traditional medical school curricula as follows: (1) the number of scheduled class hours is less than that at other medical schools in the United States (on average 72%), (2) the lack of competition fostered by ungraded examinations in basic science courses is unique, and (3) historically, the Yale MD thesis tradition has been unique, although several other schools recently initiated a similar requirement.

The School of Medicine has well-established, nationally recognized programs focused on patient-oriented clinical research, primarily at a postgraduate level. These programs include the Robert Wood Johnson Clinical Scholars Program (one of four national programs), the Investigative Medicine Program (a unique PhD program for clinicians), and initiatives associated with our NIH-supported General Clinical Research Center (which is funded through 2010). A major goal of the initiatives at the Yale Child Study Center (YCSC) herein described is to extend—in a coordinated and flexible manner—the opportunities provided by these postdoctoral programs to outstanding Yale medical students to work on childhood psychiatric disorders.

Currently, approximately 50% of Yale medical students elect to spend an additional (fifth) year of medical school devoted in full or in major part to research. This high rate of participation in 1-year pull-out programs (including the Doris Duke Clinical Research Fellowship at Yale and Yale endowed fellowships) reflects the great interest in research among Yale students.

The YCSC has established a disproportionately strong tradition of mentored theses and research opportunities for Yale medical students. Over the past 10 years (during which records have been electronically maintained and more easily accessible for query), Child Study Center faculty have served as primary research mentors for 27 medical school theses. With a median class size of 100 students per year, this amounts to almost 3 theses per year (median, 2; range, 0–8), remarkable statistics given the size of the Center as one of the smallest departments within the Yale School of Medicine. Not only has the quantity of these theses been noteworthy; their quality has been likewise singular. For example, between 2002 and 2005 alone, six YCSC-mentored theses were recipients of prestigious research prizes, and several theses have led to publication in peer-reviewed journals [24–33].

In summary, the Yale MD thesis requirement builds on existing strengths by better integrating medical students into the well-established research training programs available at Yale in general and at the YCSC in particular. Our goals are to attract the brightest medical students into careers in clinical and translational research in child psychiatry, to imbue them with a spirit of discovery and the application of new knowledge for the benefit of their patients, to inspire them to characterize and solve important problems, to teach them to work within complex research teams, and to support their professional development as future physician-scientists while at Yale and beyond.

*Extracurricular initiatives*

Most medical schools across the country have student interest groups in psychiatry, and Yale is no exception. For more than a decade, the Yale Medical Student Psychiatry Association has held regular meetings, invited guest lectures, sponsored pizza and movie nights, and established a network to connect students with mentors and like-minded peers. In addition to this established and popular initiative, we describe a more recently minted one that is specific to child and adolescent psychiatry.

*The Donald J. Cohen/Klingenstein mentorship program for medical students at Yale*

In recognition of the critical shortage of child psychiatrists available to meet national needs for clinical care, research, and education and being well aware of the fact that average medical students have minimal exposure to child psychiatry during their years of training, a program designed to increase exposure to the field was organized at the YCSC in 2002. Named after the late Donald J. Cohen (1940–2001; director of the YCSC from 1983–2001), the program was funded through the generosity of the Klingenstein Third Generation Foundation, a nonprofit organization with a commitment to children's mental health causes, of whose executive board Dr. Cohen had long been an active member.

In 2002, one of us (JFL) was invited by the Foundation to initiate a medical student program that would honor the late Donald Cohen. Two of us (MHB, JFL) developed this fellowship working with the faculty of the YCSC. Christopher Young, then a postdoctoral research fellow at Yale, was also instrumental. This fellowship program focuses on allowing first-year medical students to work directly with child psychiatric patients and serve as the direct interface between their families and their health care providers under the supervision of the treating professional. The program has attracted approximately 15 to 20 first-year Yale Medical Students each year since it was formally inaugurated in the fall of 2002.

During its first 3 years in existence, the program became a remarkable success. Sixty-five first- and second-year Yale medical students participated between 2002 and 2004 (for an 11% class participation average). Students were paired with 23 full- or part-time faculty members (most of them child psychiatrists but also some child psychologists, developmental pediatricians, and educators). Despite the lack of financial support for their efforts, mentors became actively engaged, seeing their involvement with medical students as a priority within their teaching activities. The energy and fresh intelligence of these students was a powerful incentive for the participation of full-time and clinical faculty members. Students became involved in a wide range of activities under the close one-on-one mentorship of senior clinicians. Activities ranged from the long-term follow-up and frontline clinical involvement with a single child and family to multiple clinical encounters with a diverse range of psychiatrically impaired children and adolescents to starting research projects relevant to children's mental health, spanning from basic bench science, clinical, and epidemiologic studies all the way to policy proposals. Complementing these individual working relationships, students met monthly for dinner discussions of clinical cases or research initiatives. Discussions were led and organized by students and attended (more so than moderated) by senior faculty members, including the authors and Dr. Samuel Ritvo (Yale Medical School, Class of 1948).

To date, the program has consisted of the three main elements of direct clinical experience, a monthly seminar, and exposure to ongoing research programs at the YCSC.

*Direct clinical experience.* Clinical relationships with patients and their families have been a priority and mainstay of the program. This direct clinical experience is the main selling point of the fellowship program, because Yale offers little by way of direct clinical responsibilities during the first 2 years of classes. Yale is not alone in having relatively few opportunities for students to become involved in the long-term clinical follow-up of patients. The key role of clinical immersion in the program has been emphasized when recruiting new mentors and selecting returning ones. Some students follow individual patients, do home and school visits, and participate directly in the care of the patients (under immediate supervision). They are also available by telephone to act as a liaison. Other students participate in the life of the inpatient or other clinical units by meeting patients and their families and sitting in on systematic evaluations, in-depth interviews, and clinical team discussions.

*Monthly seminar.* The monthly seminars consist of case presentations led by a medical student and facilitated by the program directors and the student's mentor. Dinner is served, and after the case presentations an open discussion typically addresses emotionally charged aspects of the case, including questions about specific interactions with the child, diagnoses, and therapies used in the child's treatment. Although the presentations are not intended to be explicitly didactic, they address the state-of-the-art with regard to assessment and treatment for specific disorders. The seminars are organized by the second-year student leaders and are designed to be a learning opportunity for all students, regardless of their previous knowledge or experience.

Independently of what students take away from clinical experiences and monthly meetings, the relationship that they develop with their mentor (or mentors) is critical. Students often rate the mentorship relationships per se as one of the more valuable parts of the program. The underlying philosophy and specific details of our approach to mentorship have been reviewed elsewhere [34], but it is worth noting at this juncture that its elements can be exportable, generalizable, and adaptable and are generally cost-effective. As a case in point, variations on the basic elements of the program (namely, mentored relationships and small group gatherings) have been adapted successfully into national [35] and international [36] mentorship programs that take place during annual meetings.

*Research education extension of the program.* Based on the 22 evaluation reports received at the end of the past academic year, Yale students gave the program an overall score of 8.7 out of a possible 10, with no student rating it lower than an 8. The most commonly cited area for improvement by students was a request to increase their exposure early to the research opportunities available at the YCSC. This request was addressed partly through the following initiatives.

*Summer electives.* Most students begin research work during the summer after their first year. For example, during the summer of 2004, 73 (of 96) first-year medical students remained in New Haven to work with faculty members on a wide variety of projects. Many students continue their research work in the afternoons, evenings, and weekends during the second year of medical school, and there is an additional 8-week block available for student research during the summer before beginning the third year. Additional 3-month blocks are available in late-third to mid-fourth years for completion of research work. A total of 6 to 9 months is currently available for research by each Yale student during 4 years at medical school. By emphasizing in the CAD course and in the monthly dinner presentations some of the available labs and areas of study in the YCSC, interested students have been increasingly able to forge partnerships and identify research mentors early in their training. In the best of circumstances, this has led to ongoing research involvement throughout their 4 (or 5) years and to a thesis project and published papers related to it.

*Yearlong research fellowships.* Yale encourages its students to consider a fifth year of medical school to devote exclusively to research. This Student Research Fellowship Program is facilitated by charging no tuition for the extra year and providing a limited number of stipends that can be paid to students. In recent years, 16 to 20 students have been supported on a stipend level of $20,772 to $27,100 per year. These stipends have been available on a competitive basis and have been mostly specific to disease or specialty, depending on the relevant funding sources (eg, National Cancer Institute, National Institute for Diabetes and Kidney Disease). All stipends are paid directly to the students and are considered taxable income. Although to date there have been no fellowship slots specifically earmarked for research in child psychiatry, students have expressed interest. We anticipate that the Cohen/ Klingenstein Third Generation Foundation Program and the increased visibility of child psychiatry research as part of the preclinical curriculum combined will lead to further interest in such fifth-year opportunities.

*Securing dedicated funding.* All programs currently require a competitive application. Summer research stipends are awarded primarily to students between the first and second years. Short-term stipends are awarded for specific blocks (1–3 months) during the academic year when full-time research is performed. These projects are supported by various organizations (NIH, Howard Hughes Program, private donors, and departmental and university funds.) Currently, a limited number of stipends are available from the Office of Student Research to support first-year summer research opportunities, but there is none for the subsequent programs, which are often critical toward developing the full potential of a first-year research experience. At the time of this writing we have submitted a research infrastructure grant (R25) to NIMH. If funded, this mechanism would provide supplemental (summer research) or currently not available (short-term or year-long) funds specifically earmarked for medical student research in child psychiatry.

A solid presence of YCSC-backed medical student research projects has been bolstered substantially by the availability of resources and opportunities. However, it is important to note that many past and currently ongoing experiences have happened in the absence of any dedicated funding support for research education in the area of pediatric mental disorders. Our hope is that through the expansion and formalization of dedicated funding streams, we may be able to expand this heretofore effective model. Two examples may serve to clarify this point. First, one of the residents in our integrated research pathway (described below) completed original research in the genetics of neuropsychiatric disorders of childhood during his fifth year of medical school [32]. As a Yale student, he was fortunate to secure fifth-year funding because of the happenstance overlap of his area of interest (genetics) with available funding sources. Rather than having funding constrained by the focus of existing sources, however, we want to ensure the availability of a similar mechanism regardless of the student's specific area of interest within child psychiatry. Second, four students recently involved in ongoing research activities at the YCSC have done so in the absence of Yale funding. In three of those four cases, students have been granted funding through the Jean Spurlock Fellowship for Minority Medical Students sponsored by the AACAP. Delighted as we are to see the involvement of underrepresented students in our research efforts, we would like to offer similar opportunities to all medical students, regardless of their minority status.

*The Klingenstein Third Generation Foundation/American Academy of Child and Adolescent Psychiatry medical student mentorship network*

As a consequence of the success of the mentorship program at Yale, and in consultation with the leadership of the AACAP, the Klingenstein Third Generation Foundation invited applications in the fall of 2004 for similar programs to be set up across the country. Eighteen institutions were invited to apply. Out of 13 applying institutions, 5 were selected (Harvard, Johns Hopkins, Mount Sinai, Stanford, and the University of California, Davis).

The Klingenstein Third Generation Foundation also allocated additional funds for the AACAP to organize a task force to assess the efficacy of this network. The AACAP established a subcommittee for the Klingenstein Programs on Mentorship, a part of the Committee for Medical Students, Residents and Early Career Psychiatrists. Led by one of us (AM), the subcommittee is charged with coordinating the AACAP's effort to organize and evaluate these and similar medical student initiatives across the country.

At a minimum, we are confident that we will be able to describe the trajectory of students involved in the mentorship programs, with special attention paid to how many students eventually pursue careers in child psychiatry in general and research activities in particular. The evaluation also will provide better understanding of the opportunities, challenges, and loci for improvement for each program and for the network as a whole. To evaluate specifically how many of the Klingenstein Third Generation Foundation participants pursue academic careers as independent physician-scientists, Dr. James Hudziak of the University of Vermont (and a member of the original Institute of Medicine Panel) has agreed to serve as an external advisor.

## Postgraduate and undergraduate initiatives

Two self-evident truths about education are that it can never start too early or ever be considered complete. We have turned these tautologies into concrete opportunities on either side of the medical school trajectory and present them briefly in reverse chronologic order. We strongly believe that all of these initiatives (ie, premed, med, postmed), whether used piecemeal or in toto by students, are fundamentally interconnected and ultimately serve shared goals.

## Postgraduate initiatives: The Albert J. Solnit Integrated Child and Adult Psychiatry Research Pathway

In the summer of 2002, one of us (JFL) was asked by Marilyn Benoit, then President of the AACAP, to chair a task force on curricular reform in the research training of child psychiatrists. The initial membership included Eugene Beresin (Harvard), Steven Cuffe (University of South Carolina), John March (Duke), Randy Ross (University of Colorado), Hans Steiner (Stanford), and Sydney Weissman (Northwestern). This task force developed the rough outline of the integrated research pathway that is currently in place at Yale and the University of Colorado. Added impetus was provided when NIMH Director Thomas Insel named one of us (JFL) in the fall of 2003 to serve as the Co-Chair of NIMH's National Psychiatry Training Council. This council was formed to implement the recommendations of the Institute of Medicine's committee report [12], which was highly critical of the existing research training opportunities within psychiatric residency programs. John Greden, Chair of the Department of Psychiatry at The University of Michigan, served as the other Co-Chair of this NIMH

Council. In the course of the next 2 years, two of us (JFL, MHE) served as the Co-Chairs of the Model Programs Task force of this council. This task force had regular conference calls and focused on areas of subspecialty training—including substance abuse and geriatric psychiatry—and child and adolescent psychiatry. During this same period, one of us (MHE) also served as the Chair of the Accreditation Council for Graduate Medical Education's (ACGME) RRC for Psychiatry and was a Director for the American Board of Psychiatry and Neurology (ABPN).

The integrated research pathway is a direct result of the deliberations of this task force and the NIMH Council and is modeled on the Triple Board Program and the American Board of Internal Medicine's Research Pathway. It meets all current ACGME requirements for adult psychiatry and child and adolescent psychiatry.

The integrated research pathway was formally endorsed by the Executive Council of the AACAP in the fall of 2004 and in the summer of 2005 by the American Board of Psychiatry and Neurology. There are currently 13 participants in the integrated research pathway (6 at Yale and 7 at the University of Colorado). To date, each of the three Yale cohorts has recruited one of its two students from the Yale School of Medicine, emphasizing the developmental aspect of the initiatives described, in that each of the students had participated in some or all of the activities outlined—curricular and extracurricular. The University of Illinois at Chicago and Johns Hopkins are likely to implement their own integrated research training programs in the near future.

At Yale, this program was named to honor the memory of the late Albert J. Solnit, a world-renowned pioneer in child psychiatry who served from 1966 to 1983 as the third Director of the YCSC. As a neuroanatomist, pediatrician, child psychiatrist, and psychoanalyst, Al's breadth and impact were enormous. Under his leadership, the YCSC became internationally recognized for its multidisciplinary programs of clinical and basic research, community outreach, and social policy. His effective leadership has been instrumental in encouraging physicians to listen to patients and their families and encouraging educators, judges, health care providers, and parents to work together to support the best interests of children and families.

The YCSC integrated research training program is funded by the generous support of a group of anonymous donors, start-up funds from the Yale University School of Medicine, and a longstanding NIH-funded Institutional Research Training Program (T32MH018268-21) directed by one of us (JFL). Two of us (DES, AM) direct the child and adolescent clinical components of this program in conjunction with the Director of Residency Training for the Department of Psychiatry at Yale (RB).

The integrated research training pathway is a 6-year research program within an integrated pairing of the established and accredited adult and child psychiatry training programs at Yale (please refer to Box 2 for a program overview and http://info.med.yale.edu/chldstdy/training/adultchild.html for

**Box 2. Program overview: the Albert J. Solnit Integrated Child and Adult Psychiatry Research Pathway**

*PG-1 internship year*

| Inpatient adult psychiatry 3 months | General pediatrics 6 months | Child and adult neurology 2 months | Inpatient child psychiatry 1 month |
|---|---|---|---|
| $1^{st}$ month call free; 5 calls in each of $2^{nd}$ & $3^{rd}$ month | Q4 call on inpatient months | Q4 call in adult month | 4 from-home evening/ weekend calls |

*PG-2 basic skills year*

| Inpatient child psychiatry 2 months | Outpatient child (1.5 days/wk) and adult (1.5 days/wk) psych, didactics/seminars (0.5 day/wk), and research (1 day/wk) 10 months |
|---|---|

*Long-term psychotherapy program and pediatric continuity experience*

| 8 from-home evening/ weekend calls | 10 months call-free |
|---|---|

*PG-3 intensive services year*

| Inpatient adult psychiatry 3 months | Inpatient adult psychiatry 3 months | Child & adult consultation/ liaison psych 1 month | Emergency psych 1 month | Child psychiatry community services selective 3 months |
|---|---|---|---|---|

*Long-term psychotherapy program & pediatric continuity experience & research seminar*

**Approximately 20–25 calls throughout the year**

*PG-4 outpatient services year*

Outpatient child (2 days/wk) and adult (2 days/wk) psych, and research (1 day/wk) 12 months

***Long-term psychotherapy program & pediatric continuity
    experience & research seminar***
Call-free year
*PG-5 & -6 research years*
Mentored research and formal coursework (4 days/wk) and
    outpatient child and adult psych (1 day/wk) 12 months
*Long-term psychotherapy program & pediatric continuity
    experience*
Call-free years

a detailed description). This program is designed to integrate training in research and clinical psychiatry for physicians who are seriously pursuing careers in academic child and adolescent psychiatry research. Similar to the American Board of Internal Medicine's research pathway (www.abim.org/ subspec/pathway), the integrated program adapts the currently available core clinical training in adult psychiatry and child and adolescent psychiatry to the needs of individuals committed to research careers.

Over 6 years, the integrated research pathway provides core clinical training in adult psychiatry and child and adolescent psychiatry, which would otherwise be available only as sequential training experiences in separate training programs. Early participation in successful research programs is another key ingredient, and the integrated research pathway includes a strong pediatrics primary care component during its first postgraduate year.

The core features of the integrated research pathway include the following components:

*Early identity formation.* A key ingredient involves direct experience in caring for children and families throughout the training experience. There is also a commitment to early identity formation as an independent physician-scientist.

*Mentorship and career development.* Trainees are assigned a research faculty mentor from their basic skills-1 (PGY-1) year onward. Their mentors are accomplished investigators with a sustained record of competitive research funding and active research programs. Mentors have a major responsibility for supervising the trainee, providing assessment and constructive feedback, documenting the trainee's research progress and performance, and assisting with career development and application for a mentored career development (K) award. Participants work closely with their research mentor and residency training director to design an appropriate sequence of clinical training and research education and experience.

*Integrative program structure.* The program integrates research with clinical training and child and adolescent clinical training with adult training by structuring these experiences concurrently and using shared group learning and faculty supervision to foster integration. Unlike traditional training models in psychiatry, research and child psychiatry training begin early and continue throughout the residency.

*Optimal focus on child psychiatry.* Wherever possible, child psychiatry rotations are substituted for adult psychiatry, as permitted by ACGME and American Board of Psychiatry and Neurology requirements for adult and child and adolescent psychiatry. For example, pediatric medicine is scheduled as the required primary care medicine rotation.

*Foundation of core clinical training.* The integrated program provides a full range of inpatient and outpatient experiences that support the acquisition of fundamental clinical skills in adult and child psychiatry. Residents achieve competencies in all six areas identified by ACGME: medical knowledge, patient care, practice-based learning, interpersonal and communication skills, systems-based practice, and professionalism. This strong clinical foundation serves as the base for evidence-based clinical practice and the development of advanced research skills for independent investigation.

*Evidence-based perspective.* The principles and practice of evidence-based medicine anchor the curriculum and training experiences in adult and child psychiatry. Regularly scheduled evidence-based medicine seminars build skills in evidence-based clinical practice.

*Early research immersion.* Early, intensive immersion in child psychiatry research during the PGY-2 year fosters early professional identity development as a child and adolescent psychiatry researcher and is expected to reduce attrition from long-term commitment to a research career.

*Formal research training.* Optimally, training in the integrated research pathway should include coursework leading to a PhD or master's degree, if this degree was not already acquired or as determined by a trainee's learning needs assessment. Supported, concurrent formal research training is available through the investigative medicine program at Yale (http://info.med.yale.edu/invmed/) and the Yale Department of Epidemiology and Public Health (http://publichealth.yale.edu/). This training begins in the basic skills PGY-2 year.

*Comprehensive research experience.* The integrated research pathway provides a research experience that is comprehensive in terms of time, formal curriculum, responsible conduct of science, mentorship, structured evaluation, and feedback. These components are essential for professional growth and development. Over the course of training, integrated research pathway trainees are guided through progressive, supervised research experiences, from critical appraisal of the literature, literature reviews, and secondary data analyses through increasingly complex research projects, independent study design, and grant-writing, culminating in the submission of an application for a career development award in the PGY-6 year.

*Debt repayment.* Scheduled research time of at least 80% in the basic skills year (PGY-2) qualifies trainees for the NIH loan repayment program. Thus far, one of our applicants has been successful in applying for this significant financial benefit.

Finally, the Residency Review Committee of the ACGME is exploring ways of maximizing the flexibility for other such programs to meet training requirements. For all programs, the securing of funding remains a major challenge to address to ensure their long-term survival.

*Undergraduate initiatives*

Not satisfied with the first year of medical school as being early enough to start recruitment and exposure to child and adolescent psychiatry, we have made major efforts on a new frontier: college students. Three different courses are currently taught at Yale College by YCSC faculty, and plans are underway to expand similar offerings.

*Love and attachment (James F. Leckman, MD, and Linda Mayes, MD).* The first of these classes is also required for the participants in the integrated training program during their basic skills (PGY-2) year. It is taught by two members of the YCSC faculty and focuses on evolutionary theory and its relevance to normal development and psychopathology [37]. At the level of subjective experience and behavior, the early phases of romantic love and early parental love share much in common and often lead to the same outcome—the formation of intimate interpersonal ties [38–40]. An examination of shared elements provides a useful vantage point for considering the evolution and neurobiology of love and its range of normal and psychopathologic outcomes. The syllabus of this course selectively reviews portions of the ethologic and psychological literature for romantic love and the early parental love before turning to an examination of the available neurobiologic data on central nervous system salience and reward pathways and their role in the initiation of pair bonds and early parental behavior [41,42]. This focus is followed by a consideration of various forms of psychopathology, including autistic disorder, obsessive-compulsive disorder, and drug dependence. Intrinsic to this course is the point of view that it is likely that certain adaptive "sets" of human mental states and behaviors are evolutionarily conserved and that this conservation is reflected in our genetic makeup, the functional neurobiology of our brains, our behavior during related developmental epochs, and our vulnerability to certain forms of psychopathology.

*Child development and language, literacy, and play (Nancy Close, PhD, and Carla Horwitz, PhD).* This course combines reading of selected material with supervised participant-observer experience in infant programs, a day-care and kindergarten center, or a family day-care program. Regularly scheduled seminar discussions emphasize theory and practice. An assumption of the course is that it is not possible to understand children—their behavior and development—without understanding their parents and the relationship between child and parents. The focus is on infancy and early childhood. Enrollment is limited to juniors and seniors. A second semester course reviews the development of curricula for preschool children— 3-, 4-, and 5-year-old children—in light of current research and child development theory. A third semester examines the complicated role that play has in the development of language and literacy skills among preschool-aged children. Topics include social-emotional, cross-cultural, cognitive, and communicative aspects of play.

*Autism and associated developmental disorders: seminar and practicum (Fred Volkmar, MD, and Ami Klin, PhD).* This course consists of weekly seminars on major topics in the etiology, diagnosis, treatment, and natural history of childhood autism and other severe disorders of early onset. Topics also include mental retardation, behavioral disorders, and childhood psychosis. A second semester provides an advanced study of the evaluation of individual children with autism and associated disorders, experience in the design of curricula, and work with individual children and groups of children with autism and similar disorders.

Apart from the recurrent theme of early exposure to the field and the specific opportunities within it, these courses have had additional and unexpected benefits. For example, the recruitment of undergraduate students in computer science and robotics into the autism laboratories has led into some of the YCSC's more creative lines of scientific inquiry: eye tracking in the early identification of autism [43,44] and clinical application of humanoid robotics to novel social training and face-processing interventions [45]. The recruitment and training of child and adolescent psychiatrists is far from the only outcome that we should be looking for. Attracting outsiders into our fold to forge novel and unexpected bridges has major potential to advance the scientific base of our discipline.

*Coda: not forgetting volunteers and research assistants.* We have made additional efforts to educate undergraduate students from other institutions besides Yale over the summer. To this end, we are offering a weekly, lunch-time, case-based overview course of child psychiatry to undergraduates volunteering or working as research assistants in the child and adult psychiatry departments. This seminar series provides an opportunity to educate future child psychologists, psychiatrists, social workers, and pediatricians even earlier in their career trajectory. It will help foster their identity formation and help them interact with more like-minded peers, students, residents, and our senior faculty.

### Acknowledgments

This article is dedicated to the memories of Donald J. Cohen (1940–2001) and Albert J. Solnit (1920–2002), visionary leaders devoted to education in child and adolescent psychiatry after whom two of the programs here described have been named.

## References

[1] Andreasen N. Understanding schizophrenia: a silent spring? Am J Psychiatry 1998;12: 1657–9.
[2] Kim WJ. Child and adolescent psychiatry workforce: a critical shortage and national challenge. Acad Psychiatry 2003;27(4):277–82.
[3] Kim WJ. Recruitment. Child Adolesc Psychiatr Clin N Am 2007;16(1): in press.
[4] Bartell A, Gray D, Anders T. Portals of entry. Child Adolesc Psychiatr Clin N Am 2007; 16(1): in press.
[5] Institute of Medicine. Research on children and adolescents with mental, behavioral, and developmental disorders. Washington, DC: National Academy Press, 1989.
[6] National Advisory Mental Health Council. Breaking ground, breaking through: the strategic plan for mood disorders research. Washington, DC: Department of Health and Human Services; 2001.
[7] Schrier R. Ensuring the survival of the clinician-scientist. Acad Med 1997;72:589–94.
[8] Pincus HA, Haviland MG, Dial TH, et al. The relationship of postdoctoral research training to current research activities of faculty in academic departments of psychiatry. Am J Psychiatry 1995;152(4):596–601.
[9] Pincus HA, Dial TH, Haviland MG. Research activities of full-time faculty in academic departments of psychiatry. Arch Gen Psychiatry 1993;50(8):657–64.
[10] Leebens P, Walker D, Leckman J. Perceived personal and institutional influences on child psychiatry research careers. Acad Psychiatry 1995;19:150–8.
[11] Leebens PK, Walker DE, Leckman JF. Determinants of academic survival: survey of AACAP poster authors. J Am Acad Child Adolesc Psychiatry 1993;32(2):453–61.
[12] Institute of Medicine. Research training in psychiatric residency: strategies for reform. Washington, DC: National Academy Press, 2003.
[13] Weintraub W, Plaut SM, Weintraub P. The role of medical school electives in the choice of child psychiatry as a subspecialty. Acad Psychiatry 1991;15(3):132–6.
[14] Mayes LC, Cicchetti D, Acharyya S, et al. Developmental trajectories of cocaine-and-other-drug-exposed and non-cocaine-exposed children. J Dev Behav Pediatr 2003;24(5): 323–35.
[15] Mayes LC. A behavioral teratogenic model of the impact of prenatal cocaine exposure on arousal regulatory systems. Neurotoxicol Teratol 2002;24(3):385–95.
[16] Abelson JF, Kwan KY, O'Roak BJ, et al. Sequence variants in SLITRK1 are associated with Tourette's syndrome. Science 2005;310(5746):317–20.
[17] Sweatt JD, Weeber EJ, Lombroso PJ. Genetics of childhood disorders: learning and memory, Part 4. Human cognitive disorders and the ras/ERK/CREB pathway. J Am Acad Child Adolesc Psychiatry 2003;42(6):741–4.
[18] Engel GL. The clinical application of the biopsychosocial model. Am J Psychiatry 1980; 137(5):535–44.
[19] McHugh PR, Slavney PR. The perspectives of psychiatry. 2nd edition. Baltimore (MD): The Johns Hopkins University Press; 1998.
[20] Henderson SW, Martin A. Formulation and integration. In: Martin A, Volkmar FR, eds. Lewis's child and adolescent psychiatry: a comprehensive textbook. 4th edition. Baltimore (MD): Lippincott Williams and Wilkins, in press.
[21] Fox G. Teaching normal development using stimulus videotapes in psychiatric education. Acad Psychiatry 2003;27(4):283–8.
[22] Falzone RL, Hall S, Beresin EV. How and why for the camera-shy: using digital video in psychiatry. Child Adolesc Psychiatr Clin N Am 2005;14(3):603–12.

[23] Venkatesh K. HIPAA or Hippocrates on the phone? Acad Med, in press.

[24] Blair J, Taggart B, Martin A. Electrocardiographic safety profile and monitoring guidelines in pediatric psychopharmacology. J Neural Transm 2004;111(7):791–815.

[25] Blair J, Scahill L, State M, et al. Electrocardiographic changes in children and adolescents treated with ziprasidone: a prospective study. J Am Acad Child Adolesc Psychiatry 2005; 44(1):73–9.

[26] Scahill L, Blair J, Leckman JF, et al. Sudden death in a patient with Tourette syndrome during a clinical trial of ziprasidone. J Psychopharmacol 2005;19(2):205–6.

[27] Bloch MH, Peterson BS, Scahill L, et al. Adulthood outcome of tic and obsessive-compulsive symptom severity in children with Tourette syndrome. Arch Pediatr Adolesc Med 2006; 160(1):65–9.

[28] Bloch MH, Leckman JF, Zhu H, et al. Caudate volumes in childhood predict symptom severity in adults with Tourette syndrome. Neurology 2005;65(8):1253–8.

[29] Bloch MH, Sukhodolsky DS, Leckman JF, et al. Fine-motor skill deficits in childhood predict adulthood tic severity and global psychosocial functioning in Tourette's syndrome. J Child Psychol Psychiatry, in press.

[30] Donovan A, Siegel L, Zera G, et al. Child and adolescent psychiatry: seclusion and restraint reform. An initiative by a child and adolescent psychiatric hospital. Psychiatr Serv 2003; 54(7):958–9.

[31] Donovan A, Plant R, Peller A, et al. Two-year trends in the use of seclusion and restraint among psychiatrically hospitalized youths. Psychiatr Serv 2003;54(7):987–93.

[32] Fernandez T, Morgan T, Davis N, et al. Disruption of contactin 4 (CNTN4) results in developmental delay and other features of 3p deletion syndrome. Am J Hum Genet 2004; 74(6):1286–93.

[33] Leckman JF, Herman AE. Maternal behavior and developmental psychopathology. Biol Psychiatry 2002;51(1):27–43.

[34] Martin A. Ignition sequence: on mentorship. J Am Acad Child Adolesc Psychiatry 2005; 44(12):1225–9.

[35] Milam-Miller S. Mentorship matters. AACAP News; January/February 2006:15–6.

[36] Martin A. Dignified returns: Berlin and Donald J. Cohen in 2004. International Association of Child and Adolescent Psychiatry and Allied Professions (IACAPAP) Bulletin 2004; 14(Suppl):2–5.

[37] Leckman JF, Mayes LC. Understanding developmental psychopathology: how useful are evolutionary accounts? J Am Acad Child Adolesc Psychiatry 1998;37(10):1011–21.

[38] Leckman JF, Mayes LC. Preoccupations and behaviors associated with romantic and parental love: perspectives on the origin of obsessive-compulsive disorder. Child Adolesc Psychiatr Clin N Am 1999;8(3):635–65.

[39] Leckman J, Hardy S, Kervene E, et al. A biobehavioral model of attachment and bonding. In: Sternberg RJ WK, editor. The psychology of love. 2nd edition. New Haven (CT): Yale University Press; in press.

[40] Leckman J, Carter C, Hennessy M, et al. Biobehavioral processes in attachment and bonding. In: Carter CS AL, editor. Attachment and bonding: a new synthesis. Dahlem Workshop Report 92. Cambridge (MA): MIT Press; 2005. p. 303–49.

[41] Leckman JF, Feldman R, Swain JE, et al. Primary parental preoccupation: circuits, genes, and the crucial role of the environment. J Neural Transm 2004;111(7):753–71.

[42] Leckman JF, Mayes LC, Feldman R, et al. Early parental preoccupations and behaviors and their possible relationship to the symptoms of obsessive-compulsive disorder. Acta Psychiatr Scand Suppl 1999;396:1–26.

[43] Klin A, Chawarska K, Paul R, et al. Autism in a 15-month-old child. Am J Psychiatry 2004; 161(11):1981–8.

[44] Klin A, Jones W, Schultz R, et al. Defining and quantifying the social phenotype in autism. Am J Psychiatry 2002;159(6):895–908.

[45] Shic F, Klin A, Jones W, et al. Swimming in the underlying stream: computational models of gaze in a comparative behavioral analysis of autism. Journal of Artificial Intelligence, submitted for publication.

[46] Klin A, Jones W, Schultz R, et al. Visual fixation patterns during viewing of naturalistic social situations as predictors of social competence in individuals with autism. Arch Gen Psychiatry 2002;59(9):809–16.

[47] Pruett KD, Pruett MK. Only God decides: young children's perceptions of divorce and the legal system. J Am Acad Child Adolesc Psychiatry 1999;38(12):1544–50.

[48] State MW, Lombroso PJ, Pauls DL, et al. The genetics of childhood psychiatric disorders: a decade of progress. J Am Acad Child Adolesc Psychiatry 2000;39(8):946–62.

[49] Marans S. Listening to fear: helping kids cope, from nightmares to the nightly news. New York: Henry Holt & Company; 2005.

[50] Himelstein BP, Hilden JM, Boldt AM, et al. Pediatric palliative care. N Engl J Med 2004; 350(17):1752–62.

ELSEVIER
SAUNDERS

Child Adolesc Psychiatric Clin N Am
16 (2007) 45–54

CHILD AND
ADOLESCENT
PSYCHIATRIC CLINICS
OF NORTH AMERICA

# Recruitment

## WunJung Kim, MD, MPH

*Division of Child and Adolescent Psychiatry, Department of Psychiatry, Medical University
of Ohio at Toledo, 3130 Glendale Avenue, Toledo, OH 43614-5810, USA*

Recruitment is a vital function of any profession for its survival, growth, and development. Child and adolescent psychiatry is a relatively young branch of medicine. Leo Kanner was the first academic child psychiatrist, appointed to the faculty of Johns Hopkins University Medical School, and wrote the first textbook of child psychiatry in 1935 [1]. An organization of the child guidance clinics, founded by multidisciplinary child mental health administrators in 1945, the American Association of Psychiatric Clinics for Children began to deliberate optimum standards of operating clinics and standards of training of multidisciplinary mental health professionals—social work, clinical psychology, and child psychiatry [2]. The American Academy of Child Psychiatry, later renamed the American Academy of Child and Adolescent Psychiatry (AACAP), was founded exclusively by psychoanalytically trained academicians of child psychiatry in 1953 and began to move the field closer to the mainstream of medicine.

The movement resulted in the establishment of a subspecialty board certification process by the American Board of Psychiatry and Neurology (ABPN) in 1957, which was also supported by the American Association of Psychiatric Clinics for Children. The credentialing requirements by ABPN eliminated the existing path taken by pediatricians to become child psychiatrists: undergoing 2 years of child psychiatry training after completing pediatric training.

The number of ABPN-certified child and adolescent psychiatrists has increased exponentially from its first examination in 1959 to a total of 5925 by 2006, far greater than the rates of increase for general psychiatrists (http://abpn.com/cert.statistics.htm). The total number of ABPN-certified general psychiatrists from 1935 to 2006 reads 43,850, of which child and adolescent psychiatrists constitute 13.5%. The exponential growth has not been able to meet society's needs/demands for qualified child and adolescent

*E-mail address:* wjkim@meduohio.edu

1056-4993/07/$ - see front matter © 2006 Elsevier Inc. All rights reserved.
doi:10.1016/j.chc.2006.09.003          *childpsych.theclinics.com*

psychiatrists, however. A lack of child and adolescent psychiatrists has been recognized within the field and by several study groups and national commissions. The Surgeon General's report in 1999 decried, "There is a dearth of child psychiatrists...Furthermore, many barriers remain that prevent children, teenagers, and their parents from seeking help from the small number of specially trained professionals who are available...This places a burden on pediatricians, family physicians, and other gatekeepers to identify children for referral and treatment decisions" [3]. It was reiterated in the Report of the Surgeon General's Conference on Children's Mental Health in 2001, "The burden of suffering by children with mental health needs and their families has created a health crisis in this country. Growing numbers of children are suffering needlessly because their emotional, behavioral and developmental needs are not being met by the very institutions and systems that were created to take care of them" [4].

The most recent national report, the President's New Freedom Commission on Mental Health in 2003, also described an inadequacy and shortage of specialists to serve children, adolescents, and older Americans [5]. This article reviews (1) the historical trend of recruitment, (2) recruitment dynamics (training programs and trainees), (3) workforce models, and (4) future direction.

**Historical trends**

In 1947, the American Association of Psychiatric Clinics for Children approved 25 child guidance clinics that met its training standards and began to certify graduates of approved training programs [2]. The first time the review committee for psychiatry and neurology (the forerunner of residency review committee for psychiatry) reviewed child psychiatry training programs in 1960, only 11 of 17 programs reviewed were approved [6]. The number of approved programs increased exponentially to 130 at its peak in the 1980s but has decreased gradually to 114 in 2006 (www.acgme.org/adspublic/accredited_programs.asp). The total number of residents enrolled in accredited child and adolescent psychiatry training programs had increased from less than 100 in the first year the residency review committee approved to 550 in 1980. The number continued to increase moderately to approximately 700 until 1990. The average numbers in the 1990s remained stagnant at approximately 700 per year, decreasing to 673 in 2002–2003. The number increased to its highest, 742, in 2005–2006. Total numbers aside, the demographic changes have been significant: a steady increase of female residents and international medical graduate residents, mirroring medical school enrollment trends and general psychiatry resident recruitment trends. At the turn of the century (2001–2002), the majority gender of child and adolescent psychiatry residents became female for the first time according to the ACGME resident census and graduate medical education track [7]. The proportion of female residents has been increasing gradually and will continue to increase further, again reflecting a steady increase of female enrollment in undergraduate colleges and medical schools in the last decade. Child and adolescent psychiatry is the only psychiatry subspecialty with a majority of female residents (56.9%), compared with addiction psychiatry (45.7%), forensic psychiatry (45.6%) and geriatric psychiatry (45.8%); general psychiatry also had a majority of female residents (52.7%) in 2004–2005 [8]. The proportion of international medical graduates in child and adolescent psychiatry was approximately 30% in 1980 and decreased to approximately 20% in 1990. The trend reversed in the 1990s until early 2000, however, which mirrored general psychiatry's recruitment trends, and reached 43.7% in 2004–2005 [8]. Most international medical graduates are Asian Americans educated in India and Pakistan.

## Recruitment dynamics

### Training programs

The child guidance clinic movement in the early twentieth century attracted a small group of physicians in pediatrics and psychiatry into a newly emerging field of child psychiatry [9]. Post–World War II prosperity and interest in children's well-being and Freudians' influence also attracted a cadre of bright physicians to child and adolescent psychiatry. The perceived lack of scientific basis by an unorganized system of diagnosis, the predominantly psychosocial treatment models of psychiatry, technologic advances, and greater specialization in medicine began to affect recruitment of medical students into psychiatry in the late 1980s throughout the 1990s. The declining pool of general psychiatry residents has affected severely the recruitment of general psychiatry residents into child and adolescent psychiatry [10]. Since inception, child psychiatry also has faced the challenges and crises by the question of whether child psychiatry is a mental health discipline or medical discipline [11]. Other factors have contributed to the decline of recruitment in general psychiatry and child and adolescent psychiatry because of weakening training programs or closures:

1. Elimination of training grounds because of deinstitutionalization and closure of state psychiatric hospitals, some of which sponsored child and adolescent psychiatry residency programs
2. Reorganization of the National Institute of Mental Health as an organization primarily supporting research rather than supporting training or clinical services
3. Advance of managed care and decrease in clinical revenues
4. Promotion of an increase in primary care physicians and a decrease in specialists by governmental agencies and medical/professional organizations

5. Reduction of direct graduate medical education funding by 50% for subspecialty training by the 1997 Balanced Budget Act
6. Competition for specialty training for the first time in history with addiction, geriatric, and forensic psychiatry fellowships

In just a 5-year period from 1995 to 2000, the total number of training programs in general psychiatry decreased from 197 to 187 and the total number of residents decreased by 16.8% [12].

The merger and closure of well-respected child and adolescent psychiatry training programs also occurred in the 1990s, including programs at Menninger Clinic, Sheppard Pratt Hospital, Georgetown University, and Lafayette Clinic. Although United States medical graduate recruitment to psychiatry and child and adolescent psychiatry has declined significantly, psychiatry and child and adolescent psychiatry have relied increasingly on international medical graduates for recruitment through the 1990s and 2000s. Although there are many excellent international medical graduate residents across medical specialties, professional organizations, medical school/university leadership, and teaching hospitals traditionally have used US medical graduate recruitment as an index of a specialty or program's viability and attractiveness.

*Trainees*

Increasing educational debt load of medical students and the burden of longer training for subspecialty certification have been cited often as factors in problems of recruiting United States medical graduates in subspecialties, especially revenue poor ones [13]. Many medical students and general psychiatry residents enter medical schools and psychiatry residency considering child and adolescent psychiatry as their career choice. Reports have indicated that positive exposure to child and adolescent psychiatry during the third-year clerkship in medical school and the second year of psychiatry residency helps to maintain or consolidate trainees' interest in child and adolescent psychiatry [14,15]. Direct clinical contact with diverse patient populations, having an interesting teacher, and observing his or her clinical skills are important aspects of students' positive experiences in child and adolescent psychiatry [16]. Other factors that predict child and adolescent psychiatry career choice include electing pediatric rotation, being female, coming from non–research-oriented medical schools, and coming from non–primary care-oriented medical schools [17]. Three decades ago at the University of Maryland, Walter Weintraub, MD and colleagues began to follow-up medical students participating in the combined accelerated program in psychiatry, a 4-year medical school track that contained a strong child and adolescent psychiatry component [18]. The program clearly documented its salutary effect on prevention of erosion of student's interest in child and adolescent psychiatry. Medical schools and the medical community in general traditionally have regarded psychiatry—especially child and adolescent psychiatry—as a soft science, dissuading many students and residents interested in child and adolescent psychiatry. It is also estimated that approximately 20% of US medical schools do not sponsor child and adolescent psychiatry residency programs and more than 30% of US medical students have minimal or no clinical clerkship exposure in child and adolescent psychiatry, a critical void in the recruitment and education of future physicians [15,19,20]. The kind of student contact with and perception of psychiatry residents also may affect medical student recruitment [10,14].

## Workforce models

Although recruitment lacked in the 1990s, a critical question arose as to whether the workforce was adequate for society's needs, (ie, the needs of mentally ill patients). The traditional need-based approach to estimate child and adolescent psychiatry workforce requirements have repeatedly documented a great shortage of workforce [20]. In 1980, the Graduate Medical Education National Advisory Council examined workforce issues based on the prevalence of child and adolescent psychiatry illnesses, severity of illness, and the need for direct child and adolescent psychiatrist care. It recommended that the number of child and adolescent psychiatrists be increased to approximately 8000 to 10,000 [21]. In 1990, the Council on Graduate Medical Education reanalyzed data used for the Graduate Medical Education National Advisory Council Report based on a combination of the "adjusted needs model" and the "requirements model," which was derived from the staffing patterns of the growing health delivery system of Health Maintenance Organizations. It estimated that the nation would need more than 30,000 child and adolescent psychiatrists by the year 2000 [22]. In 1990, there were 4212 child and adolescent psychiatrists in the US, with a mean of 6.73 child and adolescent psychiatrists per 100,000 children and adolescents under the age of 18. The distribution ranged from 0.81 in Mississippi to 18.9 in Massachusetts per 100,000 youths [23]. In 2001, there were approximately 6500 child and adolescent psychiatrists in the United States, with a mean ratio of 8.67 per 100,000 youths, ranging from 3.1 in Alaska to 21.3 in Massachusetts [24]. In translation, considering the prevalence of child and adolescent psychiatric illness and the population of "serious emotional disturbances" and "extreme functional impairment," a child and adolescent psychiatrist would have to carry a case load of 750 of the most severely disturbed children and adolescents at any given time [20,25]. The reality is that as the National Institute of Mental Health, the Surgeons General, the President's New Freedom Commission on Mental Health, and other groups have reported, only approximately 20% of emotionally disturbed children and adolescents receive some kind of mental health care, and only a small fraction of them receive evaluations and treatment by child and adolescent psychiatrists. In addition to absolute numbers, there are also factors affecting effective workforce size by reduction of work hours by aging workforce, increasing female workforce, changing life styles, and increasing demand of the socioeconomic model of workforce [26–28]. According to the data by the American Medical Association Physician Masterfile, the mean age of child and adolescent psychiatrists is 50 years.

**Future direction**

Recognizing that the critical shortage of child and adolescent psychiatry workforce amounted to a public health crisis, the AACAP formed a taskforce to re-examine the workforce status in 1999. The Bureau of Health Professions in the Department of Health and Human Services tracks specialty workforce trends based on demand-use models that project the demand of physicians required to provide health care services at the current levels of use, primarily based on the availability and health benefits. The research arm of the Bureau of Health Professions, the National Center for Health Workforce Information and Analysis, performed the data analysis for the AACAP Taskforce on Workforce Needs in 2000 and reported that the demand for child and adolescent psychiatry services was projected to increase by 100% between 1995 and 2020 [19,20]. That is, even if the funding and recruitment remain stable at the current level, there will be only 8312 child and adolescent psychiatrists, 4312 less than the 12,624 child and adolescent psychiatrists that would be needed to meet the demand in 2020. The demand for adult psychiatry services was projected to increase by 19%. In response to the sobering report of the taskforce regarding the plight of the nation's children with severe mental illness and the severe access problem, the AACAP set the recruitment of medical students and residents as the first priority of the organization and launched a 10-year recruitment initiative. The steering committee on workforce issues has been formulating multilevel efforts and multipronged strategies.

*Multiple portals of entry*

The triple board residency program, a 5-year combined program of general psychiatry, child and adolescent psychiatry, and pediatrics, was piloted by the ABPN in 1987 to capture the interest of medical students in child and adolescent psychiatry and recruit them directly into the combined residency. Seven pilot programs had expanded to 12 programs initially but decreased to 10 programs currently. The combined residency has been moderately successful by adding approximately 20 child and adolescent psychiatrists to the field each year. There is a strong movement to support and expand the triple board program and develop a new 3-year combined general and child and adolescent psychiatry residency program to attract medical students and pediatricians who have shied away from pursuing child and adolescent psychiatry partly because of the reluctance to undergo 3 to 4 years of general psychiatry training before embarking on child and adolescent psychiatry training. Similarly, another new portal has been slowly evolving: integrated residency of general psychiatry and child and adolescent psychiatry, which allows the postgraduate year 1 resident to begin a child and adolescent psychiatry learning experience [29]. This new model has been approved by the residency review committee in psychiatry, which allowed Yale University, University of Colorado, and Duke University to begin such programs in 2005 and 2006. The integrated program is hoping to produce future academic and research child and adolescent psychiatrists by emphasizing scholarly and research activities during their integrated 5 to 6 years of training that eliminates the burden of 1 to 2 years of postresidency research fellowship.

*Advocacy*

The stigma of mental illness not only limits the access of children who have mental illness but also affects recruitment. The AACAP is an active participant of the Campaign for Mental Health Reform, collaborating with 15 other national health organizations to make mental health a national priority and early access, recovery, and quality of mental health the hallmarks of the nation's mental health system. The campaign was formed as a result of the recommendations by the President's New Freedom Commission on Mental Health. With the coalition of other mental health and medical professional organizations, the AACAP has assisted to draft a legislative bill (H.R. 1106/S537 in the 2004–2006 Congress), the Child Health Care Crisis Act, which would create educational incentives in the form of loan forgiveness and scholarship to encourage the recruitment of child and adolescent psychiatrists and other children's mental health professionals. It also would restore full funding support of child and adolescent psychiatry training by Medicare graduate medical education funding for 2 years after general psychiatry training. Members of the AACAP and Society of Professors in Child and Adolescent Psychiatry (an organization of directors of child and adolescent psychiatry programs) have been active in informing and educating legislators on the critical national shortage of child and adolescent psychiatrists and other children's mental health professionals and have been able to generate bipartisan support. It has not been easy to convince most legislators to have the bill passed in its entirety, but it is hoped the bill would be approved as an amendment to the Higher Education Act and Medicare bill at the end of the 2004–2006 Congress. The AACAP also has been collaborating with the Annapolis Coalition in recommending expansion of competent mental health workforce in the nation to the government as recommended by the President's New Freedom Commission on Mental Health [5].

*Mentorship*

It is believed that talented and involved mentors make a positive difference for recruitment. The managed care involvement, graduate medical education funding cut, and evolving productivity model in the academic world may have rendered academic child and adolescent psychiatry less attentive to mentoring general psychiatry residents and medical students. Teachers may be less rewarded for their devotion to their teaching than to revenue-generating clinical and research activities. The AACAP presidential initiative by Thomas N. Anders, MD began in 2004 to fund a teaching scholars program that supports six teaching scholars to participate in an intensive program of instruction at the Harvard Macy Institute for Physician Educators. The program focuses on the latest methods of learning and teaching, curricular evaluation, leadership, and information technology. The cadre of these talented and well-educated child and adolescent psychiatrists is hoped to become master teachers to mentor and teach junior child and adolescent psychiatry faculty, residents, and medical students, thus resulting in improved recruitment. The AACAP efforts also have focused on direct contact with medical students by helping to organize the Special Interest Group Network in medical schools throughout the United States. The goal is to provide medical students with opportunities to learn about the field of child and adolescent psychiatry by arranging mentors within their medical school and in their local community. First established as a Donald J. Cohen Fellowship at Yale University, a mentoring program for medical students has expanded to a dozen medical schools across the country by the support of the Klingenstein Third Generation Foundation and the John and Patricia Klingenstein Fund. This program is described in detail by Andres Martin, MD in an article elsewhere in this issue [30].

## Summary

Positive and negative developments in child and adolescent psychiatry have provided challenges and opportunities throughout a 100-year history of its profession, from the initial child guidance clinic movement to the current expanding scientific knowledge base. The expansion of a high-quality workforce in clinical, academic, and research arenas remains to be a major goal of the field. Many complex, intertwined factors at institutional and individual levels have affected recruitment of medical students into child and adolescent psychiatry. Lack of exposure in the medical school curriculum, increasing levels of educational debt burden, long years of residency training, and relatively low income potential have been barriers of recruitment [20]. Academic child and adolescent programs have struggled in the era of managed care on top of federal and state funding cuts for support of recruiting residents and faculty. In the face of the stigma of mental illness, devalued image of the profession, and overwhelming negative environment, child and adolescent psychiatry has been able to attract small numbers of dedicated and humanistically orientated young trainees into the field and has made impressive progress in its short history. Growing scientific knowledge through basic science and clinical research—especially in neuroscience, developmental science, and clinical care (eg, neuroimaging, genetics, pediatric psychopharmacology)—has been enriching the profession's traditional biopsychosocial model of clinical care. The clinical demands for and a chronic undersupply of qualified child and adolescent psychiatrists have raised the public awareness as evidenced by markedly increasing media coverage in recent years, both print and broadcast. A report on the workforce shortage by the Associated Press in April 2006 resulted in wide coverage of the issue in more than 120 news outlets in the United States and throughout the world. The public awareness of and demand for access to appropriate child and adolescent psychiatric services have led policymakers and accreditation and health care organizations to consider support for research training, flexible portals into child and adolescent psychiatry training, and opening of new training programs. The supply-demand dynamics also have resulted in a favorable job market for child and adolescent psychiatric practitioners—especially graduating residents—in terms of flexibility in the location and kind of professional career and an increasing income potential [31]. The AACAP's 10-year recruitment initiative strives to inform and generate the support of medical/psychiatric educators, governmental agencies, and the public at large to improve the profession's recruitment efforts to provide access to quality care and needed services to the nation's children and adolescents and their families.

## References

[1] Kanner L. Child psychiatry. Springfield (IL): Charles C. Thomas; 1935.
[2] Gardner G. History of child psychiatry. In: Freedman A, Kaplan H, Sadock B, editors. Comprehensive textbook of psychiatry. 2nd edition. Baltimore: Williams & Wilkins; 1975. p. 2032–5.
[3] US Department of Health and Human Services. Mental health: a report of the Surgeon General. Rockville (MD): US Department of Health and Human Services, Substance Abuse and Mental Health Services Administration, Center for Mental Health Services, National Institute of Mental Health; 1999.
[4] US Department of Health and Human Services. US public health service report of the Surgeon General's conference on children's mental health: a national action agenda. Washington, DC: Department of Health and Human Services; 2000.
[5] President's New Freedom Commission on Mental Health. Achieving the promise: transforming mental health care in America: final report. Rockville (MD): US Department of Health and Human Services, Substance Abuse and Mental Health Services Administration, Center for Mental Health Services, National Institute of Mental Health; 2003.
[6] Schowalter J. Recruitment, training, and certification in child and adolescent psychiatry in the US. In: Lewis M, editor. Child and adolescent psychiatry. 3rd edition. Philadelphia: Lippincott Williams & Wilkins; 2002. p. 1429–32.
[7] Brotherton SE, Simon FA, Etzel SI. US graduate medical education, 2001–2002. JAMA 2002;288:1073–8.
[8] Brotherton SE, Rockey P, Etzel SI. US Graduate medical education, 2004–2005. JAMA 2005;294:1129–43.
[9] Musto D. History of child psychiatry. In: Lewis M, editor. Child and adolescent psychiatry. Philadelphia: Lippincott Williams & Wilkins; 2002. p. 1446–9.

[10] Sierles FS, Yager J, Weissman SH. Recruitment of US medical graduates into psychiatry: reasons for optimism, sources of concern. Acad Psychiatry 2003;27(4):252–9.

[11] Cohen RL. Another dangerous opportunity: child and adolescent psychiatry faces health care reform. Bull Menninger Clin 1994;58(4):462–73.

[12] Rao NR. Recent trends in psychiatry residency workforce with special reference to international medical graduates. Acad Psychiatry 2003;27(4):269–76.

[13] Jewett EA, Anderson MR, Gilchrist GS. The pediatric subspecialty workforce: public policy and forces for change. Pediatrics 2005;116(5):1192–202.

[14] Martin VL, Bennett DS, Pitale M. Medical students' perceptions of child psychiatry: pre-and post-psychiatry clerkship. Acad Psychiatry 2005;29:362–7.

[15] Stubbe D, Joshi P, Kim W. Choosing child and adolescent psychiatry as a career: a survey of key factors. AACAP News 2002;33(4):182–3.

[16] Szajnberg NM, Beck A. Medical student attitudes toward child psychiatry. J Am Acad Child Adolesc Psychiatry 1994;33(1):145–51.

[17] Haviland MG, Dial TH, Pincus HA. Characteristics of senior medical students planning to subspecialize in child psychiatry. J Am Acad Child Adolesc Psychiatry 1988;27(4):404–7.

[18] Weintraub W, Plaut SM, Weintraub P. The role of medical school electives in the choice of child psychiatry as a subspecialty. Acad Psychiatry 1991;15(3):135–6.

[19] The American Academy of Child and Adolescent Psychiatry. Report of the AAC task force on work force needs meeting the mental health needs of children and adolescents: addressing the problems of access to care. Washington, DC: AACAP; 2001.

[20] Kim WJ. Child and adolescent psychiatry workforce: a critical shortage and national challenge. Acad Psychiatry 2003;27(4):277–82.

[21] Graduate Medical Education National Advisory Committee. Report to the secretary. DHHS Publication HRA 18–651–657. Washington, DC: US Government Printing Office; 1980.

[22] Council on Graduate Medical Education. Re-examination of the Academy of Physician supply made in 1980 by the Graduate Medical Education National Advisory Committee (GMENAC) for selected specialties, bureau of health professions in support of activities of the Council on Graduate Medical Education. Cambridge (MA): ABT Associates; 1990.

[23] Thomas CR, Holzer CE. National distribution of child and adolescent psychiatrists. J Am Acad Child Adolesc Psychiatry 1999;38(1):9–16.

[24] Thomas CR, Holzer CE. Continuing shortage of child and adolescent psychiatrists. J Am Acad Child Adolesc Psychiatry 2006;45(9):1023–31.

[25] US Department of Health and Human Services. Mental health, United States. Washington, DC: US Department of Health and Human Services; 1998.

[26] Cooper RA. Weighing the evidence for expanding physician supply. Ann Intern Med 2004; 141(9):705–14.

[27] Scully JH, Wilk JE. Selected characteristics and data of psychiatrists in the United States, 2001–2002. Acad Psychiatry 2003;27(4):247–51.

[28] Dial TH, Grimes PE, Leibenluft E, et al. Sex differences in psychiatrists' practice patterns and incomes. Am J Psychiatry 1994;151:96–101.

[29] Gray D, Anders T. Portals of entry. Child Adolesc Psychiatr Clin N Am 2007;16(1).

[30] Martin A, Bloch M, Stubbe D, et al. Child psychiatry education during medical school (and before and after). Child Adolesc Psychiatr Clin N Am 2007;16(1).

[31] Kim W, Stubbe D. Good news! Survey indicates positive views of child and adolescent psychiatry. AACAP News 2002;33(5):204–11.

ELSEVIER
SAUNDERS

Child Adolesc Psychiatric Clin N Am
16 (2007) 55–66

CHILD AND
ADOLESCENT
PSYCHIATRIC CLINICS
OF NORTH AMERICA

# Triple Board Training and New "Portals" into Child Psychiatry Training

Douglas D. Gray, MD[a,*], Deborah A. Bilder, MD[a], Henrietta L. Leonard, MD[b], Thomas F. Anders, MD[c]

[a]Department of Psychiatry, University of Utah School of Medicine, 650 South Komas Drive, Suite 208, Salt Lake City, UT 84108, USA
[b]Department of Psychiatry and Human Behavior, Bradley Hasbro Research Center, One Hoppin Street, Coro-2, Providence, RI 02903, USA
[c]Department of Psychiatry and Behavioral Sciences, University of California Davis M.I.N.D. Institute, 2825 50th Street, Sacramento, CA 95817, USA

The triple board program, the combined residency in pediatrics, general psychiatry, and child and adolescent psychiatry, celebrated its twentieth birthday at the 53rd Annual American Academy of Child and Adolescent Psychiatry meeting in San Diego in 2006. Originally an experiment in medical education, the triple board program has established itself as a permanent and successful training program. It offers a viable 5-year alternative to the traditional 7 to 8 years of residency training required for board eligibility in pediatrics, general psychiatry, and child and adolescent psychiatry. In an early review, Schowalter [1] described that the field wanted to capture the medical students who were interested in medical and psychological disorders of childhood. One primary objective was to address the workforce shortage of child psychiatrists by recruiting medical students who may have otherwise pursued general pediatrics. The second objective was to bridge the gap between child psychiatry and pediatrics by training physicians proficient in the culture, language, and content of both specialty fields. Although the shortage crisis continues, both objectives were met. Some medical students who had planned a career in pediatrics were recruited into the field of child psychiatry, without regret [2]. A new breed of child psychiatrists who think differently than their child psychiatry colleagues emerged from the triple board programs [3]. The graduates often serve as role models in academic settings and attract medical students to the field.

* Corresponding author.
*E-mail address:* Douglas.gray@hsc.utah.edu (D.D. Gray).

1056-4993/07/$ - see front matter © 2006 Elsevier Inc. All rights reserved.
doi:10.1016/j.chc.2006.09.001                                   *childpsych.theclinics.com*

The success of the triple board experiment has facilitated further consideration and support for the development of other novel training portals into child psychiatry.

## Triple board history

In 1980, the Graduate Medical Education National Advisory Committee identified the acute shortage of child and adolescent psychiatrists in the United States and the need for recruitment into child psychiatry training. This report and others that delineate the workforce shortage in child and adolescent psychiatry are well summarized by Kim [4]. Two years later, Dr. Stanford Friedman published an essay describing his wishes related to child psychiatry training and proposed an alternative entry into child psychiatry [5]. This new training pathway intended to draw from a pool of physicians already committed to children's health care who would otherwise be dissuaded by their disinterest in adult psychiatry or desire to complete their residency training within half a decade. Two significant sources of child psychiatry trainees were declining: pediatricians pursuing child psychiatry training and medical students entering general psychiatry programs. The triple board program was selected after several other options were considered by the Committee on Certification in Child Psychiatry, which focused primarily on capturing students interested in the medical and psychological disorders of childhood [1–3].

The 5-year triple board curriculum includes 24 months of pediatrics, 18 months of general psychiatry, and 18 months of child and adolescent psychiatry training. Upon completion of the triple board program, graduates are board-eligible in all three disciplines [6]. The six pilot sites (Albert Einstein, Brown, Mount Sinai, Tufts, Kentucky, Utah) began training their first residents on July 1, 1986. The initial interest in, commitment to, and oversight of the triple board programs were impressive. The Pediatrics-Psychiatry Joint Training Committee was comprised of representatives from the Committee on Certification in Child Psychiatry, the American Board of Pediatrics (ABP), the American Board of Psychiatry and Neurology (ABPN), the American Academy of Pediatrics, the American Academy of Child and Adolescent Psychiatry (AACAP), and the American Psychiatric Association. There was also a National Institute of Mental Health representative and a professional educator. The National Institute of Mental Health, Center for Mental Health Services, ABP, and ABPN provided funding to support the prospective study and administration of these pilot programs by the Pediatrics-Psychiatry Joint Training Committee [3].

In the subsequent 10 years, the six pilot programs received vigorous oversight by these organizations. Annual site visits involved residents and training directors; summary site reports were generated. This process was designed prospectively to evaluate the triple board program as an experiment in graduate medical education. Recruitment data, resident performance measures, clinical reasoning assessments, and postgraduate follow-up were collected systematically. Medical students who had interviewed for triple board positions but ultimately chose to pursue more traditional training were sought for follow-up. National resident retreats held annually fostered camaraderie among residents and training directors across sites. The programs thrived under close monitoring and ownership provided by the governing committees, ABP, and ABPN. In 1995, when the fifth and last cohort of pilot project residents completed training, the triple board experiment was declared a success and awarded permanency. In effect, this achievement allowed additional training programs to add triple board tracks and allowed existing programs to increase their training slots from the two slots per year that had been permitted [3].

**Triple board outcome measures**

The pilot triple board programs were monitored and supervised carefully during the first decade. Program evaluations included analysis of data collected on the initial 109 residents who trained at the pilot sites [3]. Program directors consistently reported satisfaction with the quality of the applicants. Triple board residents performed at a level indistinguishable from their pediatric colleagues on pediatric rotations and superior to the general and child psychiatry residents on psychiatry rotations. In comparison to graduating child and adolescent psychiatry residents, senior triple board residents scored higher on a clinical reasoning assessment. In-training pediatric examination results were below the average for the postgraduate year 1 to postgraduate year 3 training levels in comparison to categorical pediatric residents but were on par for psychiatry in-training examinations. Among pilot program graduates, 96% (47/49) had at least one board certification and 86% were board certified in at least two areas, but only 37% were triple boarded. In terms of academic appointments, 45% of graduates held faculty positions at the conclusion of the evaluation period in 1995 [3].

A second analysis of triple board graduates extended beyond the pilot period and included graduates from 1991 through 2003. In 2004, Warren and colleagues [2] collected data using a structured written survey. The response rate was 81% (113/140). The importance of these data lies in the evolution of the triple board program since its inception. Although the distribution of rotations among pediatrics, psychiatry, and child psychiatry has remained unchanged, the order in which residents take these rotations has evolved significantly over time and differs at specific sites. This difference has resulted in more integration among specialties throughout the duration of training. Residents also are permitted to take the pediatric board examination during their fifth year of training instead of waiting until the completion of the residency program. A subsequent decrease in attrition and improvement in board pass rates have followed these changes.

The result of the written survey from the second analysis revealed a wide variety of career options for graduates and overall high satisfaction with triple board training. All three areas of training were equally valued. Most responders believed that 5 years was the right length for their training. Board certification rates for all graduates were highest for general psychiatry (81%), followed by pediatrics (63%) and child and adolescent psychiatry (57%). Most of the responders who had not passed a board examination had not taken the examination. Many of these responders had not yet had the opportunity to do so because of the required sequence of these examinations. For example, written and oral board examinations for general psychiatry must be passed to establish eligibility for the child and adolescent psychiatry board examinations. Among graduates who have taken board examinations, pass rates were highest for general psychiatry (96%; 91/95), followed by child and adolescent psychiatry (92%; 64/70) and pediatrics (77%; 71/92). Negative outcomes included 29% of triple board graduates reporting barriers to taking so many board examinations (eg, not perceived as important for career, expense, length of time to complete, need to recertify in all three fields) and the fact that most graduates are still not triple boarded. Of note, the pass rate for individuals who took the pediatric board examination during a later time frame (1998–2003) was 83%, compared with 70% during an earlier era (1991–1997). Although the top priority is to graduate skilled clinicians, triple board training directors also have the expectation that graduating residents will be prepared to pass all three board examinations [2].

Although critics have viewed certification in only one or two specialties as a failure or wasted training for graduates of combined training programs, this is not necessarily the case. Just as with other combined programs, graduates often pursue further subspecialization that may not require all board certifications [7]. Some graduates have pursued subspecialty fellowships in pediatrics or psychiatry and have been boarded in those as well (eg, emergency medicine, forensics).

**Program requirements**

The triple board requirements that were developed carefully by ABP and ABPN have remained unchanged over the last 20 years. A resident completes 24 months of pediatrics, 18 months of general psychiatry, and 18 months of child and adolescent psychiatry. These months include intern, intermediate, and senior levels of responsibility. For example, triple board residents must complete 4 supervisory pediatric months, which is only 1 month short of their categorical pediatric colleagues. Four pediatric intensive care rotations (three in newborn intensive care unit, one in pediatric intensive care unit) are required for graduation. The newborn care requirements (three in intensive care unit, one in nursery) are equivalent to the pediatric program requirements. Exceeding the categorical pediatric requirements, triple board residents maintain a pediatric continuity clinic throughout the duration of the 5 years of training. Inpatient/residential psychiatry treatment experiences are generally limited to 6 adult psychiatry months and 6 child psychiatry months. Triple board outpatient psychiatry experiences mirror the requirements of its psychiatric counterparts more closely because a sufficient number of patients are treated for at least 1 year. Specific requirements for adult and child psychiatry rotations are more flexible than for pediatrics [6,8].

A major programmatic issue for triple board programs is how best to integrate each of the three disciplines over the 5 years of training. Trying to make sure each discipline is approached in a focused and longitudinal manner often conflicts with the concept of integrating the training to create a separate identity and knowledge base for the resident. The various triple board program designs provide medical students several options in selecting a program that best fits their needs. Many of the training sites have different lengths for the initial pediatric training. Although the pediatric continuity clinic provides an experience across all 5 years, there have been discussions as to whether more pediatric rotations in the later years might increase the pass rate for the pediatric board examination. Another logistical issue involves preserving psychotherapy seminars and psychotherapy experience longitudinally. Each training site has dealt with this issue in a different way, but many sites have outpatient psychiatry and child psychiatry experiences that exceed requirements. Although a constant challenge, each program has balanced the programmatic issues of integration. It is understood that what the triple board resident learns is integrative and unique, not just additive.

## Career development of triple board graduates

### Specialized roles

Triple board programs were created to produce more child and adolescent psychiatrists by tapping into a pool of medical students considering a career in pediatrics. At first glance, a medical student who is considering the triple board program might assume that it would be a way to keep career options open. Some graduates practice pediatrics, psychiatry, or a combination of both. This goal misses the full potential offered by the triple board training. Triple board residents develop remarkable careers in areas that require the use of all skills gained in training. For example, graduates are perfectly trained for consult-liaison psychiatry in large university or children's hospitals. Others with subspecialty training are superb physicians in pediatric oncology, emergency medicine, and intensive care. Their training allows them to communicate well with staff in pediatrics and psychiatry. Comprehensive management in some diagnostic areas, such as eating disorders, requires several skill sets. Some triple board graduates treat anorexia across the continuum of care, including acute medical and psychiatric needs, and provide long-term nutritional and behavioral health care. This integration and continuity of services can vastly improve patient care. Triple board graduates provide outpatient psychiatric consultation in pediatric specialty clinics for patients who struggle with treatment adherence to their medical regimen (eg, for asthma, pain, and other chronic illnesses). They also may provide psychiatric consultation in a primary care setting. Triple board graduates are well trained to manage the psychiatric comorbidity of patients who have neurodevelopmental disorders. Other areas of focus for triple board graduates include adolescent medicine, juvenile court settings, emergency medicine, addiction psychiatry, and careers in public health [2]. Current triple board residents and graduates are exploring new avenues of access to medical and psychiatric treatment for vulnerable populations, such as children in foster care. The hope is that the emotional and medical needs of these populations can be met in a single clinic setting. Combining medical and psychiatric funding streams for children is one of the keys to facilitate the integrative care model.

*Research*

Despite the demands of triple board training and limited research time, one third of triple board graduates complete additional training. Forty-five percent of the graduates have faculty appointments. Many have completed research fellowships and have been successful in academic research careers. The number of triple board residents who are entering research fellowships continues to grow, which has increased the number of academically trained triple board graduates. There are many examples of triple board graduates who have developed full-time research careers, and some, such as Xavier Castellanos, MD, and Robert Findling, MD, have been acknowledged at triple board administrative meetings.

**Recent developments in and current status of triple board programs**

There are ten active triple board programs in the United States, with a total of 22 positions for the postgraduate year 1 [9]. Most programs are small, with two residency training slots in each year. A few programs have increased their capacity to three positions per year. Program designs are diverse, with some focusing initially on pediatric training and others integrating rotation blocks with residents rotating between specialties every 6 to 12 months. Residents have several options when looking for the program that best meets their style and needs. Most of the current programs are located in the eastern United States, with Hawaii and Utah being the exceptions. To increase applicants' ability to learn about triple board programs, the National Association of Pediatric, Psychiatry, and Child and Adolescent Psychiatry Training Directors developed a website in 2006 (www.tripleboard. org) that includes general information regarding all triple board programs and links to individual program websites. This website also contains the training requirements for all triple board programs, developed and approved by the ABP and the ABPN.

The Accreditation Council of Graduate Medical Education (ACGME) accreditation of a triple board program depends on the individual accreditation of its three component residencies rather than the combined program itself. The residency review committee (RRC) of the ACGME must accredit each institution's pediatrics, general psychiatry, and child and adolescent psychiatry programs for the respective triple board program to be viable. All other combined programs, such as medicine-pediatrics (the largest and oldest), share the same dependency on the accreditation of each component program. In the future, the RRC plans to establish accreditation for all combined residency training programs, starting with medicine-pediatrics. Eventually, triple board programs will receive accreditation independent of its associated training programs.

In 2002, the ABPN convened a meeting with training directors from triple board programs and representatives from relevant organizations. They addressed how current programs are meeting the new RRC requirements for general psychiatry and child and adolescent psychiatry. The meeting focused on issues related to board pass rates, recertification, and clinical competencies. They suggested projects to collect graduate and performance data and create an organization to enhance communication across programs. The meeting reviewed the unique advantages of triple board training.

The success of the triple board pilot programs ironically prompted the withdrawal of its collective leadership, the Pediatrics-Psychiatry Joint Training Committee, once permanent status was achieved. This change unwittingly led to "benign neglect" of the triple board programs. There was no structural organization between the programs, and most of the relevant professional societies did not even discuss these programs on their websites. With concern about these issues, the AACAP approved the proposal requesting Abramson funds to fund a national meeting in Providence, Rhode Island (2003) with training directors and selected residents from all of the programs [10].

The primary goal of the national triple board meeting was to address obstacles faced by current and future triple board programs. Some of the questions discussed were as follows: What is the identity of the triple board program residents and graduates? Should there be specific triple board educational experiences and specific clinical competencies? What are the measures of success for graduates? How can medical students access information about the programs? How can the programs develop a national organization that will increase information, visibility, recruitment, and programmatic issues? How can the current programs be supported and future programs encouraged? How are curriculum and programmatic issues resolved? How will the new requirements in general psychiatry and child and adolescent psychiatry be integrated?

At the AACAP Abramson meeting, the National Association of Pediatrics, Psychiatry, and Child and Adolescent Psychiatry Training was formed to address, in part, the concerns about lack of visibility and coordination across sites. A website (www.tripleboard.org) was endorsed and subsequently developed. A triple board mission statement was agreed upon as follows:

> "The five year combined residency integrates pediatrics, general psychiatry, and child and adolescent psychiatry to train physicians who synthesize the clinical knowledge and skills of these disciplines. The training provides a foundation for clinical care, education, advocacy, public policy, and research with a developmentally informed biopsychosocial approach to health, illness, and prevention. This unique program transcends the boundary between pediatrics and psychiatry to optimize the care of children, adults, and families in community and academic settings" [10].

A plan to reach medical students with information about the triple board programs was developed [11].

At this meeting, curriculum and program design issues were reviewed across programs. Recommendations were developed to specifically integrate the new ACGME requirements in pediatrics, general psychiatry, and child and adolescent psychiatry. The current ABP and ABPN requirements also were reviewed, and specific recommendations were developed on modifying the requirements, which were subsequently forwarded to the respective boards. Recommendations for integrated (triple board) electives for medical students and the need for integrated clinical competencies were developed. The goals of the AACAP Task Force on Workforce issues were reviewed, and the triple board program's impact on these issues was discussed [12]. A report on the meeting was filed with the AACAP [10].

## Future of triple board training and the new portal of entry

In 2005, the AACAP Steering Committee on Workforce Issues made a conscious effort to increase support for triple board training programs and promote the concept of triple board training [12]. Subsequent plans were made that included the appointment of a triple board training director as co-chair of the AACAP Workgroup on Training and Education and a reception at the AACAP annual meeting celebrating the 20 years of training triple board residents. The steering committee also began exploration of a new "portal" into triple board training. At the same time, the triple board training directors' organization (National Association of Pediatrics, Psychiatry, and Child and Adolescent Psychiatry) became more organized and began collecting dues from each program for use in collective projects. The first project was the completion of the national triple board website (www.tripleboard.org).

*New portal into triple board training*

Currently, the decision to pursue triple board training must be made by the fourth year of medical school. Triple board programs participate in the National Residency Match Program. Transferring into a triple board program from another residency program can be daunting and requires prospective approval of the ABP and ABPN. Exceptions are made for pediatric residents who complete a pediatric internship in a program affiliated with a triple board program. Options for other residents are limited.

Under the current system, pediatricians who want to become child psychiatrists must complete 4 to 5 years of additional training after a pediatric residency. The broad range of experience gained through a primary care residency translates into 1 year's credit (internship) toward general psychiatry requirements. The potential for a pool of future child psychiatrists is excellent, however. DeMaso and colleagues [13] studied the outcome of child psychiatry residents recruited after residency training in pediatrics alone. In comparison to their counterparts with a general psychiatry background, these residents performed favorably across measures of case formulation, ability to form empathic relationships, and overall performance. Jellinek [14] noted that "pediatrician-child psychiatrists" are uniquely positioned to draw further recruits into child psychiatry through their influence as role models in the pediatric setting.

In 2001, the AACAP Council selected the "workforce crisis" as the top priority for the AACAP for the next 10 years (2002–2012). The Steering Committee for Workforce Issues was formed, and a strategic plan was created. One of the three major strategies of the plan was to expand portals of entry into child and adolescent psychiatry. Several portals were suggested, including a new portal for pediatricians interested in child and adolescent psychiatry training. By 2005, this proposed portal was gaining momentum. The concept was an integrated 3-year psychiatry/child psychiatry program for pediatricians to become board eligible in general and child and adolescent psychiatry. Most pediatric subspecialty fellowships are also 3 years long, which allows the new portal to compete for well-qualified pediatric residents who otherwise may have pursued other subspecialties. Child and adolescent psychiatry training directors hear frequently from mid-career pediatricians who would consider a career change into child psychiatry if the right opportunity were available. The new portal takes into account overlapping requirements already completed during a physician's pediatric residency. For example, pediatric residency programs require a child neurology rotation. Thus, several requirements would be "double counted." This proposal has the support of the AACAP, the American Psychiatric Association, the American Academy of Pediatrics, the ABPN, and the American Association of Directors of Psychiatry Residency Training. The proposal was reviewed by the psychiatry RRC of the ACGME in October 2006. If approved, this portal may be operational by July 2007.

A committee is being developed that would review regional applications for pilot programs with oversight and monitoring similar to that of the pilot triple board programs at their inception. The psychiatry/child psychiatry portal requires coordination within only one medical school department, which offers an administrative advantage over traditional triple programs that must work between pediatrics and psychiatry departments. Completion of a pediatric residency program is certainly sufficient preparation for the demands of psychiatry training.

## Integrated research training programs for child psychiatrists

The inadequate opportunities for research training of psychiatry residents were discussed in the Institute of Medicine's committee report [15]. The same findings apply to the training of child and adolescent psychiatrist researchers. A task force chaired by James Leckman, MD, developed a comprehensive plan of research training for child psychiatrists. This model has been used to develop new research training programs at Yale University and the University of Colorado. These new programs include a 6-year curriculum, research mentorship, and formal research training. The adult and child psychiatry training is integrated rather than sequential. Residents begin child psychiatry and research training by their postgraduate year 2. Although all of the training requirements of the ABPN and the ACGME are met within the integrated training model, experience with children and adolescents is prioritized. For example, pediatric rotations meet the medical training requirements during the internship. General psychiatry training requirements are met with child and adolescent patient populations where requirements allow. The two programs have begun to share resources via telemedicine video conferences, and an annual summer institute is planned for all research residents in both programs. It is anticipated that more academic training sites will join the research consortium as greater resources become available. A more thorough description of the integrated research program at Yale can be found in the article by Martin and colleagues elsewhere in this issue.

## Integrated child and adolescent psychiatry clinical programs

As a result of collaborative efforts by the AACAP, American Psychiatric Association, and American Association of Directors of Psychiatry Residency Training, the ACGME has revised the psychiatry training requirements to provide more flexibility in the time requirements of general psychiatry experiences and more substitution of child psychiatry clinical activities, permitting integrated rather than sequential completion of clinical rotations. Residents receive exposure to childhood and adolescent populations at the onset of and throughout their training. This integration allows residents to develop their professional identity as child-oriented physicians at an earlier stage. Although several clinical programs identify themselves as integrated, the level of this integration varies. Some institutions choose to list their integrated program separately from their traditional program for the National Residency Match (see the article by Martin and colleagues elsewhere in this issue).

## Summary

It is hoped that increasing the number of triple board programs in the United States, making their presence and appeal more widely known among medical students, and establishing an enhanced triple board portal for board-eligible/certified pediatricians to train in general and child and adolescent psychiatry will improve the current workforce shortage of competent, practicing clinical child and adolescent psychiatrists. By providing more support to current triple board residents, graduates, and training programs, AACAP expects that the triple board programs will continue to prosper and expand.

Similarly, the Yale and University of Colorado research training programs anticipate expanding into a national network of research training programs as more telemedicine links and academic resources become available. Finally, the greater flexibility in training requirements approved by the psychiatry RRC should encourage all training programs to emphasize development, introduce child clinical experiences, and provide longer periods for continuity of care for children early in the training program.

As many as 50% of psychiatry residents who consider pursuit of a career in child and adolescent psychiatry do not follow through on their initial intentions. They lose interest in working with children or they tire of the lengthy training period. For some residents, financial concerns dictate an early entry into practice. Integrated training addresses some of these issues and hopefully will result in enhanced recruitment and better retention of students interested in careers in child and adolescent psychiatry. Integrated training with early exposure to children also may attract some medical students whose primary motivation is to work with children and their families. The bottom line is to provide high quality care to the millions of children in our country who have mental disorders and are unable to access services because of the dearth of professionally trained child and adolescent psychiatrists.

## References

[1] Schowalter JE. Triple board: Tinker to Evers to Chance [editor's note]. J Am Acad Child Adolesc Psychiatry 1989;28(1):124–9.
[2] Warren MJ, Dunn DW, Rushton J. Outcome measures of triple board graduates, 1991–2003. J Am Acad Child Adolesc Psychiatry 2006;45:700–8.

[3] Schowalter JE, Friedman CP, Scheiber SC, et al. An experiment in graduate medical education: combined training in pediatrics, psychiatry, and child and adolescent psychiatry. Acad Psychiatry 2002;26:237–44.

[4] Kim WJ. Child and adolescent psychiatry workforce: a critical shortage and national challenge. Acad Psychiatry 2003;27:277–82.

[5] Friedman SB. If you had three wishes: fantasies related to child psychiatry training. Am J Dis Child 1982;135:942–4.

[6] American Board of Pediatrics. Guidelines for combined pediatrics-psychiatry-child and adolescent psychiatry residency training. Available at: www.abp.org/certinfo/genpeds/psych.htm. Accessed July 8, 2006.

[7] Frohna JG, Melgar T, Mueller C, et al. Internal medicine-pediatrics residency training: current program trends and outcomes. Acad Med 2004;79:591–6.

[8] Accreditation Council for Graduate Medical Education. Program requirements for residency education in pediatrics. Available at: http://www.acgme.org/acWebsite/downloads/RRC_progReq/320pr106.pdf. Accessed July 8, 2006.

[9] American Medical Association. Graduate medical education directory 2005–2006. Chicago: American Medical Association; 2005.

[10] American Academy of Child and Adolescent Psychiatry. Abramson document on file. Washington, DC: American Academy of Child and Adolescent Psychiatry; 2003.

[11] Bartell A. Triple board training: so what is it all about? American Psychiatric Association Medical School Newsletter 2000;10(1):5.

[12] American Academy of Child and Adolescent Psychiatry. Task force on work force. Available at: http://www.aacap.org. Accessed July 8, 2006.

[13] DeMaso DR, Mezzacappa E, Goldman SJ. Recruitment and training of child and adolescent psychiatry residents from pediatrics. J Am Acad Child Adolesc Psychiatry 1992;31:1100–4.

[14] Jellinek M. Recruitment of child psychiatry residents from pediatrics: difficulties and options. Acad Psychiatry 1989;13:213–8.

[15] Institute of Medicine. Report on research training in psychiatry residency strategies for reform. Available at: http://www.iom.edu. Accessed July 8, 2006.

CHILD AND
ADOLESCENT
PSYCHIATRIC CLINICS
OF NORTH AMERICA

Child Adolesc Psychiatric Clin N Am
16 (2007) 67–94

# Teaching Development in Undergraduate and Graduate Medical Education

Geri Fox, MD, MHPE, FAACAP[a],*,
Debra A. Katz, MD[b],
Florence F. Eddins-Folensbee, MD[c],
Rowland W. Folensbee, PhD[c]

[a]Department of Psychiatry, Institute for Juvenile Research, 1747 West Roosevelt Road,
University of Illinois at Chicago, Chicago, IL 60608, USA
[b]Department of Psychiatry, Division of Child and Adolescent Psychiatry, University
of Kentucky College of Medicine, 3470 Blazer Parkway, Lexington, KY 40509, USA
[c]Department of Psychiatry and Behavioral Sciences, Child and Adolescent Psychiatry,
Baylor College of Medicine, One Baylor Plaza, Houston, TX 77030, USA

Teaching normal development is, from our biased perspective, the single most interesting topic in all of medicine. When taught well, its universal appeal often provides the initial "hook" for medical students to consider child and adolescent psychiatry as a career choice. All of our students, whatever their level of training, come to the subject with a lifetime of personal observations and experiences. Students recall their own childhood and adolescent experiences and those of their siblings and friends. They remember having been parented, and many wonder how they will parent their own children (or are already raising families). The study of development enriches our understanding of the most meaningful and central themes of human existence—the formation of attachments, cognition, morality, emotional relationships, our concept of self and self-esteem, and our ever-changing relationship with family and society. Great philosophical dilemmas, such as nature versus nurture, and the meaning of existence as seen from different stages of life are also addressed. Daily challenges, such as optimal parenting techniques for different phases, are debated. Curiosity is stimulated about the early experiences that shaped our adult patients' personalities. A solid grounding in

---

* Corresponding author.
*E-mail address:* foxg@uic.edu (G. Fox).

development prevents psychiatrists from overly pathologizing their patients. To formulate a diagnosis and treatment plan, a patient's symptoms must be understood in a developmental biopsychosocial context. An additional benefit of teaching development is that, as teachers with growing families, the authors take special pleasure in the mutually enriching relationship between our academic interest and our child-rearing.

This article reviews strategies for teaching normal development in undergraduate and graduate medical education. Training directors from three different institutions (GF, FEF, DAK), each with longstanding experience teaching development, share their approaches to this subject. A psychologist (RF) also discusses teaching development from the neuroscience perspective.

The first section provides a general overview of pedagogic approaches to teaching development, common to all levels of training. The relative merits of lifespan versus topical approaches are discussed. Various strategies to enhance teaching, including the use of live interviews, stimulus videotape, case vignettes, classroom exercises, and extracurricular activities, are outlined. Audiovisual, textbook, and journal resources are outlined. Evaluation methodology is discussed.

The second section provides a review of issues targeted to three different student populations: medical students, general psychiatry residents, and child and adolescent psychiatry residents. The challenges of teaching development to these groups of trainees, with different course length and expected level of competency using lifespan and topical approaches, are addressed. Licensing body requirements, goals and objectives, and sample curricula for teaching human development to these three groups are discussed in turn.

## General overview of pedagogic approaches

### Lifespan versus topical approaches

When approaching the vast subject of human development, an instructor's first decision point is whether to use a lifespan or topical approach. A lifespan (or chronologic) approach examines sequential time periods or phases of development. These phases are generally considered to include infancy, toddlerhood, preschool age, middle childhood, preadolescence, adolescence (early, middle, and late), and adulthood (early, middle, and late). In contrast, a topical approach follows central themes or developmental lines across the lifespan. Such topics include cognition, emotion, psychosocial development, psychosexual development, morality, attachment, separation-individuation, self-concept, temperament, speech and language, and gross and fine motor development. Integration of developmental neurobiology into the curriculum offers scientific underpinning that improves understanding of traditional themes.

In the authors' opinion, the ideal curriculum combines topical and lifespan approaches. By following each theme, the students understand the issues in depth. After gaining familiarity with topics, students are then pre-pared to identify various themes within each age group.

The ultimate goal is for clinicians to be able to gauge whether observed behaviors and modes of relating are "normal" for a given child's or adult's developmental phase. This ability requires an understanding of the multiple definitions of "normal" [1], which include normality as health versus path-ology, normality as utopian ideal, normality in reference to milestones within a population (expected average age as well as range) [2], and normality as a transactional system. Achieving this goal also requires a sophisticated abil-ity to integrate one's knowledge of topical developmental lines into what is expectable for a given individual within a particular societal context.

### Strategies to enhance teaching

#### Live interviews versus audiovisual or case vignettes

Seeing real children in context helps students achieve higher-order learn-ing (using Bloom's taxonomy [3] of knowledge, comprehension, application, analysis, synthesis, and evaluation). Bringing children and adolescents into the medical school classroom (or arranging for the students to observe in school settings) provides immediacy, spontaneity, and the opportunity to in-teract. Students can be assigned to interview a particular child, and when given the child's age in advance, learn a great deal from the preparation and from the interview. The downside is that the child's behavior is unpre-dictable, and cooperation is not guaranteed. Using well-chosen case vi-gnettes or audiovisual clips allows instructors to make a particular teaching point at a chosen moment. Fox [4] provides a review of the use of stimulus videotape in teaching normal development and a list of audiovi-sual resources. Most video resources provide snapshots of different children at various ages, performing specific tasks, usually in a formal interview setting. By contrast, there are few development videotapes with extended longitudinal follow-up.

One longitudinal stimulus videotape, "Normal Development in the First Ten Years of Life" [5], is designed for educators to use as a teaching resource. Created to trigger classroom discussion while illustrating concepts, this video provides examples of one child's 10-year development. Although presented longitudinally, the clips are also organized by topic in the teacher's manual and can be shown in any order, at the instructor's discretion. The DVD for-mat allows nonanalog clip selection, so that the instructor can freely select clips without fast forwarding. The 201 real-life visual anecdotes illustrate the teacher's points and provide a stimulus for discussion. Formal (psycho-logical testing) and informal (unstructured naturalistic) assessment and ob-servation have been used. Academic, social, and family arenas are portrayed, including peer group interaction, sibling issues, and parenting techniques. To keep the video from becoming outdated, commentary is re-stricted to the accompanying log, which is easily revised as new theories of

**Box 1. Teaching strategies**

*Live interviews*
- Bring in a "normal" child to discuss "what it's like being an 8, 12, 16, year old"
- Conduct a family interview with attention to attachment, family roles, and developmental issues of family members
- Take a developmental history from a current adult patient and apply the concepts under discussion (eg, separation-individuation, moral development, temperament)
- Conduct an objective structured clinical examination of children and adults of various ages with emphasis on developmental issues

*Case vignettes*
- Discuss prepared case vignettes with analysis of developmental issues

*Case write-ups*
- Integrate a developmental formulation into a case evaluation of an adult or child

*Stimulus video*
- Use video clips to illustrate clinical concepts being discussed
- Select a "mystery clip" and ask residents to observe a particular aspect of development (eg, social skills, fine motor coordination, attachment)

*Observation experiences*
- Observe children in a school or daycare setting; consider assigning specific aspects of development to be observed (eg, motor development, psychosocial issues)

*Discussion groups (during or after class hours)*
- Watch a movie or television show geared to a particular age group (eg, Barney, Harry Potter, The Incredibles) and explain why it appeals to that age group
- Read a fairy tale and discuss the universal developmental themes present
- Discuss contemporary topics that impact on development, such as the effects of daycare, divorce, media exposure to violence

*Field trips*
- Interview teachers about the kinds of developmental expectations they have for each age group they teach

- Take a group of children to a movie and discuss what they liked (or did not like) about it afterwards and how they understood the main characters and their conflicts
- Have residents get together with each other and their children of various ages for an "observation party"

*Personal experiences related to development*
- Take a detailed developmental history of a family member or fellow student or resident
- Have residents take their own developmental history from their parent(s) with attention to specific questions, such as "Who was I most attached to growing up and why?" "How did I react to a new sibling?" "When did I first want to be a doctor?" "What was my first experience of death?" "How did I react to nursery school, summer camp, or other separations?" "How did I deal with puberty and adolescence?"

development arise. The absence of voice-over narration also allows for multiple interpretations of a given scene and maintains accessibility for various student levels.

*Other strategies to enhance teaching*

Box 1 presents various suggested strategies to enhance the teaching of normal development. Because developmental "moments" are everywhere but often go unrecognized, there are myriad opportunities to use clinical exercises to reinforce material. Clinical exercises are fun and bring the material alive. They also serve to convince even the most resistant student that understanding development is an essential part of understanding ourselves and our patients. Exercises range from simple and brief to more lengthy and complex, depending on the skills and interest of the students and teacher and the time available. Tasks such as asking residents to take a detailed developmental history of a patient, observing a group of normal children, or discussing their own developmental history with their parents provide opportunities for deeper examination and integration of the material studied. Clinical exercises can be chosen for specific purposes and with specific groups of students in mind. For example, residents may welcome the opportunity to bring their own children in for "observation," whereas medical students may appreciate an evening discussion group to get to know their development teacher on a more informal basis and possibly witness parenting in action.

*Textbook, journal, and audiovisual resources*

Selecting the proper textbook for physicians-in-training is a conundrum. On the one hand, our students generally know little about the topic and require a basic review. On the other hand, their advanced level of training demands a more sophisticated text. This situation is complicated by the eternal time crunch and often limited compliance with assigned reading. Psychiatry clinician-educators often need to teach interviewing and assessment skills and developmental theory, but it is difficult to find a text that covers both areas.

There is a plethora of excellent development textbooks on the market (see Box 2 for a nonexhaustive sampling of textbook and journal resources). Undergraduate psychology textbooks are organized by lifespan or topical approach. Although these texts provide clear explanations of basic principles, thorough literature reviews, and attractive color photographs and tables, their examples and tone can be too simplistic for medical students, residents, and subspecialty residents. Bornstein and Lamb's [6] graduate psychology text provides a more sophisticated discussion of developmental science but may offer more depth than most psychiatry curricula require. Broad integration of neuroscience with other approaches to development appears to be limited in the current literature, but the field seems to be on the verge of providing such an integration [7]. There are several smaller and less comprehensive textbooks, such as Crain's [8], that provide a general overview using a tone that is well received by the students.

Reading selected classic articles by the original authors is highly recommended for child and adolescent psychiatry subspecialty residents (see sample syllabi provided later).

## Developmental neuroscience

Box 3 presents a sample outline of developmental neurobiology topics. Developmental neurobiology may be taught as part of the human development curriculum, as part of a "Brain and Behavior" course, or integrated with psychopathology didactics. The neuroscience approach provides concrete explanations for the interacting contributions of genetics and experience. Similarly, developmental neuroscience provides concrete bases that support multiple topics of development in cognitive, moral, and social areas. For example, discussing cognitive development in terms of increasing levels of neural integration available over the course of development can support the concept of increasingly abstract cognitive processing operating at successive developmental stages.

Developmental neurobiology helps new medical students establish clear connections between psychiatry and basic science and other clinical courses. Neurobiology of development can be presented in ways that highlight the relevance of brain processes to personal functioning and to the functioning of patients. Examples include individual variation in learning styles through visual-spatial as opposed to auditory-verbal channels, recognizing ways in which personal memories are triggered by sensory stimuli, recognizing ways that societal privileges, such as driving, coincide with development of brain processes such as "stop-and-think" mechanisms in the late developing frontal lobes, and considering ways in which strong emotions interfere with thinking.

Neurobiology of development can support appreciation of current brain functioning during interventions with adults while simultaneously clarifying the impact of previous development on the nature of current brain processes. In addition to offering greater depth of understanding, focus on neurobiology supports alternative conceptualizations of problems and treatment. For example, neurobiology supports recognition that explicit memory systems change quickly, which promotes insight, whereas implicit systems change slowly, which requires repetition in the course of producing change. Considering the differences between these memory systems leads to reconceptualization of the change process during treatment. Neurobiologic development also explains variations in how experiences early in life affect incorporation of experience at different stages of development. Emotional and interpersonal experiences during the first several years of life can be encoded in the absence of long-term or explicit processing, and can be unavailable to conscious recall.

Once presented, concepts related to brain development and function can be addressed by knowledgeable faculty during case conferences. The extent of integration of brain function into explanation of human behavior and development during case conferences and lectures on other topics varies widely based on the level of awareness of these issues held by various lecturers and supervisors.

Teaching the neurobiology of development supports in-depth understanding of patients throughout the life span and in conjunction with focus on either topics or tracks of development. Neurobiology can provide structure for assessing developmentally appropriate and pathologic strengths and weaknesses in cognitive functioning, emotional processing, and social relatedness. Subsequently, lectures on psychoeducational and psychological testing have been presented as elaborations within the neuropsychological framework developed during the lecture on neurobiology of function and development. For example, patterns of results of psychological assessment can reveal problems with attention, visual-spatial integration, verbal processing, and oral or written output, each of which can be considered in light of deficits in neurobiologic processing. Consideration of neural systems that support basic arousal, emotion, anxiety, and previous experiential history can help identify sources of behavioral acting out and excessive emotional reactivity. Recognition of interactions between cognitive functioning and emotionality can guide differential diagnosis and decisions regarding medical treatment, parent training, and individual psychotherapy. Schools of psychotherapy, such as cognitive behavioral therapy and psychodynamic psychotherapy, also can be considered in light of broad neurobiologically based conceptualizations of processing, so case supervision and presentation of various theories of functioning can be tied to underlying neurobiology

**Box 2. Selected textbook and journal resources that cover development**

*Psychology textbooks*

Berk L, Development through the lifespan. 4$^{th}$ edition.
   Boston (MA): Allyn and Bacon; 2006.
Berger KS. The developing person through childhood and
   adolescence. 7$^{th}$ edition. New York (NY): Worth; 2006.
Bornstein M, Lamb M, editors. Developmental science: an
   advanced textbook. 5$^{th}$ edition. Mahwah (NJ): Erlbaum; 2005.
Bukatko D, Daehler M. Child development: a thematic
   approach. 5$^{th}$ edition. Boston (MA): Houghton Mifflin, 2006.
Cole M, Cole S, Lightfoot C. The development of children.
   5$^{th}$ edition. New York (NY): Worth; 2005.
Crain W. Theories of development: concepts and applications.
   5$^{th}$ edition. Upper Saddle River (NJ): Prentice Hall; 2005.
Davies D. Child development: a practitioner's guide.
   2$^{nd}$ edition. New York (NY): Guilford Press; 2004.
Shaffer D, Kipp K. Developmental psychology: childhood
   and adolescence. 7$^{th}$ edition. Belmont (CA):
   Wadsworth/Thomson; 2006.
Siegler RS, DeLoache JS, Eisenberg N. How children develop.
   2$^{nd}$ edition. New York (NY): Worth; 2006.

*Psychiatry textbooks*

Sadock B, Sadock V. Kaplan and Sadock's comprehensive
   textbook of psychiatry. 8$^{th}$ edition. Philadelphia (PA): Lippincott
   Williams & Wilkins; 2004. Various versions of this classic text
   (concise, synopsis) cover development to varying degrees.
Tasman A, Kay J, Lieberman JA, editors. Psychiatry.
   2$^{nd}$ edition. Wiley; 2003. This book has a detailed section
   on development with excellent tables.
   It also has a useful synopsis of key figures
   in child development.

*Psychiatry texts specifically targeted to medical students*

Andreasen NC, Black DW. Introductory textbook of psychiatry.
   4$^{th}$ edition. Washington (DC): American Psychiatric Press; 2006.
Stoudemire A. Human behavior: an introduction for medical
   students. 3$^{rd}$ edition. Philadelphia (PA): Lippincott
   Williams & Wilkins; 1998. This is a really nice text, but
   because of the death of the author, is not likely
   to be updated.

> *Child and adolescent psychiatry textbooks that cover development*
> Lewis M, editor. Child and adolescent psychiatry: a comprehensive textbook. 3$^{rd}$ edition. Philadelphia (PA): Lippincott Williams & Wilkins; 2002. The 4$^{th}$ edition is expected in 2007.
> Dulcan M, Wiener J, editors. Essentials of child and adolescent psychiatry. Washington (DC): American Psychiatric Press; 2006.
>
> *Selected journals*
> *Child development.* Society for Research in Child Development Press.
> *Developmental Psychology.* APA Press.
> *Development and Psychopathology,* Cambridge Press.

throughout training. The challenge in developing such a broad neurobiologic integration is to develop in clinical faculty an appreciation for the range of connections between brain and behavior.

*Evaluation methodology*

The Accreditation Council for Graduate Medical Education (ACGME) has placed an increased emphasis on evaluation of the core competencies [9]. How do we know that our students have learned what we expect them to? Evaluation methodology that we have found particularly relevant to normal development includes written multiple choice question examinations, essay questions, objective structured clinical examinations, and observation checklists. With adequate resources, a standardized patient examination to assess developmental screening can be used. Video clips or vignettes are useful in providing a standardized stimulus for examination purposes and can help assess how well students have integrated the information. The appropriate choice of evaluation tools must, in part, be based on the desired level of competence for each group of students.

Student assessment for large group learning is most easily and efficiently accomplished through multiple choice test questioning. Although successful performance on this measure may identify top basic science students, however, it may not predict integration of material. A review session at the end of the course and a quiz on concepts covered serve to solidify knowledge. Because this material tends to show up on standardized tests, residents see the value in having a quiz or examination at the end of the course to test their knowledge. The scores of the group also give the teacher valuable feedback as to the success of the course. Adding a clinical vignette and

---

**Box 3. Sample developmental neurobiology topics outline**

- Description of a neuropsychological approach to understanding information input, integration, and output processes
- Description of neural networks that combine multiple processes throughout the brain into unique experiences and that bridge between individual experiences
- Discussion of brain processes supporting individual functions:
  Arousal
  Emotion
  Anxiety
  Patterns of experience
- Discussion of explicit and implicit memory processes
- Identification of processes of brain development
  Genetics
  Migration
  Arborization
  Synaptogenesis
  Pruning
  Myelination
- Discussion of broad themes of neurodevelopment
  Effects of experience on brain development
  Developmental windows—opening and closing
  Interactions of brain systems during development

---

asking residents to discuss it in narrative form offers a different form of feedback about how well residents can integrate and use knowledge from the course.

Setting up an objective structured clinical examination with various stations is a wonderful way to assess learning. Stations can provide live patients of various ages, standardized patients, video, or case vignettes.

## Issues specific to training level

### Undergraduate medical education

*Special issues: Recruitment into general psychiatry, addressing needs of nonpsychiatrists*

Recruitment of PGY-1 US medical school graduates into general psychiatry through the National Residency Matching Program, declined from 745 in 1988 to below 500 per year during most of the 1990's; 524 in 2001 wast the first significant increase in a decade [10]. Increasing educational debt, pressure to pursue a primary care career, a long training period, and reimbursement problems in the managed care era are some of the factors that discourage medical students from choosing a career in psychiatry. Sierles [11] reported that the proportion of students matching into psychiatry was higher in psychiatry departments with high prestige relative to the school's other departments or in which the director of medical student education in psychiatry was the recipient of a teaching award. The latter finding highlights the potential for a well-taught development course with an energetic and enthusiastic instructor to serve as an educational and recruitment vehicle. The development course is often the first contact that beginning medical students have with general and child psychiatrists. This course provides an opportunity for the instructor to provide role modeling and mentoring, First-year medical students are receptive to learning about psychiatry as a potential career and area of need and appreciate receiving informational hand-outs on this subject [12] and information about local and national psychiatry interest clubs [13,14].

Most students do not choose psychiatry. The point that such a course also will benefit future internists or surgeons was best stated by Scully [15], who wrote, "Excellence in teaching is the critical factor in recruitment. If we convey to our students the importance and the excitement of psychiatry, there are two good possibilities. Either the students will choose a career in psychiatry or they won't. If they do, we can select from the best qualified; if they don't, they will have an appreciation of the importance of psychiatry for their patients, leading to good referrals and addressing the still real problem of stigma."

*Liaison Committee on Medical Education requirements*

The Liaison Committee on Medical Education accreditation standard ED-10 [16] states: "The curriculum must include behavioral and socioeconomic subjects, in addition to basic science and clinical disciplines." Human development/life cycle is specifically listed as a topic for which "the number of formal teaching sessions (structured sessions, such as lectures, small-group discussions, lab activities) during the preclinical or clinical years where the topic is considered to be an important learning objective" must be indicated.

*Course length, expected level of competency, goals, and objectives*

Few of us are asked to design and implement a development curriculum for medical students de novo, with freedom to choose course timing (basic science versus clinical years or a combination), setting (large classroom versus small group), format (lecture versus experiential/discussion), series, and session length. Many of these influential variables are rooted in school history and tradition, the "course" often inherited by junior faculty who soon learn that desired accommodations/changes to the status quo are at best a process, not an event. Lobbying for "market share" with other specialties often involves a lengthy process with the curriculum committee in the medical school.

Typically, medical students are taught development during the first 18 months of the curriculum, with perhaps 10 to 15 dedicated sessions (expected to cover the entire lifespan). The format is traditionally a large classroom didactic setting with limited built-in opportunity for more personal student-professor interaction. With imagination, however, the instructor may be able to vary this format using small group exercises or other approaches (see Box 1).

Although we recommend specific goals and objectives for each teaching session/exercise, an overarching set of goals for student knowledge, skills, and attitudes for medical students may include the following information.

*Knowledge.* To acquire basic understanding of biologic, psychological, and social parameters of each developmental epoch and become familiar with key developmental topics/lines; to become aware of familial and extrafamilial and cultural influences on development.

*Skills.* To recognize the impact of development on disease states and disease states on development; to recognize possible deviations from expectable development; to begin to apply knowledge of developmental epochs and lines to medical assessment and treatment.

*Attitudes.* To increase curiosity about the student's own developmental processes, particularly as they influence the student's identity as a physician; to heighten interest in the impact of development on disease and disease on development; to enhance cultural sensitivity and awareness.

*Sample curricula*

The prospective instructor is well advised to consider the developmental characteristics of medical students that may inform the teaching approach. Particularly if the course is taught early in the basic science curriculum or concurrent with "killer" memorization or heavy volume courses, students may dismiss the material as "soft science." Even the psychologically sophisticated/holistically oriented student consumers may fail to appreciate the integration of biologic, psychological, and social processes and question the "clinical relevance" of the topic while simultaneously "trying on" a new identity as a physician. Early course lectures that review the neuroscience of development and address the practical application of developmental principles (cognition, emotions) in history taking and treatment planning for ill children may provide reassurance.

For this group, we favor an integrated "sample" of the topical and lifespan approaches to create a core teaching module, using teaching tools that ideally include (for each lecture or teaching exercise) written goals and objectives, an outline, lecture notes, recommended readings, a clinical correlation or case vignette, sample test questions, and the liberal use of audiovisual aids (Box 4). "Always too short" courses can be supplemented

## Box 4. Recommended audiovisual resources

*Videos*

Apted M. 49 Up. 133 minutes total running time, VHS,
First Run Features, 2006.

Craig S, Tallon K. Right from the start. Chicago (IL): Scott Craig
Productions; 1982. VHS, 53 minutes, narrated by Sada Thompson.

Finitzo M. 5 Girls: point of view. PBS documentary, 2001.

Fox G. Normal development in the first ten years of life: an
educational videotape and teacher's aid. Complete version: 201
video clips, 6 hours 40 minutes total running time. Greatest
Hits version: 31 video clips, 55 minutes total running time. VHS
copyright 2000, DVD copyright 2003.foxg@uic.edu. View clips
at http://www.psych.uic.edu/faculty/fox.htm

NOVA (PBS). Life's first feelings (1986). http://www.pbs.org/
wgbh/nova/listseason/13.html.

Wagner J, DiFeliciantonio T. Girls like us. VHS, 57 minutes total
running time. Women Make Movies, Inc., 1996.

Visit various college publishers' websites for supplemental
audiovisual resources that accompany their textbooks.

*Links to obtain various development videos*
http://www.childdevelopmentmedia.com/index.cfm
http://www.library.gsu.edu/research/
resources.asp?ldlD=42&guidelD=0&resourcelD=6
http://www.spdnetwork.org/other/childdev.html
http://www.zerotothree.org/

*Reviews and lists of resources*

Fox G. Teaching normal development using stimulus videotapes
in psychiatric education. Academic Psychiatry 2003;27:283–8.

Kaye D, Ets-Hokin E. The breakfast club: utilizing popular film to
teach adolescent development. Academic Psychiatry
2000;24:110–6.

Parkin A, Dogra N. Making videos for medical undergraduate
teaching in child psychiatry: the development, use and
perceived effectiveness of structured videotapes of clinical
material for use by medical students in child psychiatry.
Medical Teacher 2000;22(6):568–71.

Robinson DJ. Reel psychiatry: movie portrayals of psychiatric
conditions. Port Huron (MI): Rapid Psychler Press; 2003.

Sondheimer A. The life stories of children and adolescents: using
commercial films as teaching aids. Academic Psychiatry
2000;24:214–24.

(also enhancing recruitment, mentorship connections) via additional (often after-hours) discussion groups. The course coordinator or students may suggest topics of interest and reading materials and invite guest faculty members. Contemporary topics, such as the effects of daycare, divorce, and media exposure to violence, are always well received. Box 5 provides sample UGME curricula. Box 6 lists potential discussion group topics with suggested readings.

*General psychiatry residency*

*Special issues: recruitment into child and adolescent psychiatry*
Weissman and Bashook [17] found that although 30% of residents entering general psychiatry express an interest in specializing child and adolescent psychiatry, only 18% actually end up choosing to enter a fellowship. How can initial interest be sustained during the general psychiatry residency in addition to attracting others to the field? The demand for child and adolescent psychiatrists far outstrips the supply. A report by the US Bureau of Health Professions (2000) projected a need in the year 2020 for 12,624 child and adolescent psychiatrists but a supply of only 8312 [18]. It is imperative to encourage interest in the field. In addition to required clinical

---

**Box 5. First-year medical student (M-1) sample human development curriculum**

1. Course overview and organization, history, research strategies, questions, and controversies
2. Emotions and illness: perspectives of children
3. Attachment
4. Maternal employment and emotional development/ temperament
5. Language development
6. Psychosocial development
7. Cognitive development: Piaget's theory and Vygotsky's sociocultural viewpoint and cognitive development. Information processing perspectives
8. Moral development
9. Psychosexual development
10. Forging an identity
11. Brain and development
12. Familial influences on development
13. Extrafamilial influences on development
14. Cultural influences
15. Adulthood/aging

---

**Box 6. First-year medical student (M-1) discussion group topics and reading suggestions**

- Differences in the development of men and women

Gilligan C. In a different voice. Cambridge (MA): Harvard University Press; 1993 (particularly introduction and Chapters 1 and 2)

Vaillant GE. Adaptation to life. Boston (MA): Little, Brown and Company; 1977 (particularly Chapter 10)

- Mothercare/Fathercare

Pruett KD. Fatherneed. New York (NY): Free Press; 2000 (particularly Chapters 1–3)

Bornstein MH, editor. Handbook of parenting: status and social condition of parenting (volume 3). Mahwah (NJ): Lawrence Erlbaum Associates; 1995 (particularly Chapter 1, "Mothering," and Chapter 2, "Fathers and families")

Hrdy SB. Mother nature: a history of mothers, infants, and natural selection. New York (NY): Random House; 1995

- Cultural and ethnic dimensions of development

Bornstein MH. Handbook of parenting: biology and ecology of parenting (volume 2). Mahwah (NJ): Lawrence Erlbaum Associates; 1995 (particularly Chapter 8, "Ethnic and minority parenting," and Chapter 9, "Culture and parenting")

Lewis M, editor. Child and adolescent psychiatry: a comprehensive textbook. 3rd edition. Philadelphia (PA): Lippincott Williams, and Wilkins; 2002 (Chapter 38 "Effects of culture and ethnicity on child and adolescent development")

- The impact of divorce on development

Hodges WF. Interventions for children of divorce: custody, access, and psychotherapy. 2nd edition. New York (NY): Wiley Interscience; 1991 (particularly Chapters 2 and 3)

Lewis M, editor. Child and adolescent psychiatry: a comprehensive textbook. 3rd edition. Philadelphia (PA): Lippincott Williams, and Wilkins; 2002 (Chapter 109, "The child and the vicissitudes of divorce")

---

experiences in child and adolescent psychiatry during the residency, a continuing seminar in development and child and adolescent psychiatry provides an ongoing weekly opportunity to reflect on issues regarding children, adolescents, and families.

In the authors' opinion, it is crucial to offer clinical child and adolescent psychiatry experiences and an ongoing didactic component during the formative period of the PGY-1 and -2 years. By the completion of the

PGY-2 year, residents who are considering the "short route" of entering child and adolescent psychiatry subspecialty training at the end of their PGY-3 year must decide on their career choice and begin the application process. As PGY-2 residents straggle into development class after a morning of dealing with patients on adult inpatient units, something magical happens. The opportunity to see healthy children and adolescents (live and videotaped) and reflect on issues of normal growth and development (including their own backgrounds) often provides a refreshing contrast to the chronic and severe psychopathology in which they are immersed on their rotations. This positive experience often nurtures a budding interest in the field. When the development course is integrated with exposure to various child and adolescent psychiatrist role models speaking with enthusiasm about their work and challenging child and adolescent psychiatry clinical experiences, the development course instructor also may become a mentor and career advisor. To this end, the instructor should provide students with information about career opportunities in child and adolescent psychiatry [12].

### Accreditation Council for Graduate Medical Education requirements

The program requirements for residency education in psychiatry [19] stipulate that the curriculum must include "child and adult development," and "presentation of the biological, psychological, sociocultural, economic, ethnic, gender, religious/spiritual, sexual orientation, and family factors that significantly influence physical and psychological development throughout the life cycle." "(R)esidents should have experiences in determining the developmental status and needs for intervention with the children of some of their adult patients." These requirements, although extensive, do not stipulate how education in child and adult development is to be organized. Importantly, they emphasize thinking about development throughout the life cycle, how the developmental needs of children of psychiatric patients are met, and what types of interventions might be necessary. Because general psychiatry residents treat adult patients, it is important to keep these factors in mind when designing a child development course.

### Course length, expected level of competency, goals, and objectives

A good course on development stimulates students to want to learn more. Residents often approach learning about development with the expectation that they will be asked only to memorize outdated theories or recite lists of developmental milestones. The first question is often, "Why is this relevant to what I am doing"? Especially for residents who are not interested in child psychiatry, it is useful to link learning about development with how such a process can enhance their care of adult patients. An introductory session on why one takes a developmental history along with a clinical example of how that history contributes dramatically to understanding the patient and anticipating issues in treatment often convinces even the most resistant residents that there is some usefulness to the course. In our experience, beginning in this way sparks a lively discussion about individual patients whom residents have encountered along with questions about developmental issues.

The length and structure of a development course is often determined by multiple factors, including available faculty to teach, competing demands in the curriculum, the relative importance of child psychiatry within the general psychiatry program, and how clinical experience in child psychiatry is structured in the residency program. It is ideal to begin in the PGY-1 or -2 year to stimulate interest in child and adolescent psychiatry and expose residents to a way of thinking about patients that is different from DSM-IV diagnosis or other structured formats to which they are exposed on inpatient or consultation-liaison rotations. Sessions should include time for didactic and clinical material and live and audiovisual resources (see Boxes 1 and 4). Courses generally range from 6 to 12 sessions, but material also may be incorporated in other didactic sessions or in supervision of clinical work. It is ideal to have a weekly or every-other-week seminar for continuity. It is often best to combine short readings with hand-outs that summarize key concepts because, in our experience, residents do not read lengthy assignments or material with complex theoretical terminology. Readings should include clinical examples to illustrate concepts.

The goals and objectives of a development course in general psychiatry training include the following information:

*Knowledge.* Knowledge of basic developmental concepts, terminology and key figures in child development, knowledge of lifespan versus topical approaches and major developmental achievements/conflicts of each age group studied (eg, infancy, toddlerhood), knowledge of family, social, cultural, and other factors that impact on development, and understanding of different ways of defining "normality."

*Skills.* Application of developmental concepts to understanding psychopathology in children, adolescents, and adults, advocacy for the needs of children of mentally ill parents, improved ability to develop a psychodynamic formulation and integrate developmental history with current psychopathology, and enhanced observational abilities of children encountered in day-to-day and clinical settings.

*Attitudes.* Awareness of and interest in the developmental needs of children, adolescents, and adults, heightened recognition of the impact of psychiatric illness on development and the impact of development on psychiatric illness, curiosity and interest in the impact of mental illness on parenting, and awareness of and openness toward considering one's own developmental and family issues.

*Sample curricula*

A sample curriculum for general psychiatry residents is provided in Box 7. It is helpful to use a textbook or series of hand-outs as the main

---

**Box 7. Sample syllabus for general psychiatry residency**

Required text: Crain W. Theories of development: concepts and applications. 5$^{th}$ edition. Upper Saddle River (NJ): Prentice Hall; 2005.
Topics
  (1) Introduction
  Why study development?
  Overview of topical versus lifespan approaches
  Definitions of normality
  Adult case illustrating developmental contributions to
      psychopathology
  (2) Temperament and attachment
  (3) Infancy
  Parenting
  Developing mind and interpersonal neurobiology
  Developmental milestones and assessment
  (4) Toddler/preschool
  Separation/individuation
  Sibling/family influences
  (5) School age
  Cognitive development, moral development
  (6) Emotional, psychosocial and psychosexual development
  (7) Adolescence
  (8) Young and middle adulthood
  (9) Geriatric development
  (10–12) Several sessions of live interviews interspersed
              through the course with infants, toddlers,
              preschoolers, school-aged children, and
              adolescents. Either a faculty member interviews the
              children of students or faculty or the students
              prepare and do the interviews. All interviews are
              videotaped and discussed.

---

resource for didactic material. Students benefit greatly by illustration of concepts through clinical vignettes, videotaped examples, or live interviews and often say this is what "made" the course. The syllabus provided later is flexible and can be shortened or expanded depending on the needs of the group and time available for teaching. It is important to keep in mind that this course is taught to general psychiatry residents, many of whom may not be interested in child and adolescent psychiatry, and to relate material to adult patients when possible. A good child development course often sparks interest in child psychiatry. Child psychiatrists often say that their skills in adult psychiatry improved dramatically as a result of child and adolescent psychiatry training. A successful development course hopefully will illustrate the benefit of this increased knowledge to general psychiatry residents.

## Child and adolescent psychiatry subspecialty residency

### Special issues: depth of knowledge, relation to child and adolescent psychiatry psychopathology course, and clinical integration

A major goal of child and adolescent psychiatry training is to understand when a child is abnormal or impaired enough to warrant a clinical diagnosis and psychiatric intervention. To know what is truly "abnormal," residents first must understand what is "normal" or expected at a given age and developmental level. A strong grounding in child development enables residents to formulate a comprehensive understanding of a child's problems. This understanding may lead to clinical intervention or reassurance that the child is exhibiting developmentally appropriate behavior. It also allows residents to anticipate the problems a child with a psychiatric illness might have with particular developmental stages (eg, the adolescent with pervasive developmental disorder navigating increased sexual urges or wishes to have a boy/girlfriend) and how difficulties at a particular stage of development might contribute to psychiatric problems.

Although child and adolescent psychiatry residents have extensive exposure to children with psychiatric illness, they often lack perspective on the ways in which their patients have veered off a normal developmental trajectory. They frequently do not clearly know what that trajectory should be. Like general psychiatry residents, they are bombarded with tasks that on the surface take them away from thinking about normal development: managing children in crisis, prescribing and monitoring medication, making DSM-IV diagnoses, dealing with difficult parents, and interacting with children in diverse settings (eg, hospitals, correctional facilities, residential treatment). Although most child and adolescent psychiatry residents accept the value of studying child development, they do not grasp how useful it can be to their clinical work. For example, understanding a 5-year-old child's cognitive abilities and attachment experiences dramatically influences the child's adaptation to a hospital setting. Unlike general psychiatry residents, however, child and adolescent residents are typically enthusiastic about learning about child development but are unsure as to how the material might benefit their day-to-day work. Relatively early in the course, they express surprise at how skewed their perspectives have become after working with ill children on a regular basis.

Child and adolescent psychiatry residents need an in-depth understanding of child development. They should be able to think flexibly about the clinical problems they encounter in children and use their understanding of development to inform their clinical interactions and treatment decisions. Residents typically have participated in a development course as part of their general psychiatry training and often are not aware of how much more there is to learn. Because of their constant exposure to psychiatrically ill children, they must understand in a detailed way what normal development is like and, at the same time, what factors can alter it.

Ideally, a child and adolescent psychopathology course can be integrated with what is being learned in the child development seminar. For example, when studying anxiety disorders, the teacher can reinforce what types of anxieties are developmentally appropriate at different ages. The residents hopefully are then able to determine whether a child they are seeing with separation anxiety disorder truly has a disorder or may have developmentally appropriate separation anxiety given their age, attachment experiences, and cognitive level. Child and adolescent development and psychopathology courses can be designed to complement and reinforce material if instructors are able to plan accordingly. Many programs operate with independent teaching tracks, so this approach may not be possible, but having the opportunity to discuss topics such as reactive attachment disorder while learning about infancy or discussing posttraumatic stress disorder while reviewing issues of risk and resilience in children naturally integrates subjects and learning. A creative way to integrate child development and psychopathology is through the use of didactic modules [20]. These modules define an area of instruction (eg, infant psychiatry), provide a list of recommended readings sequenced from basic to advanced, and provide an outline of what areas are covered by the module (eg, history of infant psychiatry, principles of infant psychological development, assessment and diagnosis). It is easy to see how development and psychopathology could be integrated through this approach. On a practical level, some programs might have difficulty finding teachers with the expertise in development and psychopathology or the time available to commit to this undertaking.

*Accreditation Council for Graduate Medical Education requirements*

The program requirements for residency education in child and adolescent psychiatry [19] state: "Emphasis on development is an essential part of training in child and adolescent psychiatry. The teaching of developmental knowledge and the integration of neurobiological, phenomenological, psychological, and sociocultural issues into a comprehensive formulation of clinical problems are essential. Teaching about normal development should include observation of and interaction with normal children of various ages." The approach to teaching development described in this article attempts to fulfill these goals with the awareness that resources, faculty teachers, and time allotted in the schedule differ from one institution to another. The ACGME requirements serve to underscore the importance of teaching development and the need to integrate it with clinical experience.

*Course length, expected level of competency, goals, and objectives*

Teaching child development to child and adolescent psychiatry residents should be more detailed and intensive than teaching to the groups described previously. Child and adolescent psychiatry residents need time to discuss material in depth and correlate it with their clinical experience. A year-long course is ideal to foster in-depth examination of concepts and provide time for clinical exercises to enhance material. Residents have responded well to the use of a textbook (see Box 2; Boxes 8 and 9) for core readings with supplementation by additional articles. For example, Davies [21] integrates all aspects of development nicely with liberal use of real-world clinical examples that residents find familiar to their experience. There is a beginning section on topical issues related to child development (eg, brain development, risk and protective factors, attachment) followed by well-organized chapters on specific age groups from infancy through school age. The author's writing style conveys empathy and respect for children, an awareness of the complexity of clinical work with children, and an ability to explain in jargon-free language the various theories on child development. Other advantages of this text include "clinical correlation" chapters that follow sections on each period of development along with the use of numerous clinical examples throughout the text. This textbook covers all major theories in child development and provides thoughtful discussion of the pros and cons of each. Disadvantages of the book are few but include the fact that writer is a social worker and gears the book toward social work students. Although this might seem to be a significant issue, the residents who have used it enjoy the emphasis on psychosocial interventions throughout the book and the lack of attention to medication management. They report that this is a breath of fresh air in their training and often have new ideas on how to help patients they are treating from reading them.

Supplementary articles in a development course for child and adolescent psychiatry residents provide additional perspectives, augment the material in the book, and, most importantly, introduce residents to the original works of historical figures in child psychiatry. This is the first opportunity for many residents to read original articles by individuals whom they have only heard about during their training. It is often eye-opening to actually read what Bowlby said rather than review a hand-out or summary provided by a teacher. In addition to the suggested additional readings mentioned in this article, there is a comprehensive resource list of articles organized by topic (eg, social development, language development) for infant/child development [22] and adolescent/young adult development [23].

The goals and objectives of a child development course for child and adolescent psychiatry residents include the following information:

*Knowledge.* To acquire in-depth knowledge of child development, including detailed understanding of major theories and contributors, historical, contemporary and research perspectives, and developmental issues for each

**Box 8. Sample syllabus for child and adolescent psychiatry residency**

Required text: Davies D. Child development: a practitioner's guide. 2<sup>nd</sup> edition. New York (NY): Guilford Press; 2004.

- Introduction
- Why study development?
- Overview of developmental models
- Lifespan versus topical approaches
- Definitions of normality
- Risk and protective factors
  Kauai Study
  Clinical correlation with parent death (children's narratives)
- Introduction to attachment theory
  Ghosts in the nursery article
- Prenatal/newborn development and becoming a parent
  Caregiver's role
- Fetal behavior
- Newborn abilities (eg, imitation of facial expression, discrimination of smell and voice)
- Neuroscience
- Infancy I, II, III
  Daniel Stern and infant's sense of self
  Parent narratives
  Temperament (Chess and Thomas)
  Childcare Decisions and Research
  Neurodevelopment
  Psychoanalytic perspective
  Winnicott (transitional objects)
  Greenspan's basic model (six organizational
    levels of experience)
- Toddlerhood
  Kagan (biologic basis of childhood shyness)
  Fraiberg (magic years)
- Attachment and clinical correlations
- Family influences
- Separation/individuation
  Mahler (and criticism of theories from Stern)
- Preschool period
- Moral development
  Kohlberg
  Gilligan
- School-age period

Cultural influences on child development (media, sociocultural group, religion)
Family influences
Psychosocial development (self-esteem, empathy, social skills)
• Cognitive development
Piaget
• Gender identity
• Developmental lines
Anna Freud
• Erikson
• Adolescence
Cognitive developments
Psychosocial changes
Neuroscience
Daniel Offer
Clinical correlations (Anne Frank, Harry Potter, Buffy the Vampire Slayer, Stand by Me)

age group. This information includes biologic, psychological, social, family, cultural, and neurodevelopmental approaches to development and the ability to compare and contrast major developmental theories and concepts.

*Skills.* To use knowledge of development to inform residents' skills in diagnosis, treatment, and prevention efforts with children and adolescents. This goal includes learning the impact of developmental issues on psychiatric illness and vice versa and having the ability to integrate developmental information in the formulation of a child's difficulties.

*Attitudes.* To inspire an attitude of inquiry and curiosity for differences in development as they impact the individual and the family and have an awareness of other significant contributing factors (eg, cultural background, genetics, trauma).

*Sample curricula*
A suggested curriculum with topic areas and supplementary articles is presented in Box 8. Depending on time available, volume of reading for other courses, and the interest of the teacher and residents, the reading requirements for child development can be adjusted accordingly. Students tend to read only required articles, so distributing optional articles tends not to be worth the effort. Because the group of residents tends to be relatively small, the course works best if it is run like a graduate level seminar with the expectation that residents have read the material and come

**Box 9. Additional references for child and adolescent psychiatry development course**

Bowlby J. The making and breaking of affectional bonds, Parts I and II. Br J Psychiatry 1977;130–201, 441.

Fraiberg S. Ghosts in the nursery: a psychoanalytic approach to the problems of impaired infant-mother relationships. Columbus (OH): The Ohio State University Press; 1987. p. 100–36.

Werner EE. Risk, resilience, and recovery: perspectives from the Kauai Longitudinal Study. Dev Psychopathology 1993;5:503–15.

Krementz J. How it feels when a parent dies. New York (NY): Alfred A. Knopf; 1982. p. 8–15, 16–21, 42–51.

Field TM, Woodson R, Greenberg R, et al. Discrimination and imitation of facial expressions by neonates. Science 1981;218:179–81.

DeCasper AJ, Fifer WP. Of human bonding: newborns prefer their mothers' voices. Science 1980;206:1174–6.

Nelson CA, Floyd FE. Child development and neuroscience. Child Dev 1997;68(5):970–87. (Great review of imaging techniques and neurodevelopment.)

Thompson RA, Nelson CA. Developmental science and the media: early brain development. Am Psychologist 2001;56(1):5–15. (Nice discussion of neurodevelopment research versus what is widely believed and reported by the media.)

Stern D. The interpersonal world of the infant. New York (NY): Basic Books; 1985. p. 3–12, 26–46.

Tasman A, Kay J, Lieberman JA. Psychiatry, Philadelphia: WB Saunders Co.; 1997. p. 76–81. (Tables on developmental theories in the first 3 years of life.)

Jaffee SS, Viertel J. Becoming parents: preparing for emotional changes of first-time parenthood. New York (NY): Atheneum; 1985.

"At one month: the baby as a new toy." (p. 229–39)

"At one month: the Madison Avenue mother." (p. 286–92)

"At three months: infatuated with the baby." (p. 293–9)

Herschkowitz N. Neurological bases of behavioral development in infancy. Brain Dev 2000;22:411–6.

Tyson P, Tyson R. Psychoanalytic theories of development. New Haven (CT): Yale University Press; 1990. p. 94–5. (Also see table.)

Winnicott DW. Transitional objects and transitional phenomena: a study of the first not-me possession. International Journal of Psychoanalysis 1953;34:89–97.

Winnicott DW. Paediatrics and psychiatry. In: Collected papers: through paediatrics to psycho-analysis. New York (NY): Basic Books; 1958. p. 157–73.

St. Clair M, Winnicott DW: pediatrician with a unique perspective. Object relations and self psychology: an introduction. Monterey (CA): Brooks/Cole Publishing; 1996. p. 71–89.

Greenspan S. The basic model: the influence of regulatory and experiential factors on the six organizational levels of experience. Infancy and early childhood: the practice of clinical assessment and intervention with emotional and developmental challenges. New York (NY): International University Press; 1993. p. 3–28.

Kagan J, Reznick JS, Snidman N. Biological bases of childhood shyness. Science 1988;240:167–71.

Fraiberg S. All about witches, ogres, tigers, and mental health. In: The magic years. New York (NY): MacMillan; 1981. p. 3–10.

Mahler M, Pine F, Bergman A. The third subphase: rapprochement. In: The psychological birth of the human infant: symbiosis and individuation. New York (NY): Basic Books; 2000. p. 76–108.

Tasman A, Kay J, Lieberman JA. Psychiatry. Philadelphia: WB Saunders Co.; 1997. p. 425–6. (Synopsis of Margaret Mahler.)

Crain WC. Kohlberg's stages of moral development. In: Theories of development. Upper Saddle River (NJ): Prentice Hall; 1985. p. 118–36. (Also available at: faculty.plts.edu/gpence/html/kohlberg.htm.)

Moral development and moral education: an overview. Available at: http://tigger.uic.edu/ ~ lnucci/MoralEd/overviewtext.html.

Gilligan C. In a different voice: psychological theory and women's development. Cambridge (MA): Harvard University Press; 1982.

Piaget's theory of cognitive development. Available at: http://chiron.valdosta.edu/whuitt/col/cogsys/piaget.html. (Overview with nice tables.)

Piaget J. http://www.psy.pdx.edu/PsiCafe/KeyTheorists/Piaget.htm. (Many internet resources, tables, articles on Piaget.)

Tyson P, Tyson R. Psychoanalytic theories of development. New Haven (CT): Yale University Press; 1990. p. 249–92. (Gender development: a theoretical overview.)

Freud A. The assessment of normality in childhood. In: Normality and pathology in childhood. New York (NY): International

Universities Press; 1965. p. 54–106. (Discussion of developmental lines and use of regression in childhood.)

Coles R: Anna Freud: the dream of psychoanalysis. Perseus Publishing; 1993. p. 15–26. (Beautifully written summary of Anna Freud's life and work.)

Erikson E. Psychosocial theory summary. Available at: http://www.haverford.edu/psych/ddavis/p109g/erikson.stages.html.

Erikson E. Eight ages of man. In: Childhood and society. New York (NY): WW Norton and Co.; 1950. p. 247–74.

Offer D, Sconert-Reichl KA. Debunking the myths of adolescence: findings from recent research. J Am Acad Child Adolesc Psychiatry 1992;31:1003–14.

Ponton LE, Judice S. Typical adolescent sexual development. Child Adolesc Psychiatric Clin N Am 2004;13:497–511.

Schowalter JE, Towbin KE. Adolescent development. In: Tasman A, Kay J, Lieberman JA, editors. Psychiatry. Philadelphia (PA): WB Saunders Co.; 1997. p. 127–44. (Overview of biologic, social, emotional, and cognitive development in adolescence.)

Dalsimer K. Female adolescent development: a study of "The Diary of Anne Frank." Psychoanalytic Study of the Child 1982;37:487–522. (Optional paper to discuss the use of diaries, female puberty, and ordinary development during extraordinary times.)

to class prepared to discuss it. Handing out goals and objectives for each session of the course may prove to be too cumbersome, but it is often useful to distribute one or two thought-provoking questions to motivate residents to read for each session with these goals in mind. Almost every session is also supplemented by video vignettes that illustrate the material presented.

It becomes clear as the course progresses which residents are doing the reading and understanding the material. Speaking to residents individually who are not keeping up is often all that is necessary to inspire better performance. To supplement that, asking less motivated residents to present a paper or discuss a topic also serves to enhance performance. It is more helpful to have "mini-quizzes" on material covered periodically through the course rather than one "test" at the end to motivate reading and study of the material. This also provides the teacher with feedback on residents' understanding and retention of the material studied. Residents tend to rise to the challenge of this course, participate actively in the discussion, enjoy the continuity of the course and subject matter, and remark on their enjoyment of a graduate-style seminar in residency!

## Summary

Teaching normal development provides an opportunity to engage medical students and general psychiatry residents in a reflective and thoughtful conversation about the human condition. When clinical exercises are added, such as observing children at home or at school or asking students to take their own developmental history, the course becomes not only instructional but fun and useful in more meaningful ways. The subject matter is easily brought to life using various innovative teaching techniques, which have been outlined. Various textbook, journal, and audiovisual resources have been suggested, as have considerations in assessment methodology. Issues specific to undergraduate, residency, and subspecialty training levels were discussed, and sample curricula were provided for each level of training.

## References

[1] Offer D, Sabshin M. Normality: theoretical and clinical concepts in mental health. New York: Basic Books; 1966.

[2] The Denver Developmental Screening Test. Available at: http://www.denverii.com/DenverII.html. Accessed August 31, 2006.

[3] Bloom B, Englehart M, Furs E, et al. Taxonomy of educational objectives: the classification of educational goals. Handbook I: cognitive domain. New York: Longmans Green; 1956.

[4] Fox G. Teaching normal development using stimulus videotapes in psychiatric education. Acad Psychiatry 2003;27:283–8.

[5] Fox G. Normal development in the first ten years of life: a longitudinal stimulus video observation. Available at: http://www.psych.uic.edu/faculty/fox.htm. Accessed August 31, 2006.

[6] Bornstein M, Lamb M, editors. Developmental science: an advanced textbook. 5th edition. Mahwah (NJ): Erlbaum; 2005.

[7] Folensbee RW. Applying neuroscience to psychological therapies: a primer. Cambridge, UK: Cambridge University Press; in press.

[8] Crain W. Theories of development: concepts and applications. 5th edition. Upper Saddle River (NJ): Prentice Hall; 2005.

[9] Accreditation Council for Graduate Medical Education. Available at: www.acgme.org/Outcome/. Accessed August 31, 2006.

[10] The American Academy of Child and Adolescent Psychiatry Task Force on Workforce Needs: Child and Adolescent Psychiatry Workforce: A critical shortage and national challenge. Academic Psychiatry 2003;27:277–82.

[11] Sierles FS. Medical school factors and career choice of psychiatry. Am J Psychiatry 1982;139: 1040–2.

[12] Fox G. Choosing child and adolescent psychiatry as a career: the top ten questions. Available at: http://www.aacap.org/training/DevelopMentor/Content/2005Fall/f2005_a2.cfm. Accessed August 31, 2006.

[13] Available at: www.apa.org. Accessed August 31, 2006.

[14] Available at: www.aacap.org. Accessed August 31, 2006.

[15] Scully JH. Why be concerned about recruitment? Am J Psychiatry 1995;152:1413–4.

[16] Liaison Committee on Medical Education. Standards. Available at: www.lcme.org. Accessed August 31, 2006.

[17] Weissman SH, Bashook PG. A view of the prospective child psychiatrist. Am J Psychiatry 1986;143(6):722–7.

[18] Kim WJ. Child and adolescent psychiatry workforce: a critical shortage and national challenge. Acad Psychiatry 2003;27:277–82.

[19] Accreditation Council for Graduate Medical Education. Requirements. Available at: www.acgme.org. Accessed August 31, 2006.

[20] Josephson AM, Drell MJ. Didactic modules for curricular development in child and adolescent psychiatry education. Acad Psychiatry 1992;16:44–51.

[21] Davies D. Child development: a practitioner's guide. 2nd edition. New York: Guilford Press; 2004.

[22] Mayes L. Infant and child development. In: Sacks MH, Sledge WH, editors. Core readings in psychiatry. 2nd edition. Washington, DC: American Psychiatric Press; 1995. p. 647–70.

[23] Esman AH. Adolescent and young adult development. In: Sacks MH, Sledge WH, editors. Core readings in psychiatry. 2nd edition. Washington, DC: American Psychiatric Press; 1995. p. 671–80.

**ELSEVIER**
SAUNDERS

Child Adolesc Psychiatric Clin N Am
16 (2007) 95–110

CHILD AND
ADOLESCENT
PSYCHIATRIC CLINICS
OF NORTH AMERICA

# Developing a Psychopathology Curriculum During Child and Adolescent Psychiatry Residency Training: General Principles and a Problem-Based Approach

Cynthia W. Santos, MD[a,*], Andrew Harper, MD[a,b],
Ann E. Saunders, MD[a], Sonja L. Randle, MD[a]

[a]Department of Psychiatry and Behavioral Sciences, University of Texas
Medical School at Houston, 1300 Moursund Street, Houston, TX 77030, USA
[b]Harris County Psychiatric Center, 2800 S. MacGregor Way, Houston, TX 77028, USA

Curriculum development is one of the most important tasks of a residency program. There is little evidence to guide decisions about curricula, and there is an infinite variety of ways to teach any given topic. The recent emphasis on core competencies and life-long learning adds yet a new dimension to curriculum design and evaluation. Although some chapters are written on developing and monitoring psychiatric curricula generically [1–4], there is remarkably little information published in the literature on effective ways to teach psychopathology in a child and adolescent psychiatry (CAP) residency program. This article describes an approach to curriculum development and the use of this approach to devise an integrated curriculum using seminars and problem-based learning (PBL) to teach psychopathology and normal development in children and adolescents.

Kern and colleagues [5] describe a six-step approach for curriculum development that is used to outline this article. The first two steps are problem identification and needs assessment. This phase begins by examining the current approach and the ideal approach to the problem (curriculum) and is followed by a needs assessment of the learners—in this case, CAP residents. In step three, the goals and objectives for the curriculum are developed,

---

* Corresponding author. University of Texas Mental Sciences Institute, 1300 Moursund Street, Houston, TX 77028.

*E-mail address:* Cynthia.W.Santos@uth.tmc.edu (C.W. Santos).

1056-4993/07/$ - see front matter © 2006 Elsevier Inc. All rights reserved.
doi:10.1016/j.chc.2006.07.007

*childpsych.theclinics.com*

which guides the decision for which educational strategies (step 4) are best. Step 5 is implementation, which is followed by evaluation and feedback (step 6) of both the individual learner and the program.

## Problem identification and needs assessment

The primary goal of any residency program is to produce competent physicians. In developing the curriculum, however, there are several other considerations. First, programs must be familiar with the Accreditation Council of Graduate Medical Education program requirements in their specialties. The Psychiatry Residency Review Committee Program Requirements for Residency Education in Child and Adolescent Psychiatry define child and adolescent psychiatrists as "specialists in the delivery of skilled and comprehensive medical care of children and adolescents suffering from psychiatric disorders" [6]. Regarding psychopathology, the Residency Review Committee states that programs "must provide teaching about the full range of psychopathology in children and adolescents, including the etiology, epidemiology, diagnosis, treatment, and prevention of the major psychiatric conditions that affect children and adolescents" [6].

The Accreditation Council of Graduate Medical Education recently described core competencies to be taught by all residency programs, regardless of specialty [7]. These competencies include medical knowledge, patient care, systems-based practice, practice-based improvement, professionalism, and interpersonal skills and communication. The American Academy of Child and Adolescent Psychiatry Work Group on Training and Education [8] and the American Board of Psychiatry and Neurology (ABPN) [9] have described core competencies specific to CAP. The ABPN competencies for medical knowledge and psychopathology in CAP are listed in Box 1. Another important goal of CAP residency programs is for graduates to become certified by the ABPN. The 2006 ABPN CAP content outline lists "psychopathology/classification/differential diagnosis" as 20% of the overall examination [10].

Potential outlines for a psychopathology course might be found by looking at major textbooks in CAP, content outlines from the ABPN CAP examination, and content outlines from the CHILD Psychiatry Resident In Training Exam (PRITE). Many educators suggest using textbooks to guide seminar series when possible [2,3].

Developing or updating the curriculum often begins by gathering the faculty and residents to evaluate what happens currently. It is important to examine which aspects of the curriculum are effective, which areas need improvement, and what ideas there are for enhancement. Review of program/course evaluations over the past few years is the first step. Performance on CHILD PRITE and ABPN examinations is another way to assess current program strengths and weaknesses. Gathering information from graduates about the effectiveness and potential weaknesses of the program also can be helpful. Educational retreats can provide an opportunity to gather faculty and residents in an informal setting with a specific focus on curriculum review and development. A thorough overhaul probably should be done every 5 years or so, with fine tuning done on a more regular basis. The curriculum is likely to reflect more strongly those areas of interest for each individual division. It is important to involve as many people as possible in the development and implementation of the curriculum to maximize resources and provide an optimal learning experience [3].

**Develop goals and objectives**

Once a general course outline is generated, specific goals and objectives should be defined. Goals and objectives help communicate the purpose of the curriculum and suggest which learning method will be most effective [5]. Knowledge objectives, for example, are taught effectively through readings, lectures, discussion, learning projects, and PBL, whereas skills are often taught in clinical rotations [5]. Specific and measurable objectives also enable evaluation of the learner and curriculum [5]. Each residency program should have a set of overall competency-based goals and objectives that include knowledge, skills, and attitudes [6]. Didactic series must include at a minimum knowledge and attitude objectives that fit in with the program's overall core competencies [6].

**Educational strategies**

Numerous educational strategies are available for teaching psychopathology and all other areas of the curriculum. Teaching should be learner centered and emphasize adult learning principles [11]. Modern insights on learning in higher education suggest that learning should be a constructive, self-directed, collaborative, and contextual process [12]. Clinical experiences, including formal supervision and self-directed learning about the resident's patients, are perhaps some of the most important ways to learn about the psychiatric problems faced by children. Formal didactic experiences can include lectures, seminars, and PBL to further expand the residents' knowledge of psychopathology. In PBL, a clinical problem unfolds to provide a stimulus for resident learning of the basic, psychosocial, and clinical sciences. When given a clinical case scenario, the resident group identifies the current problems, discusses their current knowledge related to these problems, begins to develop hypotheses, and identifies what they need to learn to better understand the problems. When they have reached the limit of their knowledge, they identify learning issues, which they research and report back to the group at the next meeting. Continuous case presentations, case conferences, journal clubs, and other formats also help disseminate the knowledge required for the program [2]. Zisook and colleagues [13] described alternate methods of teaching psychopharmacology, including journal clubs, PBL, formalized patient-centered training, games, and modern

**Box 1. American Board of Psychiatry Neurology Child And Adolescent Core Competencies**

*Child and Adolescent Psychiatry Medical Knowledge Core Competencies*

A. General: Child and adolescent psychiatrists shall demonstrate the following:
  1. Knowledge of major disorders, including considerations relating to age, gender, race, and ethnicity, based on the literature and standards of practice. This knowledge shall include:
      a. The epidemiology of the disorder
      b. The etiology of the disorder, including medical, genetic, and sociocultural factors
      c. The phenomenology of the disorder
      d. An understanding of the impact of physical illness on the patient's functioning
      e. The experience, meaning, and explanation of the illness for the patient and family, including the influence of cultural factors and culture-bound syndromes
      f. Effective treatment strategies
      g. Course and prognosis
  2. Knowledge of healthcare delivery
  3. Knowledge of the application of ethical principles in delivering medical care
  4. Ability to reference and utilize electronic systems to access medical, scientific, and patient information
B. For Child And Adolescent Psychiatry: Psychopathology/classification/differential diagnosis
  1. Developmental disorders
      a. Mental retardation
      b. Autism/PDD
      c. Learning disorders
      d. Communication/language disorders
  2. Disruptive behavior disorders
      a. ADHD
      b. Conduct disorder
      c. Oppositional defiant disorder
  3. Mood disorders
  4. Bereavement
  5. Substance use disorders
  6. Sleep disorders
  7. Suicide
  8. Eating disorders

9. Anxiety disorders
10. Obsessive-compulsive disorder
11. PTSD/dissociative disorders
12. Personality disorders/traits
13. Schizophrenia/psychosis
14. Adjustment disorders
15. Movement disorders
16. Abuse/neglect
17. Family psychopathology
18. Somatoform disorders
19. Violence/homicide
20. Comorbidity

---

*Adapted from* The American Board of Psychiatry and Neurology Child and Adolescent Core Competencies Chart 2.1. Available at: www.ABPN.com. Accessed April 16, 2006.

technology. Most of these methods could be adapted to teach psychopathology or other topics. The use of videos and movies to depict psychopathology can be a fun and useful way to teach [14], as can field trips to specialty sites, such as autism programs or cultural centers.

PBL was first adopted in undergraduate medical education at McMaster University in the 1960s [15], and currently more than 70% of Liaison Committee on Medical Education–accredited medical schools in the United States have incorporated some form of PBL in their undergraduate curricula [16]. Despite the widespread adoption of PBL by many medical schools at the undergraduate level, only a few institutions have implemented it in their residency programs [17–19]. There are published reports of psychiatry residency programs using PBL on a smaller scale to teach ethics [20], forensics [21], and introduction to psychiatry [22]. There are also published reports on the use of PBL to teach undergraduate psychiatry [23–25]. PBL was initially designed for use in undergraduate medical education to provide a clinical context for the learning of basic sciences. In graduate medical education, residents tend to focus on the clinical aspects of education at the expense of basic science principles. PBL is an excellent way to demand the integration of knowledge of basic science and clinical principles. This is particularly important in psychiatry, in which an integrated biopsychosocial model forms the basis for clinical understanding and treatment. PBL also emphasizes adult learning principles [26]. PBL is active, learner centered, involves activation of prior knowledge, and provides elaboration of new knowledge in a clinical context.

Traditional formats also emphasize acquisition of information rather than development of skills and attitudes necessary to become competent physicians [27]. Although there has been a tendency to rely on clinical rotations for learning these skills and attitudes, many psychosocial skills critical to being a good psychiatrist can be reinforced in a PBL setting. In a review of the use of PBL to enhance the psychosocial competence of medical students, Block [24] notes that the literature suggests PBL promotes greater acquisition of psychosocial knowledge, fosters patient-centered attitudes and practices, enhances interpersonal skills, and encourages students to become engaged and self-directed learners. In particular, she notes the parallels of the process of PBL with the process of psychotherapy. "In both settings, the agenda is set by the learner or patient, the learner's or patient's goals have primacy over those of the teacher or therapist, and the teacher's or therapist's role is to facilitate learning" [24]. Residents in PBL are directed to develop good interpersonal skills and be able to work together as a group to solve a mutually identified problem. Differing viewpoints must be respected and occasionally challenged. The role of the facilitator is to listen, challenge assumptions, encourage critical thinking, guide and facilitate learning, and provide ongoing, constructive feedback. The enhanced teaching skills developed can be useful to child psychiatrists, who frequently educate families, schools, and other medical and mental health professionals about child psychiatric disorders.

A PBL format allows for much broader teaching of core competencies. Although psychopathology most logically falls in the "medical knowledge" competency and most seminar and lecture formats emphasize this aspect, PBL emphasizes several other competencies. Interpersonal and communication skills are critical because residents must communicate with each other during problem-solving activities and teach each other information related to their learning issues. The inclusion of self-directed learning as a core competency and the increasing emphasis on evidence-based medicine make PBL an attractive strategy [28]. Rather than the lecture-based emphasis on factual knowledge, residents in PBL are expected to solve clinical problems using information from literature they research and critically appraise. The clinical reasoning required in PBL is a core aspect of the patient care competency. Residents also have an opportunity to demonstrate professionalism. They are highly responsible for each other's learning, so attending PBL sessions on time and coming prepared are important.

## Implementation

Implementation of the curriculum requires an assessment and identification of necessary resources, specifically including personnel, time, facilities, scheduling, and costs. This may include a faculty development component for the learning of new educational techniques. Potential barriers to the new curriculum should be anticipated and addressed [5].

## Evaluation

Resident evaluation includes formative and summative feedback, which typically includes evaluations from clinical supervisors, scores on oral examinations, PRITE, and CHILD PRITE and can include evaluations of resident performance in didactics. A more comprehensive discussion of evaluation of competency in CAP residents can be found in the article by Sargent and colleagues [29] and in Dingle and Beresin's article [30] in this issue. In PBL, residents and facilitators are expected to provide ongoing formative feedback. Upon completion of the case, residents provide a written evaluation of the case and the facilitator and rate how well their group covered the goals and objectives. The facilitator completes an evaluation of each resident's performance during that case. Training committees in conjunction with the training director must review all resident evaluations at least biannually to review resident strengths and weaknesses and develop an educational plan [6].

Evaluation of the program consists of formal overall program evaluations, learner/faculty questionnaires, objective measures of skills and performance of its graduates, focus groups or other periodic meetings with learners and faculty, retreats and strategic planning sessions, and Residency Review Committee site visits, among others [5]. The performance of residents on CHILD PRITE and ABPN CAP examinations also provides information about the quality of the program. Scholarly activity can be built into the evaluation process, adding further incentive to clinician-educators seeking promotion.

## Curriculum development experience at one residency program

At the University of Texas Medical School at Houston, the didactic curriculum for the CAP residency program was converted to a primarily PBL format in 1996. The medical school had recently adopted this method for its second-year students, and many of the child psychiatry faculty members were involved and impressed with this teaching method. The goal was to use adult learning principles to enhance the self-directed learning of residents and promote an attitude of life-long learning. A steering committee was formed and charged with oversight of the process. The steering committee was responsible for identification of content areas to be covered in PBL, development of goals and objectives, and implementation of evaluation procedures. This committee met weekly for 3 months, then two to three times yearly for the next 2 years. The goals and objectives for PBL are listed in Box 2. Evaluations were developed for the residents' performance in PBL, the faculty facilitation skills, and evaluations of PBL as a teaching method. PRITE, CHILD PRITE, and ABPN performance would be monitored to provide another outcome measure of the program's effectiveness.

**Box 2. University of Texas at Houston problem-based learning goals and objectives for residents**

*Goals—Residents will:*
1. Develop and integrate knowledge about basic science and the clinical principles of psychopathology and normal development in children and create treatment plans based on current knowledge
2. Develop a spirit of inquiry and scholarship

*Objectives—Residents will be able to:*
1. Formulate clinical problems emphasizing the integration of knowledge of basic science and normal development with psychological theory and broader social context (K, PC)
2. Develop and demonstrate advanced critical thinking and problem-solving skills (PBI)
3. Use evidence to support medical decision making (PBI)
4. Develop and demonstrate the ability to work together as a team (IC; P)
5. Develop and demonstrate effective communication skills (IC)
6. Develop and demonstrate effective interpersonal skills (IC)
7. Demonstrate ongoing self-assessment (PBI)
8. Demonstrate self-directed, life-long learning skills (PBI)
9. Demonstrate the ability to teach others (IC)

K, knowledge; PBI, practice-based Improvement; PC, patient care; IC, interpersonal and communication skills; P, professionalism.

*Psychopathology knowledge objectives for problem-based learning/integrated curriculum*
Residents will demonstrate knowledge about the etiology, epidemiology, diagnosis, treatment, and prevention of the psychiatric conditions that affect children and adolescents, including the following topics
   1. Mental retardation
   2. Pervasive developmental disorders, including autism
   3. Disruptive behavior disorders (attention deficit hyperactivity disorder, oppositional defiant disorder, conduct disorder)
   4. Mood disorders (major depressive disorder, bipolar disorders)
   5. Anxiety disorders (obsessive-compulsive disorder, generalized anxiety disorder, posttraumatic stress disorder, separation anxiety disorder)
   6. Eating disorders
   7. Psychotic disorders (schizophrenia, brief reactive psychosis)

8. Elimination disorders
9. Somatoform disorders
10. Learning disorders
11. Substance abuse

Next, three case-writing groups were created, one for each major age group (infant/preschool, school age, and adolescence). These groups met weekly for approximately 4 months to develop three cases in each group. Nine cases were developed to represent children with a wide range of psychopathologic conditions from preschool age through adolescence. This approach allowed a natural progression of the topic of child development, which provided the foundation for the cases. Construction of each case began with an outline of goals and objectives covering normal development, psychopathology, and treatment methods. Many of the topic areas logically grouped together. For example, the psychopathology of conduct disorder includes some discussion of moral development and forensic issues. A case involving a child with attention deficit hyperactivity disorder naturally includes some discussion of the development of attention and cognition and social/peer interaction. The frequent comorbidity of learning disorders with attention deficit hyperactivity disorder fosters discussion of psychological assessment issues, education-based interventions and the laws that mandate those interventions. Cases were designed to be as realistic as possible and unfolded much as they would clinically. The first day of each case typically began with a chief complaint, encouraging discussion of normal development, initial hypothesis formation, and a clinical inquiry strategy. As more information was revealed, a diagnosis was usually reached, and the discussion turned to psychopathology and basic science issues. The end of each case generally focused on treatment issues and prognosis. Videotapes were used in several cases to enhance observational skills and make the cases more realistic. The need for residents to obtain additional information outside of the PBL session and report back to the group adds elements of self-direction, evidence-based practice, and peer teaching. Ideally, the cases build on residents' prior knowledge, enhance intrinsic interest, and assist with integration of basic science and clinical principles [31].

Evaluation of this method after several years of implementation was positive. Overall, it was well received by the residents, who admitted they were reading more and found this method of teaching helpful in their clinical work. General observations noted by the faculty facilitators were that residents were reading more than they had for seminars, and attendance and preparation for the sessions had been enhanced. The group interactions in which residents challenged each other's assumptions and provide feedback clearly emphasized interpersonal and communication skills. Although attending physicians did not notice significant change in performance on clinical rotations, the residents believed PBL was helpful in their clinical thinking and, in some cases, anticipating actual clinical situations. The residents believed that PBL was more enjoyable than traditional seminar formats. Not only did they find it helpful in their clinical decision making but they also found it helpful when taking oral examinations. They were familiar with the question-and-answer probing done during oral examinations from their PBL experience and had become accustomed to talking about their decision-making processes. On the other hand, residents worried that they might not cover content areas in the level of detail required to perform well on written examinations. The faculty members expressed similar concerns and believed that the CHILD PRITE scores were lower than expected. These potential strengths and weaknesses are similar to those identified in reviews and meta-analyses completed on PBL in medical school curricula [32–36]. Residents also wondered what they were missing from lectures. Although they admitted that they were reading more (spending on average 2–5 hours preparing for each session), they sometimes felt overwhelmed, especially if their clinical services were busy. Another concern involved what to do when one resident was less invested than the others. Because there were only three or four residents in a class, this could be problematic and had to be addressed by the group itself and the faculty early.

After 6 years of experience with PBL, in 2002, the Division of Child and Adolescent Psychiatry held a retreat to review the didactic curriculum. The needs assessment at this point included an evaluation of the strengths and weaknesses of the PBL approach and recognition that enhanced efficiency of faculty time was needed. Previously there were separate didactic series for first- and second-year residents that required 6 hours weekly of faculty time. Because there were only three or four residents in a class—one often on vacation or absent for a variety of reasons—learning in PBL was not maximized. The Accreditation Council of Graduate Medical Education core competencies had just been introduced, and so another goal was to adapt the curriculum to ensure compliance with these new requirements.

During this half-day retreat, a hybrid approach was developed that combined the first- and second-year child psychiatry residents for approximately 8 months of the year. This approach included more seminars to address the concerns about gaps in the curriculum and allowed increased depth for certain topics. The seminars focus on development and psychopathology topics not covered in the cases and theoretical and practical aspects of psychotherapy within the defined age group. In the new curriculum, the first 3 months of didactics are separate for first- and second-year residents. The first-year fellows have an introductory seminar series that includes an introduction to psychotherapy with children, psychopharmacology, interview techniques, family therapy, cultural competence, and formulation. Second-year residents have seminars during those 3 months on transition to practice/administrative issues and consultation/liaison.

The next 8 months consist of a combined curriculum that one year includes infant/preschool development and psychopathology and a neurobiology series. The subsequent year has one block of development and psychopathology in school-age children and one block of development and psychopathology in adolescents. More seminar hours were introduced, such that the seminars and PBL cases are more integrated. Each block (except neurobiology, which is entirely seminars) consists of approximately 12 to 16 seminar hours and three PBL cases that revolve around children with specific diagnoses, such that teaching of psychopathology is emphasized in the PBL cases. The PBL cases typically run three to four weekly 2-hour sessions. The expectations for each combined block are as follows, and Box 3 contains a general outline of the combined curriculum and PBL cases:

- Normal development in that age group, both cross-sectional and some longitudinal
- Psychopathology for that age group—use PBL cases for some, but augment with seminars the areas not covered by a PBL case
- Psychological theories of development, including some technical aspects of therapy for the particular age group or psychopathology being discussed
- Field trips, including at least one in each block that allows observation of and interaction with normal children of that age group; other field trips to specialty sites related to other topics covered in the block

Competency-based goals and objectives were developed for each major curriculum block, with more specific goals and objectives for PBL in general followed by goals and objectives for each individual case. Seminars have knowledge and attitude objectives, whereas PBL includes knowledge, skills, and attitude objectives. A summarized case about a patient named "Susan" follows, with associated goals and objectives shown in Box 4.

*Case example: Susan*

Susan is a 10-year-old girl brought to the outpatient clinic by her adoptive parents because she has been refusing to go to school. Further history reveals that she was adopted from Romania after the death of her parents from AIDS. Her younger sister, Robyn, was adopted along with her, but Robyn is HIV positive and was recently diagnosed with AIDS, having had several hospitalizations for HIV-related infections. Susan has spent most of her time recently caring for her sister.

The case begins on day 1 with discussion of normal development of school-aged children, focusing specifically on social development, the impact on families of having a child with a chronic medical illness, and developmental aspects of death of parents and subsequent adoption. A differential diagnosis is generated for the problem of school refusal. On

**Box 3. Outline of combined curriculum**

*Year 1*
Infant/preschool development and psychopathology
PBL cases
   Natalie
  1. Pervasive developmental disorder
  2. Mental retardation
  3. Tics and Tourette's disorder
  4. Obsessive-compulsive disorder
   John, Jr.
  1. Communication disorder
  2. Disruptive behavior in preschool children
  3. Impact of hearing impairment on language development
   Daniel Chen
  1. Selective mutism
  2. Cross-cultural aspects of psychopathology and development
  3. Etiologic factors in development of anxiety disorders

Seminars (development and psychotherapy)
Field trip to preschool
Neurobiology (seminar series)

*Year 2*
School-age child development and psychopathology
PBL cases
   Keith
  1. Attention deficit hyperactivity disorder
  2. Learning disorders
   Susan
  1. Separation anxiety disorder
  2. School refusal
  3. Grief and bereavement
   Porsha
  1. Posttraumatic stress disorder
  2. Childhood sexual abuse
  3. Impact of divorce
  4. Enuresis

Seminars (development and psychotherapy)
Field trip
Adolescent development and psychopathology
PBL cases
   Evan
  1. Conduct disorder

2. Childhood physical abuse
3. Violence
4. Substance abuse
 Sara
1. Eating disorders
2. Family psychopathology
 Bridget
1. Mood disorders
2. Psychosis
3. Suicide

Seminars (development and psychotherapy)
Field trip

day 2, further information leads residents toward a diagnosis of separation anxiety disorder, and the major learning issue is assessment, psychopathology, and treatment of separation anxiety disorder with school refusal. The residents are expected to review the AACAP practice parameters for the assessment and treatment of anxiety disorders and should review the literature on school refusal. On the final day, Susan's sister dies, and the residents discuss the impact of the death of a sibling and ways to help families cope with their grief.

Implementation of this integrated curriculum that combines both years of residents resulted in much more efficient use of faculty time—3 hours/wk for 8 months of the year and 5 hours/wk for 3 months, compared with 6 hours/wk previously. We currently have 4 years of experience with this integrated curriculum. During the most recent formal program evaluation, the residents continued to express satisfaction with PBL as a learning method but also like having more traditional seminars. Their suggestions for improvements dealt primarily with the other seminar series (transition to practice) and not with PBL. CHILD PRITE scores and ABPN CAP performance are well above the national average, and both have improved since implementing the integrated curriculum. The faculty members also have been pleased with the new curriculum. They enjoy the interactive nature of PBL but feel more confident that all major topics are being covered in sufficient depth because of seminars to complement PBL.

## Summary

Psychopathology is one of the key aspects of a curriculum in CAP. Because there is little research on effective methods for teaching this topic, an approach must be developed in each program that meets the standards set out by the Residency Review Committee and that fully prepares its graduates to be competent child and adolescent psychiatrists. Methods used for

---

**Box 4. Goals and objectives for residents in case example "Susan"**

*Normal development*
1. Understand normal social development in school-aged children (K)
2. Describe the development of attachment in children and ways in which adoption and death of parents impact it (K)

*Psychopathology*
1. Describe the differential diagnosis of school refusal (K, PC)
2. Discuss the diagnosis and epidemiology of separation anxiety disorder (K, PC)
3. Discuss etiologic factors of anxiety, including the role of contagion, temperament, and genetics (K)

*Treatment issues*
1. Develop a comprehensive treatment plan for school refusal/ separation anxiety disorder in children, including behavioral and pharmacologic interventions and discuss the evidence that supports them (K, PC, PBI)
2. Describe a plan to liaison with the schools to develop an educational approach to management of school refusal (PC, SBP)

*Other*
1. Recognize adoption as a risk factor for psychiatric diagnoses (K)
2. Understand the impact of cross-cultural/international adoption (K)
3. Describe the impact of chronic illness on families (K)
4. Understand the impact of the death of a sibling on children (K)
5. Describe ways of assisting children and families in dealing with the death of a child (PC, IC)

K, knowledge; PC, patient care; PBI, practice-based improvement; IC, interpersonal and communication skills; SBP, systems-based practice.

---

teaching psychopathology may vary widely among programs and should be based on a sound educational rationale and adult learning principles that emphasize life-long, self-directed learning. This article has described an overall approach to curriculum design and expanded on the use of PBL as an educational method. The emphasis of PBL on interpersonal skills and the integration of biologic, psychological, and social factors impacting children and their development make it a logical method for use in psychiatry. The use of this method in residency programs should continue to be explored and researched to determine its effectiveness when compared with more traditional teaching formats.

## References

[1] Yager J, Kay J, Winsead DK. Developing and monitoring the curriculum. In: Kay J, editor. Handbook of psychiatry residency training. Washington, DC: American Psychiatric Association; 1991. p. 17–47.

[2] Taintor Z, Rodenhauser P, Scully J. Planning the residency. In: Kay J, editor. Handbook of psychiatry residency training. Washington, DC: American Psychiatric Association; 1991. p. 49–81.

[3] Andrews L, Lomax JW. Developing and monitoring the curriculum. In: Kay J, Silberman EK, Pessar L, editors. Handbook of psychiatric education and faculty development. Washington, DC: American Psychiatric Association; 1999. p. 365–80.

[4] Reider RO, Mellman LA. What and how to teach in the residency program. In: Kay J, Silberman EK, Pessar LF, editors. Handbook of psychiatric education. Washington, DC: American Psychiatric Publishing; 2005. p. 143–63.

[5] Kern DE, Thomas PA, Howard DM, et al. Curriculum development for medical education: a six-step approach. Baltimore (MD): The Johns Hopkins University Press; 1998.

[6] Accreditation Council for Graduate Medical Education. Requirements for residency education in child and adolescent psychiatry, effective November 2004. Available at: http://www.acgme.org. Accessed April 6, 2006.

[7] Accreditation Council for Graduate Medical Education. ACGME outcome project. ACGME general competencies Version 1.3, 2000. Available at: www.acgme.org/outcome/comp/compFull. Accessed May 1, 2006.

[8] Sexson S, Sargent J, Zima B, et al. Sample core competencies in child and adolescent psychiatry training: a starting point. Acad Psychiatry 2001;25:201–13.

[9] The American Board of Psychiatry and Neurology. Child and adolescent core competencies Chart 2.1, 2005. Available at: www.ABPN.com. Accessed April 16, 2006.

[10] American Board of Psychiatry and Neurology. Computer-administered (formerly written) examination in child and adolescent psychiatry: 2006 content outline. Available at: www.abpn.com. Accessed June 7, 2006.

[11] Knowles MS. Andragogy in action: applying modern principles of adult learning. San Francisco (CA): Jossey-Bass; 1984.

[12] Dolmans DHJM, De Grave W, Wolfhagen IHAP, et al. Problem-based learning: future challenges for educational practice and research. Med Educ 2005;39:732–41.

[13] Zisook S, Benjamin S, Balon R, et al. Alternate methods of teaching psychopharmacology. Acad Psychiatry 2005;29:141–54.

[14] Kaye D, Ets-Hokin E. The breakfast club: utilizing popular film to teach adolescent development. Acad Psychiatry 2000;24:110–6.

[15] Barrows HS, Tamblyn RM. Problem-based learning: an approach to medical education. New York: Springer Verlag; 1980.

[16] Kinkade S. A snapshot of the status of problem-based learning in US medical schools, 2003–2004. Acad Med 2005;80(3):300–1.

[17] Foley RP, Polson AL, Vance JM. Review of the literature on PBL in the clinical setting. Teach Learn Med 1997;9:4–9.

[18] Foley RP, Levy J, Russinof HJ, et al. Planning and implementing a problem-based learning rotation for residents. Teach Learn Med 1993;5:102–6.

[19] Schwartz RW, Donnelly MB, Sloan DA, et al. Residents' evaluation of a problem-based learning curriculum in a general surgery residency program. Am J Surg 1997;173:338–41.

[20] Schnapp WB, Stone S, Van Norman J, et al. Teaching ethics in psychiatry: a problem-based learning approach. Acad Psychiatry 1996;20:144–9.

[21] Schultz-Ross RA, Kline AE. Using problem-based learning to teach forensic psychiatry. Acad Psychiatry 1999;23:37–41.

[22] McCarthy MK. Problem-based learning and psychiatry residency education. Harv Rev Psychiatry 2000;7(5):305–8.

[23] West DA, West MM. Problem-based learning of psychopathology in a traditional curriculum using multiple conceptual models. Med Educ 1987;21:151–6.

[24] Block S. Using problem-based learning to enhance the psychosocial competence of medical students. Acad Psychiatry 1996;20:65–75.

[25] McParland M, Noble LM, Livingston G. The effectiveness of problem-based learning compared to traditional teaching in undergraduate psychiatry. Med Educ 2004;38:859–67.

[26] Schmidt HG. Foundations of problem-based learning: some explanatory notes. Med Educ 1993;27:422–32.

[27] Tosteson DC. New pathways in general medical education. N Engl J Med 1990;322:234–8.

[28] Sackett D, Richardson WS, Rosenberg W, et al. Evidence-based medicine: how to practice and teach EBM. New York: Churchill-Livingstone; 1997.

[29] Sargent J, Sexson S, Cuffe S, et al. Assessment of competency in child and adolescent psychiatry training. Acad Psychiatry 2004;28:18–26.

[30] Dingle AD, Beresin G. Competencies. Child Adolesc Psychiatr Clin N Am, in press.

[31] Dolmans DHJM, Snellen-Balendong H, Wolfhagen IHAP, et al. Seven principles of effective case design for a problem-based curriculum. Med Teach 1997;19(3):185–9.

[32] Norman GR, Schmidt HG. The psychological basis of problem-based learning: a review of the evidence. Acad Med 1992;67:557–65.

[33] Berkson L. Problem-based learning: have the expectations been met? Acad Med 1993;68(Suppl):S79–88.

[34] Albanese MA, Mitchell S. Problem-based learning: a review of literature on its outcomes and implementation issues. Acad Med 1993;68:52–81.

[35] Vernon DTA, Blake RL. Does problem-based learning work? A meta-analysis of evaluative research. Acad Med 1993;68:550–6.

[36] Colliver JA. Effectiveness of problem-based learning curricula: research and theory. Acad Med 2000;5(3):259–66.

ELSEVIER
SAUNDERS

Child Adolesc Psychiatric Clin N Am
16 (2007) 111–132

CHILD AND
ADOLESCENT
PSYCHIATRIC CLINICS
OF NORTH AMERICA

# The Case Formulation in Child and Adolescent Psychiatry

Nancy C. Winters, MD[a,*], Graeme Hanson, MD[b],
Veneta Stoyanova, MD[a]

[a]Division of Child and Adolescent Psychiatry, Oregon Health and Science University,
3181 SW Sam Jackson Park Road, Mail Code:DC-7P, Portland, OR 97239-3098, USA
[b]Department of Psychiatry, University of California San Francisco,
513 Parnassus Avenue, San Francisco, CA 94143-0410, USA

Put simply, case formulation is a process by which a set of hypotheses is generated about the etiology and factors that perpetuate a patient's presenting problems and translates the diagnosis into specific, individualized treatment interventions. It is central to the practice of child and adolescent psychiatry. Even if not articulated explicitly, the case formulation guides all clinical activity. For example, how one understands a child's biologic vulnerabilities and how they interact with personality or family factors and the importance assigned to each clearly influence choices made in the assessment process and the treatment plan. Despite the widely acknowledged importance of case formulation, it is often taught cursorily in residency programs, and residents often perceive it as too challenging to actually perform [1]. Consequently, case formulation is often relegated to secondary status behind the DSM-IV-TR differential diagnosis. Such attitudes are manifested in the American Board of Psychiatry and Neurology Child and Adolescent Psychiatry certification examinations. When asked to formulate the case just presented, candidates generally return a perfunctory statement and transition quickly to discussion of DSM-IV-TR diagnoses.

How can case formulation be taught systematically and effectively to child psychiatry residents? This article reviews the various definitions of case formulation, differences between diagnosis and case formulation, how case formulation for a child patient differs from an adult patient, and case formulation in the context of residency training, including challenges for residents transitioning from adult psychiatry. It presents

---

* Corresponding author.
*E-mail address:* winterna@ohsu.edu (N.C. Winters).

1056-4993/07/$ - see front matter © 2006 Elsevier Inc. All rights reserved.
doi:10.1016/j.chc.2006.07.010                    *childpsych.theclinics.com*

a suggested structure for constructing a biopsychosocial formulation that
can be applied in a training setting. Several specialized types of psychotherapy formulation are reviewed in more detail. The article concludes with
a case example of a child psychiatry resident's case formulation before
and after discussion in supervision.

### Definitions of case formulation

If one searches the literature on case formulation in child psychiatry, one
finds a surprisingly small number of articles relative to its importance. The
indices of several textbooks in child psychiatry (and adult psychiatry) yield
no entries under formulation or any related terms. The nature of case formulation is made more ambiguous by the various terms used for it, which
reflects lack of agreement on the definition of case formulation. Commonly
used terms include clinical case formulation [2,3], diagnostic formulation [4],
psychodynamic formulation [5–7], psychotherapy case formulation [8], and
Engel's biopsychosocial approach to formulation [9].

Although these terms are used somewhat interchangeably, they have different emphases. There are, however, some areas of consensus and common-
ality. Case formulation generally refers to an integrative process that
synthesizes how one understands the complex, interacting factors implicated
in development of a patient's presenting problems. It is explicitly comprehensive and takes into account the child and family's strengths and capacities that may help to identify potentially effective treatment approaches.
The case formulation serves as a testable explanatory model that gives
rise to ideas for intervention and eliminates some options that do not fit
the model. Described most succinctly by Nurcombe and colleagues [10],
the formulation asks what is wrong, how it got that way, and what can
be done about it. The case formulation is not static. Just as a child's "story"
continues to unfold throughout the clinical process with added information,
the case formulation evolves and is continually modified. It may start as
rudimentary and become more elaborate over time.

### Case example of the "whole story"

A 14-year-old girl had been in treatment with a child psychiatrist since
age 11 for severe obsessive-compulsive disorder and generalized anxiety disorder symptoms. Numerous medication trials had only brought her partial
relief. Attempts at cognitive behavioral therapy (CBT) or other psychosocial
therapies had always met with resistance on the patient's part, and she generally seemed to be angry about having to attend therapy sessions. After 2 to
3 years of unsuccessful treatment, the patient revealed that she had a severe
phobia to elevators and heights that was making her profoundly uncomfortable during sessions. She requested that treatment sessions—previously held
on the tenth floor of the hospital—be conducted downstairs in the lobby of

the hospital. After this change was made, the patient rapidly became an active collaborator in treatment and responded surprisingly well to CBT.

The largest body of literature on case formulation is on the psychodynamic formulation. This approach is heuristically fertile in generating psychologically meaningful hypotheses that translate to psychotherapeutic interventions, but it does not adequately capture the increasingly recognized contributions of neurobiology and sociocultural influences to psychiatric illness. The biopsychosocial approach to formulation has become the most widely accepted comprehensive case formulation model. Described in 1980 by George Engel, the biopsychosocial formulation became an organizing principle for psychiatric education [9]. An internist with psychoanalytic training, Engel had a profound impact on the field of consultation-liaison psychiatry. Engel departed from the biomedical model of understanding medical illness, which he viewed as isolating components of illness, as would a bench scientist. His biopsychosocial model was based on systems theory, which conceptualized the person and the family as components of a hierarchically arranged "continuum of natural systems." He later emphasized the importance of dialogue between the patient and doctor in developing a shared narrative of the patient's private experience of illness. Through this dialogue they would discover the links between the patient's personal life and his or her experience of "falling ill" [11]. The American Psychiatric Association Commission on Psychotherapy offered the following definition:

> The biopsychosocial formulation is a tentative working hypothesis which attempts to explain the biological, psychological and sociocultural factors which have combined to create and maintain the presenting clinical problem. It is a guide to treatment planning and selection. It will be changed, modified, or amplified as the clinician learns more and more about the patient [12].

The sociocultural aspect of case formulation has received increased attention recently with the recognition that culture and ethnicity are often ignored or mishandled through ignorance, personal bias, or countertransference on the part of the therapist [13]. Cultural issues are important in child and adolescent psychiatry because they influence parenting style, developmental expectations, values and goals of the family, perception of symptoms, and attitudes about treatment. The DSM-IV attempted to improve coverage of cultural issues with inclusion of an outline for cultural formulation, although there are some limitations in its applicability to children and adolescents [14].

## Differences between diagnosis and case formulation

Diagnosis and case formulation are different processes. Diagnosis is a categorical approach to describing symptoms that occur in reliable groupings, the aim of which is to establish predictive validity for treatment outcome.

Diagnosis is atheoretical and draws on the disease concept. Case formulation reflects a more dimensional perspective in which problems are viewed as being on continua from normal to abnormal. Case formulation synthesizes information into a theory as to how problems developed and how change might unfold. Jellinek and McDermott [15] described diagnosis and case formulation respectively as the "science and art of child and adolescent psychiatry." They commented on the tension between DSM-IV structured diagnostic interviews and traditional open-ended interviews using play materials, noting that the first is quantitative and seeks accuracy, whereas the second is more qualitative and seeks meaning. Turkat [16] stated that it is problematic when a diagnosis is used as a formulation, and the term diagnostic formulation itself is confusing.

The consensus, however, is that diagnosis and case formulation complement each other and should coexist. Diagnosis by itself does not encompass the complexity of the individual case. Generally the diagnosis does not tell the clinician how two children with the same diagnosis, such as obsessive-compulsive disorder, differ in terms of strengths, vulnerabilities, precipitants of symptom exacerbations, developmental impact of the symptoms, and meaning of the symptoms to the child and family. Case formulation is seen as a vehicle to supplement and apply diagnosis to the specifics of an individual's life. Case formulation also serves as a vehicle for converting a diagnosis to a plan for treatment, especially choice of type and timing of interventions [8].

Connor and Fisher [2] maintain that case formulation must be multitheoretical because the current state of knowledge in child mental health does not endorse any one theory of causality. It must allow for biologic, psychologic, and social "multicausality." They further describe diagnostic assessment as a "divergent" activity in which information from different domains is collected and case formulation as a "convergent" activity in which information is prioritized and integrated and relationships among the data are highlighted.

## How the child and adult psychiatric formulation differ

The transition from adult to child psychiatry training presents residents not only with the challenge of learning to construct a much more complex case formulation but also of learning a whole new approach to doing evaluations. Many residents have no experience with child outpatients during their adult psychiatry training and are unfamiliar with integration of data from multiple informants and interacting perspectives. Residents have an exceedingly steep learning curve in the beginning of training as they acquire new skills in interviewing and interacting with children of different ages. New knowledge areas to master include normal and abnormal child development, common medical conditions that affect behavior, family systems theory, childhood psychiatric diagnoses, and pediatric psychopharmacology. Learning about development must include the variations in normal development, the rapid changes in childhood influenced by temperament and cognitive capacities, and psychodevelopmental issues, such as internalized object relations, identity formation, and psychosexual development. The need to master all of this material is all the more pressing because of concerns about safety of interventions in a vulnerable child population.

The first difference in the evaluation of children that bears on case formulation is the fact that children, unlike adult patients, are not self-referred but are usually referred by a parent, teacher, or some other agent. The problem is not defined primarily by the patient, and child patients may not even see the behavior expected by the parents or school as desirable. This may be an ongoing aspect of the formulation that explains limited treatment success. Externalizing problems are more often the reason for referral, although they may not be the most psychologically relevant predisposing or precipitating issue from the child's point of view. The child evaluation must use information from multiple informants, requiring an understanding of the reliability and point of view of each informant. The clinician also must form therapeutic alliances with the child and caregivers while still attempting to retain objectivity.

The chief complaint voiced by a child's parents also carries with it their expectations for normal behavior, which are filtered through their own psychology and influenced by sociocultural factors. The parent's psychological vulnerabilities also may explain why they experience the child's behavior as so disturbing. When the referring agent is outside the family it may even have different ways of labeling or defining problems based on its own internal requirements. For example, when a school refers a child it may prefer an autism spectrum diagnosis to establish eligibility for special education services. The main goal of child psychiatry interventions is to help the child return to a more normative developmental trajectory, usually defined by the parents' expectations. The child's level of development, which may differ across developmental domains, is always an essential part of the formulation. The focus of the formulation may change over time with the child's maturation, continuing and new environmental factors, and added information.

The conceptual model used to formulate the child's problems must of necessity be multifactorial and interactional. There is generally an individual component (focused on pathology within the child) and a systems-based component (focused on factors in the family or broader systems); an even more comprehensive ecologic approach is based on analysis of all contributing factors in the environment. The ecologic perspective is discussed, in more detail, in the article by Storck and Vanderstoep elsewhere in this issue [17]. Family assessment and inclusion of family factors are always necessary in the case formulation of a child. The cause of the child's problems also may be understood as circular. Family factors contribute to the child's problem, but the child's problem in turn causes more family stress, which serves to perpetuate the problem. Causative factors that are more current and immediate are most relevant, because they most powerfully alter the balance for the child, the reinforcement available for change, and the beliefs of the participants [18].

## Case example of the ecologic model

A 15-year-old girl was receiving services in a community mental health center. Her resistance to following rules and statements of suicidal ideation were causing her adoptive parents to feel so overwhelmed that they expressed concern that they could not continue taking care of her. The girl had received individual therapy for 2 months with little improvement. Attempts to add family therapy and recommendation of home visits were too little, too late, and the young woman was placed in a wilderness program and then was to go to a residential center far from her community and family. Later, it was learned that the adoptive father, a self-employed farmer, was under enormous stress and was concurrently filing for bankruptcy. This situation contributed significantly to the family's inability to grapple with rebellious behavior that represented a normative developmental challenge for this young woman.

The case formulation process assists in helping the child and adults to reach a shared definition of the problem, which is important if change is to be possible. A collaborative model in which families are partners in the case formulation process has been recommended [18,19]. Each partner in the process shares his or her formulation of the problem, comes to see some validity in the others' perspectives, and identifies what role he or she expects to play in addressing the problem. Added to the collaborative model is an emphasis on strengths-based approaches that have been embraced by system-of-care reforms and the family and consumer movement [20]. Metz [19] offered the following modifications of the American Psychiatric Association Commission on Psychotherapy's definition of the biopsychosocial formulation to reflect these perspectives (changes appear in bold):

> A biopsychosocial formulation is a tentative working hypothesis **developed collaboratively with the child and family,** which attempts to explain the biological, psychological and sociocultural factors which have combined to create and maintain the presenting clinical **concern and which support the child's best functioning.** It is an **individualized** guide to treatment planning and selection. It will be changed, modified, or amplified as the clinician **and the family** learn more and more about the **strengths and needs of the child and family.**

The involvement of multiple systems in the lives of children (eg, school, health care, neighborhoods, child care, and, for some children, child welfare or juvenile justice) also contributes to the greater complexity of the child psychiatry case formulation.

## Case formulation approaches related to psychotherapeutic models

The clinician's preferred explanatory and psychotherapeutic models have significant influence on the prominent themes and hypotheses developed in the case formulation. One of the risks in case formulation is that of eliminating what does not agree with one's theoretical orientation. This issue has lent support to use of the more structured and comprehensive biopsychosocial formulation [10].

*Case example of the role of the clinician's biases and theoretical models*

An 11-year-old boy was admitted to a child psychiatric inpatient unit for treatment of severe obsessive-compulsive disorder refractory to multiple psychopharmacologic trials. The referring practitioner, a psychopharmacology specialist, indicated that the family functioned well and family issues should not be a target of treatment, and the inpatient treatment team followed this formulation. The boy was discharged and then rapidly readmitted with continuing severe symptoms. On re-entering the inpatient setting he stated urgently "my family's all messed up!" This statement confirmed the nursing staff's observations during the prior admission. They had observed that the boy's parents were intensely controlling and not psychologically minded and that the sister also had significant emotional problems that were not being acknowledged.

Psychodynamic and cognitive-behavioral case formulations do have their place in developing the specific components of the intervention once it is chosen. The two most common types of therapeutic case formulations, CBT and psychodynamic, are described later. More extensive descriptions of case formulation approaches used in CBT, psychoanalytic therapy, brief psychodynamic therapy, dialectical-behavioral therapy, interpersonal psychotherapy, and behavior therapy are also available [8,21,22].

Psychodynamic case formulation has been written about extensively, especially in the adult literature. Psychodynamic formulations are thought to be appropriate not only for long-term or psychodynamic therapy but also to inform other modalities [7]. McWilliams [22] holds that the shorter the time to do the psychotherapeutic work the more critically important are the therapist's working hypotheses. The psychodynamic framework addresses such areas as unconscious conflicts, ego deficits, distortions in intrapsychic structures, and problems in internalized object relations [23]. Psychodynamic case formulation assumes that the goal of therapy is not only symptom relief but also development of insight, agency, identity, self-esteem, affect management, ego strength and self-cohesion, a capacity to love, work, and play, and an overall sense of well-being [22].

Cognitive-behavioral case formulation is based on premises originally set forth by Aaron Beck and colleagues about cognitive schemas and information processing errors that lead to and maintain symptoms in depression, anxiety, personality disorders, and substance abuse [24]. CBT formulations are used to identify negative core beliefs related to negative developmental events and generate cognitive restructuring and coping strategies [25]. Case formulation in cognitive therapy identifies a patient's automatic thoughts and feelings and behaviors that follow them and then identifies sources or triggers that activate the patient's symptoms. Eventually, connections are made between an incident in the child's life to core beliefs about himself or herself. Behavioral therapy formulations are particularly relevant in child psychiatry, because young children are most likely to benefit from restructuring of environmental reinforcements and may not be able to use the cognitive component of therapy. Behavior therapists focus on functional analysis of behavior and identify environmental contingencies or reinforcement and apply behavioral principles, including operant and classical conditioning, to make alterations [8].

Integrative case formulations are multitheoretical and allow for integration of components of different therapeutic modalities. Theoretical explanatory concepts are explicitly selected because of their applicability to the facts of the case and to guide individualized treatment approaches acceptable to the patient at a particular time. For example, a CBT case formulation may be most beneficial for an adolescent with generalized anxiety disorder or social phobia, but this does not exclude psychodynamic hypotheses in the case formulation to explain the meaning of specific symptoms, the readiness of the patient to address them, and developmental insults that may have played a role in symptom development. Integration occurs in the mind of the therapist as he or she develops the case formulation, not always in the therapeutic application (K. Zerbe, MD, personal communication, 2005). This perspective led to development of an integrated course on psychodynamic and evidence-based psychotherapies for children and adolescents at Oregon Health and Science University child psychiatry residency program [26]. Readings for the course are drawn from the literature on CBT, interpersonal therapy, and psychodynamic theory, paired with continuing case presentations. Review of evidence-based psychotherapy manuals is another part of the curriculum. Residents develop evolving integrated case formulations using different explanatory theories and discuss implications for selection of psychotherapeutic modalities that may vary over the course of treatment.

## Case formulation in the context of residency training

Case formulation is valuable as a teaching tool in residency programs. It strengthens a resident's understanding of the multifactorial and transactional nature of childhood psychopathology and the process of matching treatment to the individual needs of patients. It establishes hypothesis testing as the norm and can encourage investigation of the evidence base for explanatory theories and treatment interventions. Surveys suggest that psychiatry residency programs view case formulation as important but do not provide clear guidelines for how to construct formulations [8]. Even experienced clinicians may not routinely construct comprehensive case formulations, and most agree that case formulation is a poorly defined and undertaught skill [8]. Perry and colleagues [6] described five misconceptions to explain why clinicians do not regularly do case formulations: (1) the belief that case formulation is only for patients in long-term psychotherapy, (2) the view that case formulation is primarily a training experience and unnecessary for experienced therapists, (3) the belief that case formulation is an elaborate and time-consuming process, (4) the view that a loosely construed formulation "in one's head" is sufficient and does not need to be written, and (5) the worry about becoming so invested in a formulation that one will not accept information that does not fit the formulation. They counter by arguing that case formulations are just as important for short-term as for long-term treatment, are best in written form, need not be time consuming, and facilitate understanding of events that may not fit the formulation. Shapiro [7] added a sixth misconception: formulation is only useful for individuals who plan to do a dynamic therapy with a child. He emphasized that dynamic understanding also may guide a clinician toward other therapies. It is also important for understanding the significance of symptoms to children and their families and the risk of changing the dynamic equilibrium of the person treated and of the family.

Various factors contribute to resistance on the part of residents and faculty to learning and teaching comprehensive case formulations. Development of a case formulation is a longitudinal process. It requires sufficient time to get to know a child and family and the role of all the interacting contextual variables. In practice, formulations are continually revised with new information. This may be a challenge, with financial and managed care constraints leading to shortened lengths of stay in outpatient, residential, and inpatient settings. Residents need cases of sufficient duration to develop and refine good case formulations. Residents' formulations may be rudimentary early in training and should be more comprehensive as their skills expand over time. They may be more likely to focus on biologic issues early in training and gain more comfort in incorporating psychological and sociocultural issues over time. The fact that most child psychiatry residents enter child psychiatry after their third year may complicate this progression, however. In adult psychiatry they have spent much time in fast-paced inpatient settings in which there is not enough time or knowledge of the patient to go beyond differential diagnosis. They have not had the benefit of a fourth year, which generally offers added experience in longitudinal and in-depth psychotherapy. Instead, when they come to child psychiatry they are thrust into a different world in which formulations require consideration of multiple interacting contextual factors, such as the parents' own psychological issues, family dynamics, and the quality of the child's school environment. Residents who come from adult psychiatry are more accustomed to seeing a patient as an individual rather than in the context of a family or other systems. They no longer come into child psychiatry training with a predictable exposure to psychodynamic and family systems theoretical models.

When asked to formulate cases, residents may be apprehensive about "not getting the right answer," because there is no checklist or prescribed formula for case formulation. Contrast this with the more typically enthusiastic reaction to a rating scale that is easy to administer and score and yields what seems to be (but often is not) a clear answer. Teaching faculty are not immune to these factors either and may prefer to engage in discussion of areas that are perceived as more tangible and better defined, such as psychopharmacology. Residents do not understand how case formulation can be useful. They may be aware of case formulation as a requirement for the American Board of Psychiatry and Neurology oral examination, but they do not know how it can inform and guide treatment. It can become another burdensome requirement, or it may not actually be required in their clinical rotation sites. Most written documentation is driven by medicolegal or insurance requirements and includes the five-axis DSM-IV-TR diagnosis but not necessarily a case formulation. Case formulation is often not a formal part of the curriculum and the literature to support teaching it is scant. Most of the available articles are about psychodynamic case formulation in adults. The implicit message is that case formulation is not essential.

To address these problems, case formulation should be made a formal part of the curriculum in child and adolescent psychiatry. Case formulation should be taught in didactic seminars, case conferences, and supervision, and some written case formulations with supervisory feedback should be required. The process of learning to formulate is enhanced by case conferences, in which experienced clinicians demonstrate the construction of a comprehensive biopsychosocial formulation. Especially useful is the opportunity for residents to observe faculty doing case formulations "in the moment" after seeing a new case. It also can be helpful to distribute written examples of a succinct, well-written comprehensive case formulation. One way to practice formulation is to construct it as a group, having each resident take a turn contributing part of the formulation. The discussion includes how to develop specific treatment plans based on elements of the formulation, including the timing of different interventions and the prognosis. It is essential to create a nonjudgmental climate in which any formulation ideas are acceptable and seen as having merit.

Too often case formulations are taught as part of the initial assessment but not in the context of cases as they evolve in treatment. It is important to illustrate how an evolving formulation changes the treatment plan in significant ways or, in some cases, may explain a poor response to treatment. It is also helpful to revisit cases later in the course of treatment that had been formulated in case conferences. This review provides an opportunity to see whether the hypotheses generated were borne out and how new information obtained in the course of treatment modified the treatment plan. In a similar vein, the case formulation should generate hypotheses about prognosis. It should identify potential obstacles or areas of resistance that may arise in the treatment process and how to address them. A case formulation also can include consideration of issues that may arise in the therapist's reaction to the patient and family that might present obstacles to progress. For example, a resident who knows that she or he identifies with a rebellious adolescent wanting more autonomy may have difficulty developing a constructive alliance with the parent. Residents also need to learn how to integrate formulation of the parents' psychological strengths and vulnerabilities with the child formulation. This understanding is critical to engaging the parents in a constructive therapeutic alliance, without which treatment of the child is generally unsuccessful.

## Construction of the case formulation

The case formulation process begins with a comprehensive assessment that includes interviews with the child and the parents together, the parents alone, the child alone, and review of ancillary sources of information. The order of these components varies depending on the age of the child, the presenting problems, and other contextual factors. Broad-band and specific symptom rating scales can augment the data collected and may be an easier way for participants to share some information. Information should be gathered in the areas needed to identify a DSM-IV-TR diagnosis and construct a comprehensive biopsychosocial formulation as described in Table 1 and Box 1. The chief complaint and goals for treatment should be ascertained from each participant, and the signs and symptoms should be elicited and characterized with respect to onset, precipitants, severity, observable patterns, the contexts in which they occur, and their effect on the child and family. A complete medical, developmental, and educational history should be taken, as should a family assessment and information about the patient's social functioning and sociocultural or environmental factors contributing to the problems. Strengths in the child and family should be identified and acknowledged throughout the interview and data collection process.

In the assessment of a child there is a need for balance between direct observation and inference from limited or indirect information. This balance is especially important in children with less ability to verbalize and about whom more inferences are made. The mental status examination is an opportunity to directly observe and assess areas of the child's functioning needed for the differential diagnosis and biopsychosocial formulation. The mental status examination in child psychiatry uses multiple assessment methods, including verbal interaction, play, and drawing or other expressive activities. Each modality provides information about the child's capacities, thought content, and way of relating to others. Areas in the mental status examination relevant to the case formulation include observable signs, such as psychomotor

Table 1
Biopsychosocial formulation grid with examples of predisposing, precipitating, perpetuating, and protective factors in each of the formulation domains

| Domains / Factors | Biologic / Genetic, developmental, medical, toxicity, temperamental factors | Psychological / Cognitive style, intrapsychic conflicts and defense mechanisms, self-image, meaning of symptoms | Social — Social-Relationships / Family/peers/others | Social — Social-Environment / Culture/ethnicity, social risk factors, systems issues |
|---|---|---|---|---|
| Predisposing (vulnerabilities) | Family psychiatric history, toxic exposures in utero, birth complications, developmental disorders, regulatory disturbances | Insecure attachment, problems with affect modulation, rigid or negative cognitive style, low self-image | Childhood exposure to maternal depression and domestic violence, late adoption, temperament mismatch, marital conflicts | Poverty, low socioeconomic status, teenage parenthood, poor access to health or mental health care |
| Precipitating (stressors) | Serious medical illness or injury, increasing use of alcohol or drugs | Conflicts around identity or separation-individuation arising at developmental transitions, such as puberty onset or graduation from high school | Loss of or separation from close family member, family move with loss of friendships, interpersonal trauma | Recent immigration, loss of home, loss of a supportive service (eg, respite services, appropriate school placement) |
| Perpetuating (maintaining) | Chronic illness, functional impairment caused by cognitive deficits or learning disorder | Use of self-destructive coping mechanisms, help-rejecting personality style, traumatic re-enactments | Chronic marital discord, lack of empathy of parent, developmentally inappropriate expectations | Chronically dangerous or hostile neighborhood, transgenerational problems of immigration, lack of culturally competent services |
| Protective (strengths) | Above-average intelligence, easy temperament, specific talents or abilities, physical attractiveness | Ability to be reflective, ability to modulate affect, positive sense of self, adaptive coping mechanisms | Positive parent-child relationships, supportive community and extended family | Community cohesiveness, availability of supportive social network, well-functioning child/family team |

Adapted from Barker P. The child and adolescent psychiatry evaluation: basic child psychiatry. Oxford, UK: Blackwell Scientific, Inc.; 1995.

---

**Box 1. Construction of the formulation and generation of a treatment plan**

1. Brief summarizing statement that includes demographic information, chief complaint, and presenting problems from child and family's perspective and course (onset, severity, pattern) of signs and symptoms
2. Precipitating stressors or events
3. Biologic characterization
4. Psychological characterization
5. Family and other interpersonal factors
6. Sociocultural and environmental factors
7. Role performance, including level of functioning in major areas of daily life
8. Strengths and protective factors of the child, family, and system
9. Differential DSM-IV-TR diagnosis
10. Integrative statement: how the factors interact to lead to the current situation and level of functioning, prognosis, and potential openings for intervention
11. Problem list
12. Treatment plan

Note: the four "Ps" should be included in steps 3 to 8.

---

abnormalities, the child's description of his or her symptoms, the child's affective states throughout the interview and predominant mood as observed and described, language and motor functioning, cognitive functioning, thought process and thought content or perceptual abnormalities, wishes, self-concept; view of the family, developmental conflicts and other psychological themes, judgment and the capacity for self-observation and insight, and motivation to change and availability to engage in treatment. Of significant importance in the assessment of a child is the identification of strengths and protective factors. Strengths in the child and family can be used as foundations for treatment interventions; they generate motivation for working on the challenging areas through formation of a positive therapeutic alliance and instillation of hope. The child and family's views of the problem and its causes and areas they identify as strengths are cornerstones in building a collaborative evolving case formulation.

The biopsychosocial formulation grid in Table 1 adapted from Barker [27] provides a structure that can be useful for residents. The information gathered in the assessment is put into a biopsychosocial framework, which addresses each of the three domains—biologic, psychological, and social—with regard to the following factors, which have been called the four "Ps" [27,28]:

1. Predisposing factors are areas of vulnerability that increase the risk for the presenting problem. Examples of biologic predisposing factors include genetic loading for affective illness and prenatal exposure to alcohol.
2. Precipitating factors are typically thought of as stressors or other events (they could be positive or negative) that have a time relationship with the onset of the symptoms and may serve as precipitants. Examples of psychological precipitating factors may include conflicts about identity or separation-individuation that arise at developmental transitions, such as puberty onset or graduation from high school.
3. Perpetuating (or maintaining) factors include any conditions in the patient, family, community, or larger systems that serve to perpetuate rather than ameliorate the problem. Examples include unaddressed parental conflict, in which a child becomes an identified patient, a poor match between the educational services, and the child's learning needs.
4. Protective factors (strengths) include the patient's own areas of competency, skill, talents, and interest and supportive elements in the family and the child's extrafamilial relationships. Examples in the social domain might include the child having a good relationship with an understanding elementary school teacher or a favorite uncle. In the biologic domain, the child might have a talent in sports or music that can be helpful in engaging him or her in treatment and enhancing self-esteem.
5. Prognosis and potential for change is an additional "P" that should be included in the case formulation. This includes identification of areas most amenable to change and potential obstacles to successful treatment, such as when a youngster with school avoidance is rewarding by being allowed to stay home for long periods of time.

This grid can be used to facilitate comprehensive examination of areas needed for a biopsychosocial formulation. After these factors have been reviewed, the formulation should be used to develop a problem list, differential diagnosis, and generation of a treatment (see Box 1). This content can be translated into a succinct narrative as illustrated in Box 2 using the resident's case formulation example.

### Using supervision to co-develop and refine a case formulation: a child psychiatry resident's case example

The following formulation presented in two parts followed by a postscript illustrates the interactive, evolving co-development of a case formulation in supervision. The resident developed the first formulation after 2 months of treatment and revised the formulation to incorporate additional elements after discussing the case with the supervisor.

*First case formulation*

A 17-year-old girl was referred for her first psychiatric evaluation after 8 months of unsuccessful treatment for pain of unclear origin. The immediate reason for referral was the patient's worsening symptoms of depression and new onset of visual hallucinations. These symptoms had developed gradually after a febrile illness (presumed to be viral) that presented with vomiting and diarrhea. Her vomiting failed to resolve after the infection cleared, however, and had led to a 25-pound weight loss. No medical cause had been found for the intractable vomiting.

Relevant prior history included additional gastrointestinal difficulties. She had had multiple diagnostic procedures, which were ultimately inconclusive. In the initial interview the patient did not express any distress about her persistent vomiting, although she did report feelings of overwhelming depression and being scared by "visions of people in my room." Her mother, whose primary concern was her persistent vomiting, brought a calendar and a diary to the interview that contained detailed documentation of her vomiting. It was not learned until the sixth visit that the patient's vomiting had started insidiously approximately 6 months before the presumed viral infection. Around that time she had a major conflict with her biologic father and decided to stop contact with him.

She also had a history of academic underperformance. A school psychologist's evaluation, performed before the onset of her medical problems 4 years ago, did not qualify her for special education but recommended counseling. The patient's mother decided at that time to home-school her to improve her academic performance. Initially, they were part of study groups with other home-schooled children. Because of the patient's multiple medical problems, low energy, and inability to get out of bed on most days, however, the mother withdrew her from the groups. The patient's social interaction with peers her age has been limited to a weekly youth group at church. She reported that she has never been able to have a friendship lasting more than a month. She is overly sensitive to others' comments and often loses interest in friends after they disappoint her.

There seemed to be significant enmeshment and ambivalence in the mother-daughter relationship. The patient uses somatization as a way to express her feelings. Although her visions are clearly distressing, they have a phobic, rather than psychotic, quality. She was offered the option of an antipsychotic medication and later reported relief of her fear but continued to have the visions. Although the information gathered indicated that she met the diagnostic criteria for bulimia nervosa after the first visit, the diagnosis of an eating disorder was not introduced until the fifth visit. It was felt that presenting this diagnosis could interfere with forming a therapeutic

**Box 2. Construction of the formulation and generation of a treatment plan: case example**

The patient is a 17-year-old girl who lives with her mother and stepfather. She was referred by her primary care physician for evaluation of new onset visual hallucinations and worsening depression. She has had intractable vomiting with a 25-pound weight loss after a viral illness 6 months ago; no explanation has been found despite repeated diagnostic procedures. She also has a history of multiple other medical symptoms and pain without identified causes. The patient's main concern is her worsening depression, whereas the mother's main concern is her vomiting. A possible precipitating event concurrent with the onset of vomiting was that the patient had a significant conflict with her biologic father and decided to end contact with him.

The patient has been home-schooled for the past 5 years because she was underperforming academically, although psychological testing revealed no cognitive deficits. This situation has led to some social isolation. Currently, her mother closely monitors and keeps records of her medical symptoms, and the two spend much of their time together. Mental status examination reveals a normal appearing but thin young woman with significant depressive symptoms; her "visions" are more consistent with anxiety than psychotic hallucinations. Her sense of self-worth is linked to her appearance, particularly of thinness. She feels she has no friends and is not secure about her relationship with her mother. She finds it difficult to verbalize her emotions and seems to use somatization as a vehicle for emotional expression.

The patient has several biologic risks for psychiatric difficulties, including being exposed in utero to psychotropic medications, likely including alcohol. She seems to have an anxious temperament, which was likely exacerbated by an insecure attachment related to her mother's emotional unavailability during her infancy when the parents' marriage ended and her mother began a new relationship with the patient's stepfather. Psychologically, she had difficulty with affect modulation in infancy, which has persisted. She is highly reactive to interpersonal slights and subsequently has not been able to form trusting relationships with adults or peers. Her sense of self-worth seems to be invested in her appearance, which puts her at risk for an eating disorder.

Her medical symptoms have particular significance within the mother-child relationship and seem to serve the function of engaging her mother's attention. Her mother oscillates between being overly attentive to her daughter's medical systems and being unattuned to her psychological needs and desire for autonomy. There is a secondary gain to the daughter's medical complaints because they elicit the mother's attention and prevent the mother from leaving the house, thereby maintaining the mother-daughter enmeshment. In addition to somatization, she uses the defense mechanisms of displacement (onto her body), isolation of affect, repression of anger, and some psychotic distortion of reality to cope with conflicted emotions and distressing affects. Psychodynamically, the patient seems to need to be ill or mirror her mother's medically oriented perception of her problems to stay connected to her mother. Socioculturally, her family is religious and has concerns about her acceptance of their value system. Currently the patient's functioning is impaired in all her major life roles, including academic, peer relationships, and behavior in the family setting.

The patient also has notable adaptive interests and capacities. Lately, she has been learning to drive and expresses interest in spending time with people her age. She is an attractive young lady who expresses interest in making changes in the way she approaches life. These motivations, if supported by her mother, could help her to relinquish her physical symptoms. It is unclear, however, whether the closeness of the patient and her mother currently based on her medical symptoms can shift to a healthy adolescent separation-individuation process.

Diagnostically, she meets criteria for major depressive disorder with possible psychotic features, bulimia nervosa, and somatoform disorder not otherwise specified. The problems to address in treatment include her depressive and anxiety symptoms, her vomiting, her social isolation, and psychological barriers in mother and daughter to the daughter's normative adolescent separation-individuation process. The treatment plan includes (1) pharmacotherapy with an antidepressant and short-term use of an atypical antipsychotic, (2) individual psychotherapy with supportive and cognitive-behavioral components to help the patient develop more adaptive ways to express psychological needs and conflicts and advance toward normative age-appropriate goals, and (3) family

> therapy to help the mother-daughter relationship support
> the daughter's age-appropriate separation-individuation.
> The initial goal of family therapy would be to develop a
> constructive alliance with the parents, which requires respect
> and validation of their goals and values and their concerns
> about the daughter's ability to handle more autonomy.

alliance with the mother and patient, because they were very invested in other medical explanations. When it was presented, the patient's mother was reluctant to accept this diagnosis and continued to insist that the patient was vomiting because of a medical reason that had not been identified. The mother became distraught when family therapy was recommended and insisted that treating her daughter's depression would lead to an improvement of her appetite and resolve the vomiting. The patient did report dramatic improvement in her energy when her antidepressant dose was increased. She was continuing to "spit up" in the middle of the night but had not vomited in 2 weeks. They continued to come for weekly appointments.

*Additions made after the case was discussed in supervision*

The patient has several biologic risks for psychiatric difficulties, including a history of being exposed in utero to psychotropic medications, likely including alcohol. She seems to have an anxious temperament, which was likely exacerbated by an insecure attachment related to her mother's emotional unavailability during her infancy when the parents' marriage ended and her mother began a new relationship with the patient's stepfather. Psychologically, the history suggests that the patient had difficulty with affect modulation in infancy, which continued through her childhood. She is highly reactive to interpersonal slights and subsequently has not been able to form trusting relationships with adults or peers. Her sense of self-worth seems to be invested in her appearance and the desire to change her weight, which increases her risk of developing an eating disorder.

The patient also had developmental problems that manifested in academic problems in elementary school 4 years ago. After an unrevealing educational assessment, she was home-schooled, which further limited her opportunities to develop peer relationships. In the past 5 years she endured multiple medical evaluations and procedures and four hospitalizations for medical problems, which further interfered with her schooling. She is not able to verbalize her anger, and her vomiting seems to correlate with emotional distress in place of verbal expression.

Her medical symptoms seem to have particular significance within the mother-child relationship and seem to serve the function of engaging her mother's attention. Her mother's response to her oscillates between being overly involved and attentive to her medical symptoms and being unsupportive regarding her psychological vulnerabilities and desire for autonomy. She emphasizes medication as a solution to psychological problems, which minimizes the importance of her own and the patient's psychological involvement in the treatment process. There is a secondary gain to the daughter's medical complaints because they elicit the mother's attention and prevent the mother from leaving the house, thereby continuing the mother-daughter enmeshment.

In addition to somatization, she uses the defense mechanisms of displacement (onto her body), isolation of affect, repression of anger, and reaction formation to cope with conflicted emotions and distressing affects. The patient's comment that she never felt "connected" to her mother suggests that the use of somatization is associated with what Winnicott referred to as a "false self" [29] incorporating the need to be ill or mirror her mother's symptom-oriented perception of problems to stay connected to her mother. At times, she also uses the defense of psychotic distortion of reality. Another possible contributor to her anxiety, affective, and psychotic-like symptoms could be trauma related to multiple invasive medical procedures or possible physical abuse as a child.

Alongside these constitutional and psychological vulnerabilities, the patient also has some adaptive interests and capacities. Lately, she has been learning to drive and started expressing interest in spending time with people her age. She is an attractive young lady who expresses interest in making changes in the way she approaches life. These motivations, if supported by her mother, could help her to relinquish some of her physical symptoms. It is unclear, however, whether the closeness of the patient and her mother currently based on her medical symptoms can shift to a healthy adolescent separation-individuation process. The treatment plan includes individual psychotherapy with supportive and cognitive-behavioral components to help the patient develop more adaptive ways to express psychological needs and conflicts and help her advance toward normative age-appropriate goals. Family therapy has been recommended to help support the mother and daughter to reconfigure their emotional involvement to support age-appropriate separation-individuation. The mother's need for the daughter to remain dependent by being medically ill may be difficult to address without the mother receiving her own individual therapy, however.

The resident used the Defensive Functioning Scale in the DSM-IV-TR [30] to consider the patient's symptoms in terms of their defensive functions. The addition of an expanded psychodynamic formulation helped the resident more fully understand the patient's extreme dilemma. Her desire for age-appropriate autonomy was directly in conflict with her ongoing need to repair a historically weak emotional connection with her mother. Relinquishing her physical symptoms would require her mother's willingness to work to accept a less enmeshed form of relatedness with her daughter, with the attendant psychological risk (for both of them) of her daughter feeling free enough to develop other intimate relationships.

After developing the expanded case formulation, the resident felt she was working more successfully to help the daughter develop age-appropriate interests and greater autonomy. The last part of this evolving formulation occurred when she received a letter from the mother indicating her intention to end the treatment because her daughter was becoming more disobedient at home and not embracing the values of the family. In debriefing with the supervisor, additional information was shared and integrated into the formulation—that the patient's mother had become emancipated as a teenager because of a difficult family situation. With her own potentially unresolved adolescent separation, helping her daughter navigate these challenges would understandably generate internal conflict. By reviewing the case formulation and its prediction of obstacles, the resident understood that an earlier formulation of the mother's dilemma would have helped her work more effectively with both partners. She recognized that it would have been helpful to put more therapeutic time into working directly with the mother and stepfather to fully understand their goals and develop a collaborative formulation and treatment plan.

## Summary

Case formulation plays a central role in guiding treatment planning in child and adolescent psychiatry. It helps synthesize many complex factors into hypotheses about the cause of the problem. This comprehensive, individualized picture helps to translate the diagnosis into the choice of where to put therapeutic resources at a particular stage of treatment. The biopsychosocial approach to formulation is the most comprehensive and facilitates the clinician's attention to all the major domains. The case formulation is an ongoing and dynamic process, an evolving "story" or narrative that is modified as more information is added. Because children must be seen in the context of their families, schools, neighborhoods, and larger ecology, the case formulation in child and adolescent psychiatry is more contextual and relies on multiple perspectives gleaned from a lengthier interview process. In general, case formulation has not been taught extensively in psychiatric residency programs, and even experienced clinicians do not routinely construct comprehensive case formulations. Most clinicians agree that more time should be spent teaching and modeling construction of the formulation in didactics, supervision, and case conferences. Including the child and family in the construction and ongoing revision of the formulation and addressing their strengths and needs—not just problems or pathology—promotes the therapeutic alliance. Integration of multiple theoretical and explanatory perspectives can be useful in teaching and applying the case formulation process. Clinical examples in the article illustrate aspects of the case formulation and residents' use of supervision to develop more elaborated and comprehensive case formulations.

# References

[1] McClain T, O'sullivan PS, Clardy JA. Biopsychosocial formulation: recognizing educational shortcomings. Acad Psychiatry 2004;28(2):88–94.

[2] Connor DF, Fisher SG. An interactional model of child and adolescent mental health clinical case formulation. Clin Child Psychol Psychiatry 1997;2(3):353–68.

[3] Bergner RM. Characteristics of optimal clinical case formulations. Am J Psychother 1998; 52(3):287–300.

[4] Nurcombe B, Fitzhenry-Coor I. Diagnostic reasoning and treatment planning: I. Diagnosis. Aust N Z J Psychiatry 1987;21(4):277–83.

[5] Kassaw K, Gabbard GO. Creating a psychodynamic formulation from a clinical evaluation. Am J Psychiatry 2002;159(5):721–6.

[6] Perry S, Cooper AM, Michels R. The psychodynamic formulation: its purpose, structure, and clinical application. Am J Psychiatry 1987;144(5):543–50.

[7] Shapiro T. The psychodynamic formulation in child and adolescent psychiatry. J Am Acad Child Adolesc Psychiatry 1989;28(5):675–80.

[8] Eells TD, editor. Handbook of psychotherapy case formulation. New York: Guilford Press; 1997.

[9] Engel GL. The clinical application of the biopsychosocial model. Am J Psychiatry 1980; 137(5):535–44.

[10] Nurcombe B, Drell M, Leonard H, et al. Clinical problem solving: the case of Matthew, part 1. J Am Acad Child Adolesc Psychiatry 2002;41(1):92–7.

[11] Engel GL. From biomedical to biopsychosocial: being scientific in the human domain. Psychosomatics 1997;38(6):521–8.

[12] American Psychiatric Association Commission on Psychotherapy. Definition of the biopsychosocial formulation. Washington, DC: American Psychiatric Association; 1996.

[13] Mellman L, Beresin E. Psychotherapy competencies: development and implementation. Acad Psychiatry 2003;27(3):149–53.

[14] Novins D, Bechtold DW, Sack WH, et al. The DSM-IV outline for cultural formulation: a critical demonstration with American Indian children. J Am Acad Child Adolesc Psychiatry 1997;36:1244–51.

[15] Jellinek MS, McDermott JF. Formulation: putting the diagnosis into a therapeutic context and treatment plan. J Am Acad Child Adolesc Psychiatry 2004;43(4):913–6.

[16] Turkat ID. The personality disorders: a psychological approach to clinical management. New York: Pergamon; 1990.

[17] Storck M, Vanderstoep A. Fostering ecological perspectives in child psychiatry. Child Adolesc Psychiatr Clin N Am 2007;16(1):in press.

[18] Lane D. Context focused analysis: an experimentally derived model for working with complex problems with children, adolescents and systems. In: Bruch M, Bond FW, editors. Beyond diagnosis: case formulation approaches in CBT. West Sussex, England: John Wiley & Sons, Ltd.; 2003. p. 103–40.

[19] Metz P. The child psychiatric formulation: process and content considerations from a systems-based perspective. Presented at the Annual Meeting of the American Academy of Child and Adolescent Psychiatry. Toronto, October 24, 2005.

[20] Winters NC, Pumariega AJ, American Academy of Child and Adolescent Psychiatry Work Group on Quality Issues. Practice parameter on child and adolescent mental health care in community systems of care. J Am Acad Child Adolesc Psychiatry, in press.

[21] Bruch M, Bond FW. Beyond diagnosis: case formulation approaches in CBT. New York: Wiley & Sons; 1998.

[22] McWilliams N. Psychoanalytic case formulation. New York: Guilford Press; 1999.

[23] Mellman L. The psychodynamic formulation. Presented at the annual meeting of the American Association of Directors of Psychiatric Residency Training (AADPRT), March 9, 2002.

[24] Beck A. The current state of cognitive therapy: a 40-year retrospective. Arch Gen Psychiatry 2005;62:953–9.

[25] Sudak D, Beck J, Wright J. Cognitive behavioral therapy: a blueprint for attaining and assessing psychiatry resident competency. Acad Psychiatry 2003;27:154–259.

[26] Winters NC, Hanson G, Colman L, et al. Integrated teaching of psychodynamic and evidence-based psychotherapies in child psychiatry. Presented at the Annual Meeting of the American Association of Directors of Psychiatric Residency Training. San Diego, March 10, 2006.

[27] Barker P. The child and adolescent psychiatry evaluation: basic child psychiatry. Oxford, UK: Blackwell Scientific, Inc.; 1995.

[28] Nurcombe B. Developmental psychopathology and the diagnostic formulation. Presented at the Annual Meeting of the American Academy of Child and Adolescent Psychiatry. Washington, DC; October 1992.

[29] Winnicott DW. The maturational process and the facilitating environment. New York: International Universities Press; 1965.

[30] American Psychiatric Association. Diagnostic and statistical manual of mental disorder. 4th edition. Washington, DC: American Psychiatric Association; 2000. p. 807–13.

**ELSEVIER
SAUNDERS**

Child Adolesc Psychiatric Clin N Am
16 (2007) 133–163

CHILD AND
ADOLESCENT
PSYCHIATRIC CLINICS
OF NORTH AMERICA

# Fostering Ecologic Perspectives
# in Child Psychiatry

## Michael G. Storck, MD*, Ann Vander Stoep, PhD

*Division of Child and Adolescent Psychiatry, University of Washington School of Medicine,
Children's Hospital and Regional Medical Center, W3636, 4800 Sand Point Way NE,
Seattle, WA 98105-0371, USA*

For clinicians who devote their professional lives to young people, the quest to appreciate the vulnerabilities, strengths, and developmental tasks of children can yield an abundance of wonder and perplexity. Our goal is to help foster in clinicians an abiding enthusiasm and intrigue for the breadth and nuances of humanity and for the contexts in which they may be engaged over the course of a career. Although our primary audience for this article is trainees and teachers in child and adolescent psychiatry, we hope that the principles presented herein are valuable to all pediatric and mental health providers.

Children, as they grow, take part in a world that is dynamic and ever changing. They are brought to healing professionals because someone thinks they are not adequately adapting to their world. When a child is brought to a child psychiatrist, what is the clinical unit of study? Is it a behavior, a constellation of behaviors, or a biologic challenge that the child and parents are facing? Is it the body and the mind and soul of the child? Is it the family unit? Does it include the culture and community within which the child is adapting? Child psychiatry is at once a medical subspecialty dedicated to appreciating the complex biologic workings of children and an art in which the relationships of an individual living within multiple levels of affiliation and influence are examined and reworked. In this article we offer a framework to help child psychiatry trainees explore, understand, and savor the nexus of contextual complexities that affect children's mental health and adaptive functioning. We consider children as participants in a broad diversity of community domains that, taken together, comprise a child's "village." These domains include health and social service

* Corresponding author.
*E-mail address:* storck@u.washington.edu (M.G. Storck).

1056-4993/07/$ - see front matter © 2006 Elsevier Inc. All rights reserved.
doi:10.1016/j.chc.2006.09.005
*childpsych.theclinics.com*

institutions, schools and related normative activities of childhood, and familial, cultural, spiritual, and religious spheres of influence.

What are the optimal lenses through which child psychiatrists, as scientists, artists, and healers, can evaluate a child's domains of influence? This article presents an ecologic perspective on child psychiatry and discusses implications for the child psychiatry training process. We suggest tools for making sense of the systems involved in shaping the mental health of children. Methods for exploring families' perspectives on illness and healing are presented. The mutual benefits of fostering teamwork and a co-investigator spirit between patient and provider are illustrated.

## Case vignette 1

*Sean is a preadolescent boy living in a long-term psychiatric residential treatment program. He has been diagnosed with pervasive developmental disorder and posttraumatic stress disorder. His mother has major mood instability and enduring psychosocial insecurity complicated by ongoing prostitution. Sean has had multiple foster placements and numerous father figures, and all but the youngest of five siblings have been removed from his mother's custody. One evening Sean is seemingly inconsolable and lashes out at his counselors, threatening to harm himself and others. As he is guided to an area for calming, he throws himself on the floor sobbing and muttering unintelligibly. Ultimately he sits up, tears streaming down his face, looks at his gathered team, and yells, "I don't know how to be that number!" Unclear as to his meaning, his psychiatry resident waits for Sean to gather his speech and asks him to try to say more. "I don't know what to do when I'm that number!" cries Sean. It dawns on his team that the next day is Sean's birthday. Several of his birthdays have been spent in foster and residential care. Earlier in the day Sean expressed his fear that his mother would not remember to visit him on his birthday. Being the number "eleven" was very hard, and being the number "twelve" loomed distressingly.*

Who is this boy? What are his adaptive challenges? What are the unique variables (biologic, psychosocial, institutional, and cultural) that define and color his life and the way he is struggling to grow up? In this clinical moment, the focal points might be his immediate behavior, his developmental stage, notions he has acquired about acting one's age, his family matrix, his life in the milieu on the inpatient unit, and his future adaptive challenges in the community. Is his community, including his current treatment milieu, a safe and good enough place for him to figure out how to be 12 years old? How would this boy's task (of learning how to be 12) be different in other settings? What variables shape the readiness of his providers to work with this boy? What variables shape Sean's readiness to work with his care team? How can medical (clinical) education be structured and shaped so that providers provide optimal therapeutic support in this demanding treatment moment?

## Case vignette 2

*A pediatrician asks a child psychiatrist for consultation in the care of Nadia, an 8-year-old Hispanic girl with depressive symptoms and attention deficit hyperactivity disorder. Nadia has been maintained on a regimen of stimulant medication. The psychiatrist learns from Nadia's family and teacher that a special behavioral and educational program is in place at school to address her learning and attentional disorders. The parents reluctantly share that they are also providing their daughter with an over-the-counter herbal/vitamin regimen and that her grandparents are skeptical of medications. The grandparents have sought guidance and prayer from the family's minister and the congregation. The parents are worried that the medication may be interfering with Nadia's appetite and energy and with her participation on her local soccer team, an activity that she relishes.*

We can ask many of the same questions about Nadia that we did of Sean. What are her adaptive challenges? What are the unique variables (biologic, psychosocial, institutional, and cultural) that define her life and the way she is growing up? In this clinical consultation, what should the focal points for the psychiatrist be? What does Nadia think is going on for her? How do the grandparents and the minister figure into the evaluation and treatment planning? What variables shape the readiness of providers to work with this girl and her family? Who is she to her family, her teachers, and her soccer teammates? How does the family's ethnicity influence the treatment relationship? How do we make sense of the other systems of care to which she belongs? How do we formulate and communicate our treatment recommendations? How do we modify them in the face of family concerns?

To serve these children and their families, providers likely use many standard child psychiatric treatment modalities, including psychopharmacology, individual, family, and group psychotherapies, and school- and community-based interventions. How do we help trainees to build treatment plans and clinical relationships that are optimally informed by an appreciation of the constellations of influences that children face? In the famous, at times politically controversial, aphorism: "It takes a village to raise a child," there are many roles served by many people in the process of guiding a child to adulthood. An implication within the aphorism is the idea that each village might have its own unique sociocultural forces (sometimes different from the next village up the road) that shape the development of children who are its members. When invited into a village to help solve a child's (and family's and—sometimes—community's) distress, how do psychiatrists discern and implement their most salutary impact?

We suggest that for the trainee, it is helpful to cultivate three types of understanding—ecologic, ethnographic, and attributional—to broaden, enliven, and enrich the palette they use in their work with patients and families. Each type of understanding can serve as a kind of focusing device that can enhance formulative thinking and intervention skills to address the distress experiences of children and families and enhance appreciation of the perspectives of other providers involved in the treatment process.

## Ecology

For more than 30 years, academic medicine has acknowledged the use of a "biopsychosocial" model for conceptualizing influences on health [1]. Wilkinson and O'Connor [2] endeavored to carry the biopsychosocial approach into intervention constructs they termed "ecopsychiatry" by positing that treatment and prevention were activities best driven by "observing the individual in whatever life contexts appear relevant to clinical issues and the presenting problem." *Ecology* is a term coined in the nineteenth century by evolutionary biologist Ernst Haeckel, and it refers to "the branch of biology concerned with the total complex of interrelationships among living organisms, encompassing the relations of organisms to each other, to the environment, and to the entire energy balance within a given ecosystem" [3]. Bronfenbrenner [4] argued that ecologic perspectives are central in conceptualizing a child's development. According to Bronfenbrenner, "The ecology of human development is the scientific study of the progressive, mutual accommodation, *throughout the life course*, between an active, growing human being and the changing properties of the immediate settings in which the developing person lives, as this process is affected by the relations between these settings, and by the larger contexts in which the settings are embedded."

The basic assumption of an ecologic approach is that behavior can only be understood fully when it is regarded within its naturally occurring context. Bronfenbrenner has suggested conceptualizing human ecologic systems as having four levels:

1. "A *microsystem* is a pattern of activities, roles, and interpersonal relationships experienced by the developing person in a given face-to-face setting with particular physical and material features and containing other persons with distinctive characteristics of temperament, personality, and systems of belief." Homes, classrooms, and peer groups may be thought of as microsystems.
2. "The *mesosystem* comprises the linkages and processes taking place between two or more settings containing the developing persons (eg, the relations between home and school, school and workplace). In other words, a mesosystem is a system of microsystems."
3. "The *exosystem* encompasses the linkage and processes taking place between two or more settings at least one of which does not ordinarily contain the developing person, but in which events occur that influence processes within the immediate setting that does contain that person (eg, for a child, the relation between the home and the parent's workplace...)."

4. "The *macrosystem* consists of the overarching pattern of micro-, meso-
   and exosystems characteristic of a given culture, subculture, or other
   broader social context, with particular reference to the developmentally
   instigative belief systems, resources, hazards, lifestyles, opportunity
   structures, life course options, and patterns of social interchange that
   are embedded in each of these systems. The macrosystem may be
   thought of as a societal blueprint for a particular culture, subculture,
   or broader social context."

Understanding the adjustments that occur between a child and family,
peers, schoolmates, teachers, and other aspects of the child's ecology enable
us to see the factors that have caused, shaped, or sustained his or her illness
and distress. Knowing the location of the child within her or his ecology and
how he or she got there enables us to plan a course of action on which the
patient and family can embark along a path toward healing and more optimal adaptation. In ecologic interventions, rather than only targeting the suffering child, dimensions in the child's world become the focus of treatment.
Contingencies within family, school, and community systems are reshaped
to support a mutual progressive accommodation toward more adaptive
moods, thoughts, and behaviors [5,6]. In ecologic interventions, the frameworks around the child are shaped and molded to be more consistent, more
authoritative, and more supportive of the child's healthy behavior and development. Making sense of and reshaping a child's habits and symptoms
involve active consideration of the multiple levels of forces at work from
the elemental molecular to the complex community level, from the
"microsystem" to the "macrosystem."

In working with distressed children, how do we learn about these forces,
and how can we understand their influences? We introduce ethnography as
a method of inquiry that can be used by healers to develop an understanding
of children within micro-, meso-, and macrostrata of their ecologic
framework.

## Ethnography

As with many fundamental elements of modern science, the ethnographic
method reportedly has its roots in ancient Greece. The fifth century histo-
rian Herodotus wrote of the differences in laws, customs, religions, and ap-
pearances among the dozens of different peoples he encountered in his
travels. "Ethnography" is a term brought to qualitative health research by
Spradley [7] in his monograph "The Ethnographic Interview." Initially
referring narrowly to anthropologic observations of cultural practices and
beliefs among specific ethnic groups, ethnography has come to identify
a process of inquiry wherein the anthropologist (and, we suggest, the clinician) adopts a participant-observer status within the group being studied.
This process involves the observer's immersion in the culture.

In psychiatry, ethnographic perspectives are gained by learning the language, dialect, meanings, currencies of exchange, and community affiliations and linkages of children and their families. With eyes and ears open, psychiatrists may engage in ethnographic fieldwork while attending family meetings, while consulting at the bedside in an intensive care unit, or while walking the high school halls to consult with a treatment team. Families often need to engage in the same type of "ethnographic" work to understand their child and understand our hospitals and clinics. Some families need extra coaching to engage enthusiastically and skillfully in these pursuits. To this end, in many treatment facilities, cultural and language interpreters and parent advocates are offered to families to help the provider (and the provider's institution) broker the clinical process. As ethnographers, clinicians and parents are wondering "what is it like for my patient/child to navigate this setting?"

In child psychiatry, the invitation to meet and get alongside a child is usually initiated by families, guardians, or teachers. They often are eager for a clinician to have direct experience of a child's struggle so as to appreciate the forces and factors that can help to define essential features of a problem. The ethnographic approach not only involves clinicians putting themselves in the midst of that struggle but also encourages an effort by clinicians to recognize the impact of their own frameworks and biases in the midst of a child's clinical field. This process calls for the observer to step back to have, as Piaget might have said, an "abstracted view" of oneself in the midst of the clinical field and of the doctor-patient transaction. Taking the participant-observer role in dynamic moments in the life of a child enables clinicians to understand more realistically a child's dilemmas and challenges and more usefully frame the therapeutic recommendations.

Therapeutic work with children affords many opportunities for a psychiatrist to be an ethnographer. The ethnographic method, although perhaps not often labeled as such, is pervasive in clinical inquiry under various guises, such as in the formulative approaches used in family systems therapy [8] and the psychodynamic paradigm [9,10]. The ethnographic method can serve as a complementary construct for the processes already used by clinicians (eg, the diagnostic interview) for cataloguing their observations and formulating a treatment plan. Clinical perspectives can be gained from many different styles and types of participant-observation. What follows are a few examples of ethnographic data gathering by psychiatry trainees who serve as primary clinicians in community sites.

- *Walking alongside the dilemma.* A psychiatry fellow walks the hospital grounds with a 14-year-old girl who re-experiences her previously professed commitment to run away and kill herself. The fellow supports the patient in re-evaluating her feelings and choices. The patient turns around instead of fleeing the hospital grounds.
- *On the team in the social matrix.* A 13-year-old boy with major learning disabilities, posttraumatic stress, and Asperger's disorder invites his

physician to share a two-on-two game of basketball with two other patients. The boy works on passing skills, appropriate in-game language,
and teamwork. The psychiatry fellow guides the boy and his peers through
progressively skillful basketball games...and, in an act of true empathy,
suffers a sprained ankle while making a rebound.

- *The quintessential family place.* A psychiatry fellow and several other
  members of the treatment team accompany a 16-year-old boy who has
  attention deficit hyperactivity disorder and bipolar disorder to his family
  home for a therapeutic family meeting. In attendance are the boy's parents, two younger sisters, and a family pet, all of whom are highly lively,
  distractible, impulsive, and good humored in their struggles. The living
  room and kitchen, although inviting, look well lived in and highly
  cluttered.
- *Hearing in a new language.* A 16-year-old boy, son of Southeast Asian
  immigrants, sits down with the child psychiatry fellow for an interview
  in a juvenile corrections facility and speaks in a "gang dialect" about his
  childhood and family history.

The child psychiatrist's aim is to help a child successfully navigate his or
her world. To accomplish this aim, we must ensure that our intervention
strategies work effectively not only within the confines of the office or hospital but also in the child's real world zones. In vivo observation of the
adaptive repertoires of a young person in day-to-day realms broadens the
provider's understanding of the variables (ecologic forces) that influence
the patient's thoughts, emotions, and behaviors. Observations made in family, treatment, and community settings form a collection of supportive evidence and data that can yield important perspectives for case formulation
and treatment planning. These observations can provide epiphanies and developmental milestones for clinicians young and old. They are the nutrients
and fuel for clinicians as they build a professional repertoire of generalizable
understandings, behavioral skills, and shareable vignettes that may be useful
for decades to come. Helping patients to develop their own ethnographic
skills also can improve *their* life navigation abilities.

### Attribution

"All forms of healing are based on a conceptual scheme consistent with the
patient's assumptive world. The scheme prescribes a set of activities and
helps sufferers make sense out of inchoate feelings, thereby heightening
their sense of mastery..."—Frank and Frank, 1991 [11]
    "Meaning is derived through the structuring of experience into stories...
and the performance of these stories is constitutive of lives and
relationships"—White and Epston, 1990 [12]

In Plato's parable "The Myth of the Cave (Plato's Republic)" [13], Socrates chides his student Glaucon for assuming that humans can see the true

nature of the world. Socrates relates a myth in which humans are chained to a wall inside a cave where they can only make inferences about the world from shadows they see in front of them. "How could they understand anything but the shadows," queries Socrates, "if they were never allowed to turn their heads?" The humans in Plato's cave make attributions (causal assumptions) about the world based on their limited knowledge.

All humans "see" the world through lenses ground via their experiential reference points, cultural schemata, beliefs, language constructs, and unique cognitive make-up. We are all, to some degree, "chained" to the wall of our own provincial experiences and at the same time capable of traversing new territory to expand our world view. The term *attribution* is proposed as a short-hand reference to the labels and explanatory schema or models that patients, family members, psychiatrists, and fellow providers use to make sense of or assign causal links to a given symptom, disorder, or behavioral repertoire. Derived from cognitive motivation models, "attribution theory" concerns the judgments people make about what causes behavior [14]. Patient attributions about their behavior provide insights as to how and why they may or may not seek to change. Likewise, a provider's diagnostic statements often suggest to the patient and family underlying cultural ramifications and causal mechanisms and foretell treatment implications.

Examples of attributional statements from within child psychiatry are often overheard and include such assertions as

"Methylphenidate fixed my hyperactivity."
"No one will ever take me into their foster home if I'm on these medications."
"I can't control my behavior because my mom drank alcohol before I was born."
"You remind me of my father, and that's why I'm sad."
"My minister told me that God will protect me so, I feel safer now."
"I found out on the web chat group that my child has Asperger's disorder. I feel better now that I know what's wrong."
"Your son meets full diagnostic criteria for major depressive disorder. I would suggest an SSRI."

For clinicians and patients, hearing these statements can, at times, be reassuring as well as vexing. Such statements often reveal the gateway to a patient's or a fellow clinician's lively internal dialogue and a beginning for a shared dialogue in a clinical interchange.

Families, cultural communities, and professional groups may acquire or maintain common sets of attributions that shape how they view members of another group. Although there may be benefits for group members, "group attributions" also can be perilous. Challenges occur when families work with provider groups that each use different attributional schema. Within the world of biomedicine, attributional biases can differ substantially between medical specialties and even between members of the same subspecialty group. Patients may perceive one provider group as having unique understandings, limitations, or powers compared with another provider group. These concerns should be fair game for discussion between a clinician and patients. It is important to evaluate the attributions a child has formed about his or her powers and problems.

According to Piaget, an important milestone in human development is achieving the ability to "see" and construe the world from another's perspective. One of the roles that the clinician-observer can serve for patients is to provide a forum whereby multiple attributions can be displayed and compared. The process of shedding new light on a clinical phenomenon can lead to attributional shifts for patients and providers. Once two sets of attributional and explanatory models are elucidated, they can be evaluated for the degree to which they may complement or argue against each other. Helping individuals reflect on the factors that influence assignment of causation (attributions) can enhance understanding of their possibilities for and pathways to change. Searching for a common ground for illness explanations and a shared roadmap of treatment goals should drive this sometimes lively and, hopefully, collaborative process. The renowned physician and anthropologist Arthur Kleinman suggests these steps for helping achieve a shared view of attribution/causation [15–17]:

- eliciting the patient's model of illness explanation
- articulating the clinician's own explanatory/attributional model
- comparing models and negotiating a shared model

This collaborative process relies on the establishment of a trust relationship in which the patient and provider feel safe enough to share their reflections on causation and treatment goals and motivated and energetic enough to negotiate differences and find common ground.

## Case vignette 3

*Dee is a 13-year-old Navajo girl who completed eighth grade at a boarding school outside her home state. While at the boarding school, she developed distressing homicidal and suicidal thoughts. She was losing ground in academic, social, and recreational activities. Upon her return home, her family sought consultation from a child psychiatrist and a traditional Navajo healer. Dee's psychiatrist diagnosed her as meeting criteria for posttraumatic stress disorder related to the death of her beloved older sister 3 years earlier. The psychiatrist recommended a course of cognitive behavioral therapy and medication to help Dee manage her anxiety, despondency, and feelings of powerlessness. The traditional Navajo healer diagnosed Dee's distress as resulting from harmful exposure to the dead (the boarding school was located near a cemetery) and suggested that her extended family arrange for a 3-day healing ceremony to undo the pernicious influence of the graveyard exposure, strengthen the family's ties with each other, and restore Dee's role as a young woman within the Navajo community. The family arranged a team meeting of child, family, traditional healer, and psychiatrist to share understandings and forge a complementary treatment approach. At this meeting, the psychiatrist learned more about Navajo traditional healing constructs and specific symbols and stories central to the family's understanding of Dee's difficulties. At the team meeting he was able to describe a place in the healing plan for medications and cognitive behavioral therapy strategies.*

Although the clinician may help patients to modify and enlighten their causal explanations, our patients, if we are open, help us to expand our explanatory constructs so that we can become more skilled, seasoned, sensitive, and effective physicians and providers. Through carefully sharing agendas and understandings with children and families (principles essential to all good medical practice) [18], we strive to find sufficient common ground from which to move effectively toward formulation and treatment strategies that include the voices of all parties.

As we prepare to more systematically explore the worlds of our patients, Epstein's reflections on "Mindful Practice" may be a resource for boosting a clinician's readiness for the meaningful moments of patient communication and shared inquiry [19]. Through a balancing of peripheral vision, introspection, and humility for what one does and does not know, mindful practice encourages active observation of oneself and helps to cultivate a comfortable presence and curiosity in the moment with each patient and family. To stave off the sense of being overwhelmed with the mission of child psychiatry, a book such as Ann Lamott's "Bird by Bird: Some Instructions on Writing and Life" offers refuge in which clinicians can gain perspective and appreciate the goals that they hold in common with the novelist [20]: "...to help others have this sense of —please forgive me—wonder, of seeing things anew, things that can catch us off guard, that break in our small, bordered worlds." "When this happens," Lamott contends, "everything feels more spacious."

## Understanding the child in the village: domains of influence and systems of care

The ecologic, ethnographic, and attributional lenses are offered as tools to be used by providers to appreciate a child's community or "village" and the zones of influence that shape a child's life. In the partnership of health care, patients visit doctors' worlds and doctors visit patients' worlds. The tools can be used in patient-centered and doctor-centered arenas. The remainder of this article is a fieldtrip into the worlds that patients and their clinicians navigate. Our itinerary includes three different but interrelated zones:

1. The health and social welfare system zone, in which we tour the day-to-day world of the provider and try on the viewpoint of a child and family as they navigate these formal service areas.

2. The child development and activity zone, in which we explore the day-to-day world of a child, including school, peer-cultures, and recreational pursuits.
3. The cultural, spiritual, religious, and historical zone, in which we consider the determinants and the expectations of a child's behavior and development as influenced by the family's social, ethnocultural, and religious affiliations.

This topography is offered as a basis for navigating the salient areas of influence within a child's village; however, this three-zone tour is not exhaustive of a child's village grid, and the zones are not easily separable or mutually exclusive. Within the human experience there is an overarching fluidity of forces, as Bronfenbrenner acknowledges in his conceptualization of the macrosystem. As examples, a child's cultural identity may substantially influence school and activity affiliations, and a family's use of conventional and alternative healing approaches may be closely tied to its religious affiliations. A family also may shift economic classes in the course of a generation, which potentiates changes across multiple zones.

A child's symptom presentation and treatment progress are influenced by factors in many domains. For Nadia, the 8-year-old girl in case vignette 2, and Dee, the teen in case vignette 3, cultural, religious, alternative medical, recreational, and school system forces influence their emotional health status and should be taken into account in developing effective treatment strategies. For many children, particularly children with complex needs, as many as four to six healing/helping systems may be involved simultaneously. Each system may have its own explanations and attributions for the etiology of the child's problems and specific ideas as to how to help the child overcome them. Over the years, veteran clinicians get tuned to the idea that a treatment plan might involve multitasking for this multiplicity. For teachers, a central task in the mentoring process for our trainees is to help them be lively of spirit and enthused for a diversity of complex challenges as we help them collaboratively bring to light the workings and meanings of these various systems. These pursuits may take them well beyond the literal and metaphoric confines of the psychiatric office setting.

## Health and social welfare systems

### Health care institutions

What do a child and family experience as they enter and become acquainted with health care institutions? How does the health care provider, for whom the institutional zone is more familiar, see this zone through the eyes of the child and family? Intervention strategies that fall under the rubric of psychiatric treatment can be as divergent as the antibiotic penicillin for immune system-generated behavioral disorders, the chemical element lithium for mood instability, and individual and group dialectical behavioral therapy for emotional dysregulation and interpersonal relationship instability. Patients and families who receive psychiatric care may be startled by the breadth of (at times contradictory) attributions and treatment modalities offered within biomedical psychiatry alone.

Hospitals and clinics may present their own myriad microzones—from the emergency room to the continuity clinic—with distinctly different language, dialect, meanings, and "currencies of exchange." Medical student education in the clinical years provides widely divergent training milieus from clerkship to clerkship. Training within medical specialties provides divergent cultures for trainees, too. Consider the different ways a patient's problems may be interpreted in a "psychopharmacology clinic" versus a "family therapy clinic". Each clinic's culture may have its own spoken and unspoken codes regarding elements as mundane as "appropriate dress" (white coat or not?) and as esoteric as clinic assignment based on diagnostic coding. Residential treatment centers, a training zone in some child psychology residency programs, are also likely to be divergent in program philosophy and treatment team organization [21,22]. The work of Moos and colleagues [23,24] provides rich testimonials and research data regarding the impact of microcultural (milieu) dynamics on treatment outcome. If a trainee is not sure about such nuances as whether to wear a white coat or a tie or how he or she should incorporate a patient's worries about homelessness into the treatment plan, it is safe to assume that patients and their families likely will have their own uncertainties and understandable anxieties as they decode and negotiate the specific customs and expectations of our clinical cultures. On a mundane level, one family may feel discounted that the doctor has not worn a white coat, whereas a particular child may feel heightened anxiety upon seeing the doctor's white coat. On a more pervasive level, Ann Fadiman's cautionary ethnographic case study "The spirit catches you and you fall down: A Hmong child, her American doctors, and the collision of two cultures" provides a powerful portrayal of how even earnest and complex efforts by families and providers to collaborate do not fully prevent fateful misunderstandings [25].

In our first case vignette we met Sean in a moment of crisis within a hospital setting. His experience and the experience of the psychiatry fellow were shaped by the routine response patterns presented by the child care staff. This 12-year-old boy's aggressive impulses might trigger substantially different treatment approaches in a different setting. Even within a facility, the spoken and unspoken rules of the treatment culture can vary substantially from shift to shift, which affects the patient's and the psychiatry fellow's progress through the moment of crisis. One of our expectations for trainees is that they be able to consider how their patients experience these nuances. What is at stake for the patient and the trainee in these unique ecosystems? Compare how different the patient and provider's attributions may be if the treatment culture's dominant philosophy treats the boy's struggle (to figure out how to be "twelve") as "antisocial acting out" versus treating it as "an awkward struggle to develop more adaptive distress tolerance." Through the use of ecologic, ethnographic, and attributional mindfulness, trainees learn to empathize with children and families who navigate these health care arenas. Also, there is no substitute for developing relationships with patients and front-line staff members of the treatment team that facilitate shared viewing of the forces at work in the life of the child...and the work life of the treatment team. Looking for perspective on how the hospital unit is perceived by the public at large and by other treatment facilities is also critical. The usual methods of public data and news gathering apply. What printed brochures, web-based information, and word-of-mouth data are available? Clinicians should be knowledgeable regarding the availability of translator and cultural commentator services, family support and parent advocacy teams, chaplain services, clinic and hospital ethics committees, and legal counsel. To observe the health system terrain that our patients are navigating, mentors and supervisors and hospital programs themselves should have formalized ways to help young clinicians develop a big picture view of the facilities and programs in which they serve.

## Complementary and alternative medical systems

Many consumers of allopathic medical care are simultaneously consuming alternative health care. Although patients may be reluctant to share with their conventional providers their health care habits outside of conventional medicine, this is an ever-expanding part of the landscape of American health care. A recent survey found that 21% of parents had used complementary and alternative medicine (CAM) treatment for their children [26]. For children who have ongoing mental health concerns, such as attention deficit hyperactivity disorder, pervasive developmental disorder, chronic depression, or anxiety, the percent of families using CAM treatments may range as high as 64% [27,28]. Patients and families often cite as a reason for using CAM treatments the fact that the experience of the "doctor-patient" relationship can feel more supportive than that routinely associated with allopathic treatment.

CAM is a group of diverse medical and health care systems, practices, and products. For a broader and more authoritative perspective on CAM treatment practices and research findings, the reader is referred to the National Institute of Health's National Center for Complementary and Alternative Medicine (http://nccam.nih.gov/). Examples of CAM providers include holistic allopathic physicians, osteopathic physicians, naturopathic doctors, homeopathic doctors, chiropractors, acupuncturists, massage therapists, religious healers, and herbalists. Many CAM remedies are available over the counter in retail establishments, whereas other CAM therapies are prescribed and administered only by licensed CAM providers. As with the latest allopathic remedies, patients often cite the internet as a primary information source. Discussing CAM with children is also further complicated by the reality that a child or teen may not have formed the notion that one treatment modality is considered conventional and that the others are considered unconventional.

Whatever the allopathic clinicians' views of alternative therapies may be, it is important that we help our patients and families feel safe to share with us their CAM experiences and pursuits [29]. The interactions between alternative modalities and conventional treatments may affect potency, modify efficacy, and possibly potentiate dangerous side effects. The opportunity for capitalizing on the complementary contributions of these alternative therapies in the care of future patients may be lost if we do not know they are being used. Finally, the understanding of patient and family attributional viewpoints is limited without this information.

With the recognition that most of our families are using multiple strategies to address their child's mental health needs, how do we help a child and family feel comfortable to reveal and discuss their healing grid? What if the multiple treatments or different attributions are not complementary (that is, do not add to each other's strengths)? The reader is referred to such recent reference books as "Handbook of Complementary and Alternative Therapies in Mental Health" to learn about CAM and its evidence base [30]. Later we suggest specific questions that clinicians can ask to elicit information from families about the alternative treatments they have sought.

*Social welfare systems*

Our patients who are difficult to manage at home, at school, or in the community may be involved in various service systems, such as special education, child welfare, or juvenile justice. Currently, more than 500,000 children in the United States live in foster homes [31], and most of these children are affected by psychiatric illness [32]. When a patient is a foster child, an ethnographic approach helps the provider to consider the grid of influences in which this child is situated. What home cultures has the child inhabited? Has the child been separated from a sibling group and from parent figures? Has the child moved between kinship homes? How differently does the child construe the parent figures from one home to the next? Does he or she know how long he or she will stay or where he or she will be going next? Does a term such as "time-out" have different meanings in one home compared with the next? We should also put ourselves in the shoes of the foster care providers. What are the unique challenges for a family to foster, in succession, children who are uniquely complicated and needy? How might abuse experiences in a previous home shape a child's experience in the current home [33]? To serve the complex health needs of children in foster care, the child welfare system, in concert with social work and child mental health researchers, has developed therapeutic foster care models [34–37]. Psychiatrists can be better advocates for children if they are familiar with evidence-based models for treatment of special needs youth in foster care.

As with the foster care system, there is a substantial overlap in target populations between juvenile justice and mental health systems. A high proportion of adolescents with psychiatric disorders become involved in the criminal justice system [38], and an estimated 80% of adolescents who are involved in the juvenile justice system have psychiatric disorders [39]. Recognizing how mental health conditions complicate the process of successful rehabilitation, the juvenile justice system has, like the child welfare system, developed evidence-based interventions to reduce criminal recidivism and improve reintegration to home, school, and community [40–42]. These evidence-based interventions may be available to and helpful for child psychiatric patients within the local community.

Foster care and corrections environments may have their own customized perspectives on child development and the essential tasks of childhood. Success in each environment may have specific criteria. As in any of the institutional cultures, a child or teen may define success based on values that are at least hidden from—if not antithetical to—the program's goals and philosophy. For example, some youth may view a stay in detention as an opportunity to cultivate gang affiliation powers or perhaps avoid an abusive home rather than an opportunity to atone for misdeeds and modify behavior. To be an effective clinical force in such youths' paths, the clinician must be able to see the youth's and the program's reward and reinforcement structures. Peer culture rules are almost inevitably distinctly different from the rules laid out in the program's policy manual. If we do not understand how a child interprets the rules and values and assigns meanings to the structure of the foster home, correctional setting, or whatever living zones he or she inhabits, we miss vital data and possibly are compromised in our effectiveness to help motivate therapeutic change for the youth.

## Child activity zone

We shift from the institutional zone of treatment, services, and professional supports that may be at the far reaches of a child's day-to-day ecology to realms that may be so close and personal to a child that they are very challenging for the clinician to access.

The ecology of the home and the characteristics of the family system are the most fundamental determinants of a child's sense of strength, security, identity, community adaptation, and overall well-being. The reader is referred to other salient references that complement the ethnographic treatment approaches to such dimensions of family life as the family life cycle, attachment forces, emotional tone, transgenerational perspectives, and ethnocultural influences [43–46].

Although family and home represent the core in the concentric circles of influence in a child's life, at the point a child begins to gaze at strangers and toddle into uncharted territory, he or she becomes a participant in the great world beyond. When faced with clinical questions of the adaptiveness or dysfunction of a child's behavior, how do we gain access to view the realms of influence for a child beyond the household? It is important to understand the out-of-home arenas in which the child has built his or her sense of identity, mastery, and competence, such as sports, academics, clubs, and other peer group connections, socially sanctioned activities (eg, music events), and socially "unsanctioned" activities (eg, all-night dances [raves] and gang affiliations). It must be stated that what is sanctioned and what is not depends on the eye of the beholder.

When a child is evaluated for a mental health condition, the psychiatrist provides a five-axis DSM diagnosis [47]. On axis V the clinician may rate the child's functioning on the Child Global Assessment Scale [48]. The rating score is based on intuiting or measuring the child's adaptive success at home, in school, and in other community venues and take into account how he or she functions in the clinician's office. How do we gather the data to achieve an accurate intuition or measurement? The ecologic and ethnographic approaches point us to several means of data gathering. They are applied by developing a comfortable alliance with a child and family and then maintaining an open eye for the invitation by the child and family to be a co-investigator of a particular youth arena.

## Case vignette 4

*Rudy, a 13-year-old boy who had been struggling with depressive symptoms in school and at home, was quiet and sullen during his first two office-based sessions with his new therapist. On the third visit, when they left the office to walk the clinic grounds, the boy, perhaps triggered by gazing upon the surrounding ranchlands in the community, proudly began discussing his involvement in the local youth rodeo. The rodeo was the one place, he said, where he did not feel "stupid," where he did not have time to worry about his father's health, and where others looked up to him.*

We can imagine this boy having at least three distinctly different identities (at home, school, and rodeo) in the course of his day. His comfort and conflict in each of these zones figures into his "symptom profile," as does his evolving sense of efficacy in the world. We should be curious as to how his attributions about his abilities vary across these zones. To what extent are his positive attributions of himself from the rodeo useful or transferable into the classroom or home zones? The clinician's Child Global Assessment Scale score for this boy might vary considerably depending on how much the clinician knows of his functional status in the rodeo.

The adaptiveness and often coincidental maladaptiveness of the child's thoughts, emotions, and behaviors can be appreciated more fully within a contextual grid. In "The Geography of Childhood," Nabhan and Trimble [49] discuss the situation of a young man who, in his neighborhood, had learned to discriminate between the sounds of a half dozen different types of automatic weapons. "He did not see this as an unusual piece of discriminatory knowledge for someone his age. These were the sounds he'd learned and sensed to be vital to his own existence. In another place or era he would have spoken as matter-of-factly about the calls of six common species of hawks and owls." The clinician might help this young man to see how being able to know the type of gunfire is useful for him in some arenas, whereas this same ability might complicate his adaptive functioning in others. In "Fist Stick Knife Gun," Geoffrey Canada muses autobiographically that a child's sense of efficacy and adaptation can shift significantly across a small space. "The ranking order on your neighborhood block meant nothing to the children from other blocks" [50]. In how many domains of the day can a child's adaptive repertoire—his or her identity—be differentially challenged? How can our patients reveal this possibly bewildering complexity to us?

A doctor can be a participant-observer with a child. Although this relationship begins in the office and in the midst of family interviews, we should move beyond the confines of the health care zone when possible. Visiting day care programs and school classrooms provides quintessential opportunities to gather in vivo data on the adaptive repertoire of a child. A 4-year-old child's newly acquired aggressive streak at the day care center may make much more sense to a provider when directly witnessed. Watching a young girl try out for her middle school basketball team provides perspective on her abilities to reign in oppositional behavior at home or in the classroom. Walking to the corner grocery store to purchase an ice cream cone with a young child who has autistic spectrum problems may yield valuable data on the child's ability to negotiate normative (although not necessarily simple) social challenges. For a 10-year-old child who struggles with obsessionality and perfectionism, there may be no better moment to observe day-to-day life than when the child is at bat in a baseball game for his little league team.

Ethnography and sharing attributions can be conducted in an office armchair and while walking the clinic grounds. A provider may not need to literally be in the field of influences with children to tap into children's observations of themselves in their realms. Knowing which video games are played by a boy with conduct dysregulation, what songs a teen with juvenile diabetes and depressive struggles has on his *ipod,* or which internet sites a girl with anorexia visits can be critically informative for conceptualizing the youth's risk grid.

The clinician's alliance with the child's family is essential to the process of knowing which community realms are relevant to a particular child's sense of struggle or well-being. The complexity of setting agendas and gathering informed consent for gaining knowledge and access to a child's world is of no small concern. The more a young person feels that he or she is helping to prescribe the treatment agenda and consenting to the process of inquiry (and feels like a clinical co-investigator), the more likely he or she is to welcome the clinician's direct involvement in these regions. If a child grants us access, we must be ready with open ears to hear the attributions regarding the meaning of that region.

Ethnographic methods are at work in several of the innovative therapeutic approaches developed over the last decade. Some treatments are tailormade for making sense of child and adolescent community risk management skills. Motivational interviewing is based on facilitating the therapist's role as vicarious witness to the risks and in vivo challenges a patient faces [51,52]. Adventure-based therapy, used in many school and hospital programs and popularized in the last several decades in such community programs as Outward Bound, Project Adventure, and NOLS (National Outdoor Leadership School), helps teens to build self-awareness and team mindedness through participation in mentored group risk-taking activities [53–55]. Facilitation of self-awareness in the process of managing interpersonal and community risks is also a core focus of Dialectical Behavioral Therapy, widely regarded as a paradigm-shifting breakthrough in helping young people manage intense emotional struggles and high-risk behaviors [56,57]. These therapies, like the walk for ice cream or the discussion of the rodeo, provide vital glimpses into how a child adapts and help to identify child-specific levers for change and opportunities for intervention.

## Ethnocultural and spiritual-religious and historical dimensions

> *Clinician*: "What a pretty name you have. Does it have a special story?"
> *Patient*: "In my language, my name Unathi means 'from the hands of Jesus'."

Unathi, a 12-year-old immigrant child from South Africa, has been referred as a new patient to the clinic by her middle school counselor, who has concerns about her low mood and lack of engagement in school. Often when we ask a child her name and how she received it, a story emerges that unveils meaningful cultural and religious facets of the child's family life and family story.

In our third destination zone we consider the determinants and clinical presentation of a child as influenced by the family's ethnocultural and religious affiliations and the broad family stories that shape these influences. In our previous two destination zones, health systems and child activity, we visited specific geographic locations, schools, and other institutions, neighborhoods, and soccer fields within which we could conduct our clinical ethnographic data gathering and use our ecologic and attributional lenses. The third zone of culture, ethnicity and spirituality, is comprised of uniquely mapped pathways and indistinct boundaries. Culture, ethnicity, and religion are woven as tightly into the soul and identity of the child as is his or her name. Sentinel works of Erik Erikson and Robert Coles are richly descriptive oases for contemplating the developmental and existential facets of these parameters in the life of a child [58,59].

Many clinicians may not be aware that the American Psychiatric Association's "Diagnostic and Statistical Manual of Psychiatric Diagnoses" (DSM-IV) Appendix 1 invites clinicians to craft a narrative summary for categories of cultural identity including cultural explanations of the individual's illness, cultural factors related to the psychosocial environment and levels of functioning, and cultural elements of the relationship between the individual and the clinician [47]. Harper worries that the dominant role of DSM-IV as a "culture-*blind* classificatory system" [our emphasis] overshadows the rather limited DSM acknowledgment of cultural factors in psychiatric diagnoses [60].

There are risks that cultural and religious variables may be clinical afterthoughts, except perhaps in exotic clinical situations. We encourage the reader to perhaps consider that every patient brings to the clinical setting a narrative with deep ethnocultural and religious/spiritual roots. Consider the following possible roster of appointments that one might have in the course of a clinic week in many parts of America:

- a biracial 8-year-old girl with learning problems who is living with her biologic parents
- a deaf child of hearing parents or, conversely, a hearing child with deaf parents
- a boy with an Islamic stepfather and Pentecostal grandmother
- a Korean adoptee being raised in an Anglo home
- a farm girl whose family has recently moved to the city
- a boy who is a gang leader by day and a church choir member at night
- a first-generation American-born daughter of Southeast Asian refugee parents
- a girl who is class clown in second period language arts and first chair trumpet player in fifth period band (here each class can be construed as having its own culture)

Each situation calls for taking stock of the micro and macrocultural forces in the lives of these children and their families.

At the macrosystem level, America is metaphorically referred to as a "melting pot" society. Forces that guide a coalescence and homogenization of youth experiences and identities may be at work. The "melting pot" forces are also said to influence healing practices, attributions, and perspectives on child growth and development. Batts and colleagues have proposed replacing the metallurgical metaphor with a culinary one to describe the American experience [61,62]. They maintain that the values and guidelines shaping the development of youth are not "melted" into one uniform code. Instead, a "salad bowl" may better portray how they are all living in a pluralistic multicultural, nonreducible mix of values and identity experiences. Children, particularly adolescents, experience discretely different cultural identities in the daily bowl of their broadly defined community. Our clinical task is to earn access to the child and family's sharing of the discrete and interwoven identities and cultures and the transgenerational stories within which they and their kinship group define themselves.

Spradley [7] defines culture as "acquired knowledge that people use to interpret experience and generate social behavior." One facet of culture is ethnicity, which may be thought of as a group identification, a belonging to a "people" who, when viewed from within or outside the group, are regarded as sharing elements of such community dimensions as history, language, art, and values. Cultural, ethnic, racial, spiritual, religious, and historical facets, which shape and mold a child's identity, may each add different overtones to clinical relationships. These overtones are in turn shaped by such macrosystem variables as majority/minority status, recent and past political developments, renown or notoriety of specific group members, and economic shifts within the larger community. Also to be considered are a family's transgenerational experiences of such political forces as concepts of child rights in the family's cultures of origin, gender socialization, religious and ethnic persecution, and racial oppression. We should listen in for the possible family experiences of such international legacies as the Holocaust, sectarian genocide in Southeast Asia and Africa, and such American institutional legacies as slavery and segregation, in the twentieth century, of such social violations as the Tuskegee experiments, Stonewall, and the policy of sending American Indian children to boarding schools. These cultural and historical practices and events may not be far from the mind of the child and family in the room and likely will influence how they regard medical institutions and professionals. For in-depth perspectives on the rich complexity of these variables, the reader is referred to Canino and Spurlock [63] and McGoldrick and colleagues [64].

In our earlier case dialogue, the young girl, Unathi, hints at an essential role for Christianity in her life story. Religion and spiritual beliefs and practice are aspects of our patients' cultural lives that strongly affect their health-related attitudes and behaviors. For many adults and children, religious beliefs and practices may strongly influence their concepts of etiology and attributions regarding their current emotional distress. Most families credit spiritual or religious practices as resources for addressing distress [65]. In a recent survey, 60% of individuals reported using "prayer specifically for health reasons" [66]. Dell and Josephson [67] outline four approaches that may be helpful for clinicians to consider when addressing a child's and family's spiritual and religious perspectives. The clinician may

1. simply acknowledge that religious and spiritual factors can have a role in a child's problems
2. help a family to clarify religious and spiritual concerns and consider a referral to a therapist who can help provide a professional religious counseling focus

3. enjoin the family and child in an inquiry related to "philosophy of life" and "worldview" perspectives
4. in some situations directly help the child and family with their religious and spiritual concerns

Puchalski and Romer [68] proposed the mnemonic FICA, which frames a set of questions with which to address the family's spiritual and religious life as it relates to emotional health:

Faith and belief: Do you consider yourself spiritual or religious? Do you have spiritual beliefs that help you cope with stress? What gives your life meaning?

Importance: What importance does your faith or belief have in your life? Have your beliefs influenced how you take care of yourself (or your child) in this illness? What role do your religious beliefs play in regaining your health?

Community: Are you part of a spiritual or religious community? Does the community support you and, if so, how? Is there a group of people you really love or who are important to you?

Address in care: How would you like me, your health care provider, to address these issues in your health care?

A child's readiness for exploring the role of his or her personal spiritual and religious frameworks certainly depends on the child's developmental level and on the child and family's willingness to share such personal dimensions of life. A clinician's readiness to proceed is likewise related in part to his or her own personal religious and spiritual framework in life.

Returning to the issue of the ethnic identities and affiliations of our patients, a clinician wonders how and how well a child adapts across the divergent ethnic and spiritual/religious self-identifications he or she encounters in the course of a day or week. What are the risks to the child's mental health of overidentification with one of the cultures and underidentification with another? How do we define successful adaptation? Research suggests that although the prevalence of problem behaviors may be somewhat similar across cultures, the explanations for child behavior problems in families from minority racial and ethnic groups can be expected to be intriguingly varied if not discordant with "dominant culture" attributions [69]. A young person may be seen, by one observer, as acting in concert with certain cultural-familial values and life-path expectations while being regarded by another observer as odd, eccentric, deviant, or delinquent [70]. Whose judgment is most critical to a teen's path: family, community elders, teachers, or peers? In their own time and place, both may play essential roles in the guidance that shapes a young person's successful passage into adulthood. Pumariega and Cross [71] aptly describe the risks of marginalization, overidentification, identity diffusion, and negative identity formation for youth striving to cross back and forth between cultures. They also acknowledge the unique strengths and skills to be won by the young person's efforts to fit in cross culturally. "Youths who are biculturally competent demonstrate greater flexibility in roles and cognitive styles as well as adaptability to use cultural norms appropriate for a given context or situation." The culturally competent, ecologically informed, and ethnographically oriented clinician is better adapted to serve in multiple roles as broker, translator, coach, and risk management specialist as a child and family strive to decode the distinct rules and meanings found in a specific cultural zone.

Cultural variables also can have profound influences on how an individual or family believes treatment relationships should be conducted [72]. For various reasons, families may be reluctant to share their culturally mediated and intimately meaningful life-guiding perspectives with their physician. Trust must be built before they can be shared. Helping a child and family build and share their agenda and become comfortable in the health care relationship can be influenced by a host of micro-, meso-, and macrosystem factors. On the macrosystem level, since the publication of the 1989 Child and Adolescent Service System Program (CASSP) report "Towards a Culturally Competent System of Care" [73,74], many institutions and training programs have adopted new standards for health care service delivery in an effort to improve the experience for the diversity of peoples served. The CASSP report has served as a guidepost for defining an ascending level of skill and sensitivity for providing health care across cultural boundaries from cultural destructiveness and blindness to token services, to openness, innovativeness, and shared clinical missions. Cultural competence is the expectation for health care institutions and providers. The reader is referred to Kim's pertinent description of model training guidelines for cultural competence in child and adolescent psychiatric residencies [75]. His educational objectives for developing cultural competencies in child and adolescent psychiatry residency training serve as a springboard for teaching ecologic perspectives.

On the microsystem, indeed the microcultural level, we can expect each family to have its own unique sensibilities for the building of trust in a clinical relationship. Tervalon and Murray-Garcia [76] proposed a construct they term "cultural humility" that defines a heightened level of provider dedication, one family at a time, to principles of cultural sensitivity. "Cultural humility...incorporates a life-long commitment to self-evaluation and self-critique." When practicing cultural humility, the clinician strives to be mindful of power dynamics in the clinician/patient relationship, historical legacies, and political realities. Clinicians are encouraged to reflect on how their own personal cultural roots may weave through their attitudes toward cultural variables (eg, race, class, and religion) encountered in care relationships.

For the 12-year-old immigrant child and perhaps every child we are asked to help, the ethnocultural and religious considerations figure in not as appendices to our assessments and treatments plans but instead as vital, germane, and complementary influences on our clinical understandings and the roles we serve. If we engender the enthusiasm of the child and family (and the complementary providers they deem appropriate) to help us to appreciate the historical and cultural forces, unique strengths, challenges, and hopes that can shape their pathways to improved health, then we are rewarded with clinical insight. Just as we hope that our patients will appreciate our service in their lives as clinical healers, we also hope that each child and family will be comfortable to serve as mentors for us. The benefits of these lessons accumulate in the lives of clinicians and can be offered to the diversity of children and their diverse villages that lie ahead.

## Training tool

For building the clinical relationship we offer the following menu of questions which can be customized based on such factors as a child's development level, diagnostic status, and stage of treatment. This menu may guide clinicians in making ethnographic inquiries to gain information that is vital to the therapeutic process:

- *Assets and strengths*: What are you good at and what do you like to do? How do these activities help you? How are you (and your family) trying to help improve your health?
- *Worry zones*: What are your biggest worries? In what part of your life do they most show up? Which worries do you want me to help you with? What should I know about the worries of others in your family?
- *Identity*: Can you tell me about your cultural background and family customs? To what cultures and communities do you feel you belong? How do you see yourself in your family? In what settings and activities do you feel most comfortable? How do people see you in your world?
- *Attributions*: How do you explain your problems? How do others in your family and community explain your problems?
- *Provider*: How do you think I can help you? What special hopes or fears do you have related to your coming to my program here?
- *Consultants*: In addition to our work together, who else have you consulted with, such as family members, teachers, a minister, a naturopath, or a traditional/cultural healer? How do they see you, including your strengths and challenges? What concerns do you think they have about how you're doing? How do they understand, explain, and treat your difficulties? How have they been helpful to you?
- *Resources*: What other sources do you turn to for help, such as friends, coaches, church members, support groups, the library, or internet? What would they tell me about you? Have you been to any ceremonies to help you or your family? Would you like to share any articles, websites, or questions about the effectiveness of their recommendations?

- *Whom should I contact*: Would you like me to contact any of your other consultants? What information would you like me to share or obtain?
- *How can I help*: How would you like me and the treatment strategies I offer to fit in to your current treatment? How might I help you assess the benefits and risks of the various treatment strategies?

Appendices 1 and 2 are provided as guidelines for training programs to augment core educational objectives that pertain to ecologic perspectives in child and adolescent psychiatry.

## Summary

This article has presented the following tenets:

- Each child grows and develops within a complex matrix of ecological forces.
- Ethnographic methods, exploration of attributional grids, and zone visitation facilitate understanding of the child's ecology.
- The child's emotional health affects the skill and ease with which the child embraces his or her world. How children are situated in and encounter their ecologic zones affects their abilities to deal with emotional distress and influences the ways that distress is manifested.
- Understanding how a child navigates and adapts to his or her ecology can enable clinicians to develop more useful customized case formulations and treatment strategies.
- Enthusiastic and humble engagement with child and family (and their extended support system) in their natural world can lead to more effective healing and enrichment of a clinician's practice of psychiatry.

With steady and deliberate effort, clinicians can gain cultural, zonal, and cross-systemic competence that will enable them to work more effectively with a splendid variety of children from a broad assortment of villages. Making ethnographic inquiry an integral part of daily practice enables child psychiatrists to guide children and families more optimistically and adaptively on their way. The mindful quest to become multiculturally competent and ecologically oriented fosters in clinicians a sense of enrichment, enthusiasm, and readiness for intrigues to follow with the next child that comes through the door.

## Acknowledgments

The authors wish to gratefully acknowledge the editorial assistance of Rebecca Allen, PhD, ARNP, and Susan Storck, MD.

## Appendix 1

Educational objectives for developing cultural competencies in child and adolescent psychiatry residency training are as follows:

- Knowledge: The resident should be able to demonstrate an adequate understanding of the following topics:

  The cultural diversity of the children and adolescents in the United States depending on country of origin, language, religion, socioeconomic status, and other cultural factors.

  Ethnic characteristics of family structure, family values, intergenerational relationships, gender roles, and extended families.

  Ethnocultural characteristics of child rearing practices and expectations and psychosocial, academic, and other developmental tasks.

  Development of ethnic identity: bicultural identity.

  Stressors, such as premigration, migration, and postmigration stressors, often accompanying recent immigrants or refugees, as do poverty and racial stereotyping.

  Characteristics of acculturation, ethnic community, and resources for different ethnic groups.

  Ethnic attitudes toward mental health problems include identification and interpretation of symptoms and help-seeking behavior.

  Diagnosis of validity and reliability of psychiatric diagnostic systems, such as DSM-IV, for ethnic minority children and adolescents.

  Treatment considerations, such as (1) pharmacologic differences between ethnic groups, (2) modification of psychotherapy, such as family therapy, according to cultural uniqueness, and (3) the role of traditional healers and healing methods for different ethnic groups.

  Cross-cultural variations of clinical course and outcomes.
- Skills: The resident should demonstrate competencies in the following areas:

  Interviewing children and families from different ethnic groups with openness and sensitivity to cultural differences and communication.

  Interviewing non–English-speaking children and families through the use of an interpreter in an optimal fashion.

  Diagnosing and assessing children with an understanding of possible cultural differences in psychopathology.

  Providing clinical information to children and families in language understandable to them while recognizing intergenerational language and cultural gaps between them.

  Formulating treatment plans that are culturally sensitive to a child and parents' concept of mental illness.

  Providing psychotherapeutic and psychopharmacologic interventions with an understanding of possible cultural differences in treatment expectations.

- Attitudes: Residents should demonstrate in their behavior and demeanor with the following characteristics:
  Sensitivity to existing cultural, ethnic, and racial stereotypes and willingness to learn how to counteract them in their contacts with patients.
  Sensitivity to their own attitudes toward minority children and families, including countertransference and transference issues as they affect the doctor-patient relationship.
  Compassion and respect for the minority child and parents and concern about their special problems.

*From* Kim WJ. A training guideline of cultural competence for child and adolescent psychiatry psychiatric residencies. Child Psychiatr Hum D 1995;26(2):125–36; with permission.

## Appendix 2

*Fostering ecologic perspectives in child psychiatry*

*Knowledge skills attitudes for child psychiatry training programs*

From the broader ecologic perspectives of this article, we offer this summary of additional educational objectives to complement Kim's foundation of objectives addressing cultural competence for child and adolescent psychiatric residencies:

- Knowledge: The child and adolescent psychiatry resident should be able to demonstrate adequate understanding of the following topics and concepts:
  Micro- to macrosystem ecologic influences in the clinical phenomena presented by patients and families
  Use of ethnographic methods for data gathering observation in the clinical challenges
  Dialectical roles for patient and provider attributional and explanatory constructs
  Roles and influences of community systems of care and child activity zones in the development of broad-based formulations and treatment planning for children
  The nature of ethnocultural and religious and spiritual dimensions (including ceremonies) at work in the lives of patients and their families
  Methods for discerning historical and transgenerational influences on a community
  The role of complementary and alternative health care practices in the lives of patients and families

Methods for approaching each family with open curiosity and humility with the goal of actively bringing children and families into the co-investigator role in their health care

Methods for maintaining provider resilience and enthusiasm to be ready for the complexities of the next child

- Skills: The child and adolescent psychiatry resident should be able to demonstrate clinical competencies in the following areas:

Connecting with children in a way that fosters a comfortable eagerness for safe collaboration and shared adventure in the clinical mission

Developing communication and networking skills for building alliances with all children and families and their community resources

Conducting diagnostic interviews that facilitate ethnographic access to diverse realms of clinical data, including family legacies

Constructing grids, with families, across time and space that help show historic and current nodal points of community influences (including complementary healing practices)

Integrating each child and family's unique illness explanations into a broad-based formulation grounded in ecologic perspectives

Building communication strategies, based on cultural humility, customized to the language, ethnocultural, community variables, and religious affiliations of the child and family

Being able to step back from one's biases, if necessary, to facilitate the awareness of otherwise hidden, tacit, or guardedly offered perspectives from patients, families, and other informants

Participating in team meetings in schools, corrections facilities, foster homes, day care centers

Observing children in community settings in a fashion that is comfortable for provider, family, and community

- Attitudes: The child and adolescent psychiatry resident should be able to demonstrate the following attitudes in their manner and mindset:

Readiness for having a fresh set of eyes and ears for the unique story and village of influences that each child brings to the clinic and the nuances that emerge each day

Sensitivity to one's own family background, training story, and clinical knowledge base and how it is brought to clinical encounters

Openness to self-mentoring and mentoring by senior colleagues to maintain the capacity for curiosity and humility

Openness to children and families serving as teachers regarding the skills needed for negotiating the village challenges and the customized teamwork that each clinical mission requires

Readiness to look for clinical perspectives in such disparate zones as the internet, a baseball field, a day care lunch, a home visit, in service of one's mission with a child and family

# References

[1] Engel GL. The need for a new medical model: a challenge for biomedicine. Science 1970;196: 129–39.

[2] Wilkinson CB, O'Connor WA. Human ecology and mental illness. Am J Psychiatry 1982; 139(8):985–90.

[3] Encyclopædia Britannica Online. Available at: http://www.search.eb.com.offcampus.lib. washington.edu/eb/article-9110583. Accessed July 1, 2006.

[4] Bronfenbrenner U, editor. Making human beings human: bioecological perspectives on human development. Thousand Oaks (CA): Sage Publications; 2005. p. 6.

[5] Stormshak EA, Dishion TJ. An ecological approach to child and family clinical and counseling psychology. Clin Child Fam Psychol Rev 2002;5(3):197–215.

[6] Henggeler SW, Schoenwald SK, Borduin CM, et al. Multisystemic treatment of antisocial behavior in children and adolescents. New York: Guilford Press; 1998.

[7] Spradley J. The ethnographic interview. New York: Holt, Rinehart & Winston; 1979.

[8] Kramer DA. The biology of family therapy. Child Adolesc Psychiatr Clin N Am 2001;10(3): 625–40.

[9] Shapiro T. The psychodynamic formulation in child and adolescent psychiatry. J Am Acad Child Adolesc Psychiatry 1989;28(5):675–80.

[10] O'Brien JD, Pilowsky D, Lewis OW, editors. Psychotherapies with children and adolescents: adapting the psychodynamic process. Washington, DC: American Psychiatric Press; 1992.

[11] Frank J, Frank J. Persuasion and healing: a comparative study of psychotherapy. Baltimore (MD): Johns Hopkins Press; 1991. p. 112.

[12] White M, Epston D. Narrative means to therapeutic ends. New York: Norton; 1990.

[13] The Dialogues of Plato, The Seventh Letter. Chicago: William Benton, Encyclopedia Britannica, Inc; 1952.

[14] Graham S, Folkes VS. Attribution theory: applications to achievement, mental health, and interpersonal conflict. Hillsdale (NJ): Lawrence Erlbaum Associates; 1990.

[15] Kleinman A. The cultural meanings and social uses of illness: a role for medical anthropology and clinically oriented social science in the development of primary care theory and research. J Fam Pract 1983;16(3):539–45.

[16] Kleinman A. Patients and healers in the context of culture: an exploration of the borderland between anthropology, medicine and psychiatry. Berkeley (CA): University of California Press; 1980.

[17] Kleinman A, Eisenberg L, Good B. Culture, illness, and care: clinical lessons from anthropologic and cross-cultural research. Ann Intern Med 1978;88(2):251–8.

[18] Participants in the Bayer-Fetzer Conference on Physician-Patient Communication in Medical Education. Essential elements of communication in medical encounters: the Kalamazoo consensus statement. Acad Med 2001;76:390–3.

[19] Epstein RM. Mindful practice. JAMA 1999;282(9):833–9.

[20] Lamott A. Bird by bird: some instructions on writing and life. New York: Anchor; 1994.

[21] Whittaker JK. The re-invention of residential treatment: an agenda for research and practice. Child Adolesc Psychiatr Clin N Am 2004;13(2):267–78.

[22] Epstein RA Jr. Inpatient and residential treatment effects for children and adolescents: a review and critique. Child Adolesc Psychiatr Clin N Am 2004;13(2):411–28.

[23] Moos RH. Situational analysis of a therapeutic community milieu. J Abnorm Psychol 1968; 73(1):49–61.

[24] Timko C, Moos RH. Outcomes of the treatment climate in psychiatric and substance abuse programs. J Clin Psychol 1998;54(8):1137–50.

[25] Fadiman A. The spirit catches you and you fall down: a Hmong child, her American doctors, and the collision of two cultures. New York: Noonday Press; 1997.

[26] Ottolini MC, Hamburger EK, Loprieato JO, et al. Complementary and alternative medicine use among children in the Washington, DC area. Ambul Pediatr 2001;1:122–5.

[27] Chan E. The role of complementary and alternative medicine in attention-deficit hyperactivity disorder. J Dev Behav Pediatr 2002;23:S37–45.
[28] Bussing R, Zima BT, Gary FA, et al. Use of complementary and alternative medicine for symptoms of attention-deficit hyperactivity disorder. Psychiatr Serv 2002;53:1096–102.
[29] Gralow JR. Combining complementary and conventional therapies in medical practice: a medical oncologist's perspective. Northwest Physician 1996;7–11.
[30] Shannon S, editor. Handbook of complementary and alternative therapies in mental health. San Diego (CA): Academic Press; 2002.
[31] Perez A, O'Niel K, Geserich S. Demographics of children in foster care. Pew Commission on Children in Foster Care; Georgetown University, Washington, DC: 2003.
[32] Clausen JM, Landsverk J, Ganger W, et al. Mental health problems of children in foster care. J Child Fam Stud 1998;7(3):283–96.
[33] Chapman MV, Wall A, Barth RP. Children's voices: the perceptions of children in foster care. Am J Orthopsychiatry 2004;74(3):293–304.
[34] Kutash K, Rivera VR. What works in children's mental health services? Uncovering answers to critical questions. Baltimore (MD): Brookes; 1996.
[35] Evans ME, Armstrong MI, Dollard N, et al. Development and evaluation of treatment foster care and family-centered intensive case management in New York. Journal of Emotional and Behavioral Disorders 1994;2:228–39.
[36] Evans ME, Armstrong MI, Kuppinger AD, et al. Preliminary outcomes of an experimental study comparing treatment foster care and family-centered intensive case management. In: Epstein MH, Kutash K, Duchnowski A, editors. Outcomes for children and youth with behavioral and emotional disorders and their families. Austin (TX): Pro-Ed; 1998. p. 543–80.
[37] Chamberlain P, Reid JB. Using a specialized foster care treatment model for children and adolescents leaving the state hospital. J Community Psychol 1998;19:266–76.
[38] Vander Stoep A, Evens CC, Taub J. Risk of juvenile justice systems referral among children in a public mental health system. J Ment Health Adm 1997;24(4):428–42.
[39] Teplin LA, Abram KM, McClelland GM, et al. Psychiatric disorders in youth in juvenile detention. Arch Gen Psychiatry 2002;59:1133–43.
[40] Borduin CM, Henggeler SW, Blaske DM, et al. Multisystemic treatment of adolescent sexual offenders. Int J Offender Ther Comp Criminol 1990;35:105–14.
[41] Henggeler SW, Melton GB, Smith LA. Family preservation using multisystemic therapy: an effective alternative to incarcerating serious juvenile offenders. J Consult Clin Psychol 1992; 60:953–61.
[42] Borduin CM, Mann BJ, Cone LT, et al. Multisystemic treatment of serious juvenile offenders: long-term prevention of criminology and violence. J Consult Clin Psychol 1995;63:569–78.
[43] Nichols M, Schwartz R. The fundamental concepts of family therapy. In: Family therapy: concepts and methods. 5th edition. Boston: Allyn and Bacon; 2001. p. 103–36.
[44] Rothbaum F, Rosen K, Ujiie T, Uchida N. Family systems theory, attachment theory, and culture. Fam Process 2002;41(3):328–50.
[45] Waters E, Cummings EM. A secure base from which to explore close relationships. Child Dev 2000;71(1):164–72.
[46] McGoldrick M, Carter E. The family life cycle. In: Walsh F, editor. Normal family processes. New York: Guilford; 1983. p. 167–95.
[47] American Psychiatric Association. Diagnostic and statistical manual of mental disorders: DSM-IV. Washington, DC: American Psychiatric Association; 1994.
[48] Shaffer D, Gould MS, Brasic J, et al. A children's global assessment scale (CGAS). Arch Gen Psychiatry 1983;40(11):1228–31.
[49] Nabhan GP, Trimble S. The geography of childhood: why children need wild places. Boston: Beacon Press; 1994. p. xiii.
[50] Canada G. Fist stick knife gun (excerpted). The Sun. August 1996: 10–14.

[51] Miller WR, Rollnick S. Motivational interviewing: preparing people to change addictive behavior. New York: Guilford; 1991.

[52] Sindelar HA, Abrantes AM, Hart C, et al. Motivational interviewing in pediatric practice. Curr Probl Pediatr Adolesc Health Care 2004;34(9):322–39.

[53] Gass M. Adventure therapy: therapeutic applications of adventure programming. Dubuque (IA): Kendall/Hunt Publishing Company; 1993.

[54] Moote GT Jr, Wodarski JS. The acquisition of life skills through adventure-based activities and programs: a review of the literature. Adolescence 1997;32(125):143–67.

[55] Jelalian E, Mehlenbeck R, Lloyd-Richardson EE, et al. Adventure therapy combined with cognitive-behavioral treatment for overweight adolescents. Int J Obes (Lond) 2006;30(1): 31–9.

[56] Linehan M. Cognitive-behavioral treatment of borderline personality disorder. New York: Guilford Press; 1993.

[57] Katz LY, Cox BJ, Gunasekara S, et al. Feasibility of dialectical behavior therapy for suicidal adolescent inpatients. J Am Acad Child Adolesc Psychiatry 2004;43(3):276–82.

[58] Erikson EH. Childhood and society. 2$^{nd}$ edition. New York: Norton; 1963.

[59] Coles R. The spiritual life of children. Boston: Houghton Mifflin; 1990.

[60] Harper G. Cultural influences on diagnosis. Child Adolesc Psychiatr Clin N Am 2001;10(4): 711–28.

[61] Batts VA. Keynote address. Presented at the Annual Meeting of the National Association of School-based Health Centers. Portland, OR, June 15, 2006.

[62] Batts VA. An experiential workshop: introduction to multiculturalism. In: Stricker G, Davis-Russell E, Bourg E, et al, editors. Toward ethnic diversification in psychology education and training. Washington, DC: American Psychological Association; 1990:9–16.

[63] Canino IA, Spurlock J. Culturally diverse children and adolescents: assessment, diagnosis, and treatment. New York: Guilford Press; 2000.

[64] McGoldrick M, Giordano J, Giordano J, et al, eds. Ethnicity and family therapy. New York: Guilford Press; 2005.

[65] Josephson AM, Dell ML. Religion and spirituality in child and adolescent psychiatry: a new frontier. Child Adolesc Psychiatr Clin N Am 2004;13(1):1–15.

[66] Barnes PM, Powell-Griner E, McFann K, et al. Complementary and alternative medicine use among adults: United States, 2002. Adv Data 2004;343:1–19.

[67] Dell ML, Josephson AM. Working with spiritual issues of children. Psychiatr Ann 2006; 36(3):176–81.

[68] Puchalski CM, Romer AL. Taking a spiritual history allows clinicians to understand patients more fully. J Palliat Med 2000;3:129–37.

[69] Mohler B. Cross-cultural issues in research on child mental health. Child Adolesc Psychiatr Clin N Am 2001;10(4):763–76.

[70] Fisher PA, Storck M, Bacon JG. In the eye of the beholder: risk and protective factors in rural American Indians and Caucasian adolescents. Am J Orthopsychiatry 1999;69(3): 294–304.

[71] Pumariega AJ, Cross TL. Cultural competence in child psychiatry. In: Noshpitz JD, Greenspan S, Wieder S, et al, editors. Handbook of child and adolescent psychiatry. New York: Wiley; 1997. p. 473–84.

[72] Schwab-Stone M, Ruchkin V, Vermerien R, et al. Cultural considerations in the treatment of children and adolescents. Child Adolesc Psychiatr Clin N Am 2001;10(4): 729–43.

[73] Cross TL, Bazron BL, Dennis KW, et al. Towards a culturally competent system of care. In: Child and adolescent service system program (CASSP) report. Washington, DC: Georgetown University Child Development Center, CASSP Technical Assistance Center; 1989.

[74] Stroul BA, Friedman RM. A system of care for children and youth with severe emotional disturbances, revised edition. Washington, DC: Georgetown University Child Development Center, CASSP Technical Assistance Center; 1986.

[75] Kim WJ. A training guideline of cultural competence for child and adolescent psychiatric residencies. Child Psychiatry Hum Dev 1995;26(2):125–36.
[76] Tervalon M, Murray-Garcia J. Cultural humility versus cultural competence: a critical distinction in defining physician training outcomes in multicultural education. J Health Care Poor Undeserved 1998;9(2):117–25.

ELSEVIER
SAUNDERS

Child Adolesc Psychiatric Clin N Am
16 (2007) 165–181

CHILD AND
ADOLESCENT
PSYCHIATRIC CLINICS
OF NORTH AMERICA

# Teaching Evidence-Based Medicine Pediatric Psychopharmacology: Integrating Psychopharmacologic Treatment into the Broad Spectrum of Care

Allan K. Chrisman, MD*, Harry T. Enderlin, MD,
Kerry Lee Landry, MD, Jennifer S. Colvin, MD,
Matthew R. DeJohn, MD

*Department of Psychiatry and Behavioral Sciences,
Duke University Medical Center, Duke Child & Family Study Center,
718 Rutherford Street, Durham, NC 27705, USA*

Pediatric psychopharmacology is taught at the Duke University Hospital Child and Adolescent Psychiatry (DUHCAP) Residency Training Program within the context of an evidence-based medicine (EBM) model. Psychopharmacology is embedded within a series of seminars, one of which has the primary emphasis of a systematic review of psychotropic medications. The basic goal of the course is to develop competence in the psychopharmacologic management of psychiatric problems of children and adolescents as part of a biopsychosocial/developmental model of care. Associated with this overarching goal the following attitudes, knowledge, and skills are required for the demonstration of competence in the practice of evidence-based pediatric psychopharmacology. A) Attitudes, which are intended to (1) develop confidence in using psychotropic medications flexibly within a hierarchy of evidence to accommodate the needs of patients with concurrent psychiatric

Financial disclosure: Allan K. Chrisman, MD, receives funding from: Speaker Bureaus of Shire US, Inc.; Novartis; McNeil and Research Funding: Shire US, Inc.; Novartis; Lilly; McNeil and Pfizer.

* Corresponding author. Duke Child and Family Study Center, 718 Rutherford Street, Durham, NC 27705.

*E-mail address:* chris014@mc.duke.edu (A.K. Chrisman).

illnesses, (2) demonstrate an analytic and investigatory approach to clinical situations (ie, independent pursuit of knowledge as indicated by literature searches, other investigative work, and research), (3) indicate willingness to obtain information from electronic data bases and scientific literature with recognition that the scientific literature must be integrated in an evolutionary manner (ie, no one study or theory is likely to address all clinical situations), (5) show respect for the complexity of any patient's presentation-interacting factors that influence the presentation, treatment, and response to pharmacotherapy, (6) show respect for other members of the mental health delivery team, and (7) indicate awareness of the limits of knowledge, both individual and collective, which recognizes how gaps may be filled by education or research. B) Knowledge, which is intended to (1) understand indications for psychotropic medications in child and adolescent psychiatric disorders and their basic pharmacokinetic and pharmacodynamic features at each developmental phase, (2) understand target symptoms and associated impairments of psychiatric disorders that are amenable to psychopharmacologic interventions, (3) know the common phases of psychopharmacotherapy (acute, maintenance, and monitoring), (4) know the safety issues for psychotropic medications, (5) know factors attributable to the rates of adherence to pediatric psychopharmacologic treatments, (6) know the role of pediatric psychopharmacology in community agencies and local mental health delivery systems and organizations, and (7) know the collaborative role of a child psychiatrist in providing psychopharmacotherapy with other child mental health disciplines. C) Skills, which are meant to (1) provide comprehensive psychopharmacologic consultation, (2) provide formulation of an understanding of psychiatric disorders amenable to psychopharmacologic treatment, including biologic, social/cultural, educational, and psychological factors, (3) show formulation of an appropriate, evidence-based psychopharmacologic treatment plan, which considers available resources, risk/benefit ratios of treatments offered, and likely outcomes of treatments delivered, (4) provide the delivery of a range of pharmacologic treatments alone or in combination with psychosocial therapies to patients of different gender, culture, and ethnicity, in a range of settings and clinical urgency, (5) understand the formation of successful working relationships with other members of the outpatient multidisciplinary team, (6) indicate the articulation of research issues that are relevant to psychopharmacologic treatments, and (7) assess personal knowledge using a systematic methodology.

Decades from now, the reasons that children and adolescents present to psychiatrists will not have changed significantly [1]. The art of engaging patients and motivating them to change will remain the same. Advances in neuroscience and genetics [1], an expanded evidence base for psychosocial and pharmacologic treatments, and novel targets for pharmaceuticals will alter how psychiatrists evaluate and treat patients [2]. Training a workforce of child and adolescent psychiatrists to keep pace with and implement these changes presents significant challenges. At DUHCAP we are trying to develop a curriculum to meet these challenges.

A critical aspect of this curriculum is integrating EBM into all aspects of patient assessment and treatment. Teaching psychopharmacology from an EBM perspective requires the essential EBM skills, which include developing appropriate clinical questions, searching the literature, and critically appraising studies. Equally important is integrating EBM psychopharmacology into real-time care of patients and being able to apply the best available clinical evidence when the perfect study has not been done [3,4]. We begin each EBM conference with a focused patient-centered clinical question and end each conference with a discussion of how the evidence would direct care of the patient to ensure that trainees practice each of these skills. Trainees are prepared for real world evidenced-based practice, which begins and ends with an individual patient [3]. A common criticism of EBM, particularly in child psychiatry, is that there is not enough evidence in some areas to use EBM. Developing an EBM approach teaches one to think critically about each case, to update continually one's knowledge base, and to identify clinical questions that need further investigation. Active input from clinicians is needed to ensure that the most relevant clinical issues and populations will be studied.

There is legitimate concern about the influence of drug companies on practicing clinicians. This influence is of particular concern in child and adolescent psychiatry, in which most prescribing is off label, without US Food and Drug Administration approval. This particular situation is a product of the limited number of scientific studies of psychotropic medications in children and adolescents [5]. Child and adolescent psychiatrists are left to extrapolate findings from adult studies of these medications. Although the recent developmental epidemiologic studies have demonstrated that the psychiatric disorders originally identified in adults are also present in youth with continuity to adulthood [6], the developmental psychological and physiologic differences require distinct studies to determine the efficacy and effectiveness of the medications used in adults. Daily use of critical evaluation skills will better prepare trainees to objectively analyze pharmaceutical representatives' materials [7] and biases in pharmaceutical trials [8]. An EBM outlook is increasingly important because patients are making requests based on direct advertising. To incorporate the latest scientific information at the point of a clinical encounter, ready electronic access to literature searches and journals are needed to use EBM skills. Role modeling by clinical faculty is also essential for the reinforcement of the use of EBM in daily practice.

Fellows come to child psychiatry training with different backgrounds and aspirations. DUHCAP is working to offer nontraditional tracks through child psychiatry training to address the shortage of child psychiatrist clinicians and researchers. Some flexibility in choosing clinical and research electives in our program allows trainees to gain more experience in areas of relative weakness and pursue specialized training suited to their career aspirations. Adult learning theory tells us that trainees will assimilate more fully and retain knowledge that is directly relevant to their life goals. The EBM model for teaching psychopharmacology is readily suited simultaneously to accommodate different levels of knowledge. Similarly, associating teaching of psychopharmacology with clinical case conference modules motivates adult learners because they can see directly how the pharmacology knowledge is applicable to patient care [3]. Some flexibility in the choice of clinical modules further allows the addition of specialized sessions to address current trainees' particular interests and current topics in psychopharmacology (eg, monitoring for cardiovascular risks and critically assessing the increase in atypical antipsychotic prescriptions for children).

The critical thinking skills and habits fostered by EBM are essential to life-long learning [9]. In this approach to patient care, the patient encounter stimulates acquisition of new knowledge [3]. In the adult learning theory model, fellows are motivated to acquire knowledge by the relevance of the knowledge to real-life tasks and they take responsibility for their learning [3]. Adult learning theory in medical education is reflected in problem-based learning [3]. Our curriculum includes case-based modules in which child residents work together to develop differential diagnoses and treatment plans. Problem-based learning conferences have been shown to correlate positively with in-training examination scores, whereas traditional didactics have shown no correlation [10].

Another key feature of the didactics and clinical care in the context of the Duke Child and Adolescent Psychiatry Residency is an emphasis on providing complete care, including evidenced-based psychosocial treatments. As studies continue to demonstrate efficacy of psychotherapy alone or in combination with drug treatment for child psychiatric disorders, standard of care requires integration of psychotherapeutic treatment strategies [2]. Trainees must be prepared to provide such treatment or collaborate closely with practitioners who provide these treatments [11]. A detailed knowledge of evidenced-based therapies is critical for child psychiatrists, who must be able to recommend a comprehensive treatment plan and determine when to augment ongoing drug or psychosocial treatment with another modality. Several aspects of the curriculum under development at Duke teach trainees to coordinate psychosocial and pharmacologic treatments. In case-based modules, treatment plans developed by fellows most often include psychosocial treatments. Expert clinicians who facilitate the modules are drawn from psychology and psychiatry faculty. Child psychiatry residents attend a didactic for the psychology interns on evidence-based psychotherapies. In this didactic, case conferences presented by child residents or psychology interns alternate with lectures. At New York University School of Medicine, adult psychiatry residents and psychology interns reported benefit from a shared case conference [12]. The combined didactic at Duke has been received positively by trainees and has fostered cross-referrals between the psychiatry and psychology clinics.

Graduate medical education has become competency based [13]. What to require in psychiatric training has been the subject of protracted debate. Even within the narrower field of child psychopharmacology, determining what to require of trainees is difficult because there is too much basic and clinical knowledge to cover in a 2-year fellowship. Ultimately, decisions about required competencies should be driven by experimental validation of benefit to patient care of particular educational programs [8]. Until evidence-based teaching becomes a practical reality, a useful proxy is to require trainees to develop the skills needed to practice psychopharmacology using the EBM paradigm. Such practice is informed by the standard of assessment and treatment required in studies validating the treatments. For example, wherever possible, treatment decisions should be driven by diagnoses informed by validated rating scales. Treatment response should be tracked with rating scales for psychiatric symptoms and side effects [2].

Alternative methods of teaching psychopharmacology have been proposed [14]. Increased retention has been associated with more active learning [14]. Trainees' knowledge of current psychopharmacology may be assessed by pretests and posttests associated with content modules and by PRITE scores. Given the rapid change in the field of psychopharmacology, however, an emphasis on the process of assimilating new knowledge rather than traditional lecture formats will prepare trainees to remain current as the field advances [14]. Rapid developments in neurobiology and clinical psychiatry make this an exciting time for the field of child psychiatry. The question of how to prepare trainees to provide the best possible care for patients is being addressed by many programs. In the following discussion we review the principles and pragmatics of the curriculum being developed at Duke.

### Learning modalities: basics of curriculum development

As with most educational experiences, development of curricula for teaching psychopharmacology is driven by various specific goals. Kern and colleagues [15] describe a systematic approach for developing a curriculum that can be applied to psychopharmacology curriculum for trainees. Steps in this process include problem identification and general needs assessment, needs assessment of target learners, determination of goals and measurable objectives, development of educational strategies or interventions, implementation, and evaluation and feedback. Ideally, this process would take place in a dynamic fashion, with input from all participants, from instructors to trainees to patients and patient families, consistently incorporated for further development of the curriculum. Although each unique program will have certain areas of interest and goals, all programs will have some core goals and objectives that are driven by supervising and certifying agencies, such as Accreditation Council of Graduate Medical

Education and Accreditation Board of Psychiatry and Neurology. Some of these areas are discussed in later sections and are important to keep in mind during curriculum development. Most programs likely would agree that one overarching goal for their child and adolescent psychiatry trainees is to develop a skill set that will enable them to continue on the path of lifelong learning that will best allow them to provide optimal patient care throughout their careers in our rapidly changing and evolving field.

Once these goals have been established, the next step in development is to determine specific measurable objectives that can be used to drive the creation of educational methods and allow for the assessment of progress toward the achievement of the established goals. As for educational methods and interventions, a wide variety of modalities are available and each has different strengths and weaknesses [8]. Ideally, a curriculum for teaching psychopharmacology would incorporate several different types of educational methods. Use of various methods can allow for better accommodation of different learning styles, maintenance of learner interest, and possible reinforcement opportunities that could deepen learning, improve knowledge retention, and improve application of knowledge. We describe in this article specific examples of how our training program has structured a curriculum for psychopharmacology. Other examples from various programs across the country can be found in works by Zisook and colleagues [14] and Georgiopoulos and colleagues [16].

## Collaboration of care

Appropriate application of psychopharmacology is an essential skill for child and adolescent psychiatrists to have and continually develop. Similar to our patients, however, psychopharmacology does not exist in a bubble. Our patients exist in a world of expanding systems, from internal processes to a wide array of external interactions, which include not only areas under the direct purview of mental health systems but also families, school, social service, community groups, legal systems, health care systems, and beyond. Understanding the influences these systems have on a given patient and coordinating care within these systems are crucial to the development and implementation of treatment plans. Other authors in this collective work discuss this aspect of training in its entirety. For the purpose of this article, we focus on collaboration within mental health systems, specifically regarding the coordination of psychopharmacology and psychotherapy.

Increasing amounts of evidence support the use of specific types of psychotherapy in the treatment of certain types of psychiatric disorders. As discussed in more detail in subsequent materials within this collective work on training, the rigor of evidence-based practice has been applied to the assessment of various psychotherapy modalities with and without combined psychopharmacotherapy. For example, evidence has shown that certain types of cognitive behavior therapy and behavior therapy combined with pharmacotherapy may play an important role in the appropriate management of attention-deficit hyperactivity disorder, obsessive-compulsive disorder, and depression [17–20]. Additional studies are currently underway to evaluate the role of cognitive behavior therapy with and without pharmacotherapy in the treatment of adolescent suicide attempters, treatment-resistant obsessive-compulsive disorder, and separation anxiety, social phobia, and general anxiety disorder [20–22]. These initial studies have helped to guide not only the practice of mental health care but also the training of providers. Training programs—by choice and by competency requirements—provide some training in various psychotherapy modalities. This rise in evidence-based psychotherapy not only helps in the curriculum design for psychotherapy but also highlights the importance of skill set development by child and adolescent psychiatry trainees in the areas of recommending, providing, and collaborating with others in the provision of psychotherapy. Although the unique environment of training allows for the opportunity for one provider to administer pharmacotherapy and psychotherapy, this can be less easily accomplished after training for various reasons, including managed care, practice limitations, and an inadequate access to good supervision, among others. A common real-world experience is for a child and adolescent psychiatrist to provide pharmacotherapy with another clinician providing psychosocial treatment. This type of arrangement can allow for optimization of resources (more therapists available than child and adolescent psychiatrists) via review/discussion of evidence-based psychotherapeutic modalities, initial assessment processes, and interval assessment of treatment effects. It also can result in disjointed and inadequate care if not conducted in a collaborative and integrated fashion. It is crucial for trainees to acquire the skills to administer/ensure a collaborative, integrated treatment for their patients.

What should this "collaborative skill set" include? Ellison [11] describes it as including the abilities to feel and convey a receptive and respectful attitude toward collaborating providers, identify appropriate providers, adequately document issues pertinent to collaborative care, and communicate periodically with co-providers to monitor patient progress and changes in treatment plan. Ellison's work indicates some specific educational modalities (didactic, practical experience, supervision, and evaluation) with an emphasis on collaborative care. These exist in the goals and objectives of our curriculum.

The DUHCAP Residency Training Program strives to meet these goals and objectives related to collaborative care through various educational modalities, similar to Dr. Ellison's recommendations. Within training clinics, initial assessment and continued treatment process involves sharing of information between the child and adolescent psychiatry trainee and family, schoolteachers, and psychosocial treatment providers. In an ongoing biweekly evidence-based psychotherapy seminar, discussion of the most current psychotherapy research includes psychiatrists and psychologists.

Psychologists and child psychiatrists for the development and review of treatment plans also attend bi-weekly case conferences. Trainees collaborate regularly on cases with PhDs and licensed clinical social workers under the supervision of MDs and PhDs. Trainees are also given the opportunity to participate as psychotherapists or pharmacotherapists in multimodal treatment studies [20,21] with video supervision and group supervision. Overseeing the trainees' performances in all these settings, the program director collects feedback from each trainee's supervisors, collaborating providers, and 360-degree evaluations from patients for biannual evaluations.

Although this work speaks specifically to the importance of collaboration with psychotherapy providers, most of the skill set required to collaborate effectively with psychotherapists easily transfers to working with different types of individuals from different fields and systems. The coordination of care that can exist in a collaborative environment has the potential to improve patient outcomes while optimizing efforts of pharmacotherapists, psychotherapists, and beyond.

## Role of evidence-based medicine

The use of EBM has permeated medical education, from first-year medical school to fellowship. In teaching pediatric psychopharmacology, its application brings up several unique issues, which are the focus of this section. Child and adolescent psychiatry is a field relatively bereft of high-quality quantitative data, especially related to the use of psychotropic medications [5]. For this reason, rigorous evaluation of treatment studies and a reasonable prediction of benefit and harm, particularly when extrapolating from adult studies, are crucial.

The proper evaluation of a psychotropic treatment study in an evidence-based model requires education in the key aspects of methodology and the level of evidence obtained. The teaching of EBM in child psychiatry in general was addressed in a thoughtful and comprehensive manner by March and colleagues [9] in "Using and Teaching Evidence-Based Medicine: The Duke University Child and Adolescent Psychiatry Model." They defined EBM as "a set of processes that facilitate the conscientious, explicit, and judicious integration of individual clinical expertise with the best available external clinical evidence from systematic research in making decisions about the care of individual patients." Although the review of specific EBM procedures is beyond the scope of this article, March and colleagues also make the pertinent point: "Whether for specific care of individual patients or for decisions regarding systems issues such as specifying treatment options in a mental health center or managing a drug formulary, the essence of applying available evidence to patient care involved assessing the validity, clinical importance, and applicability of the evidence..." This is the "end game" of EBM: application to the individual patient. This premise holds true for the specific case of teaching psychopharmacology. EBM should assist the pediatric psychopharmacologist by informing decisions regarding individual patient care when using medications.

In teaching psychopharmacology, the role EBM has in clinical care is emphasized. The central importance of translating the results of a medication study into a framework of understanding regarding risks and benefits for the patient and his or her family is an overarching theme embedded in the curriculum. Patients and their families must understand that when efficacy (therapeutic effect) or harm (severity and seriousness of adverse effects compared with the benefits from the medication and the impairments from the illness) is addressed, one is speaking of percentages/chances and not guaranteed results. Although the statistical terms and concepts are taught and used in discussions in seminars, the use of these terms and concepts is not as helpful in the clinical encounter. What patients/parents must know are the chances for improvement given the particular problems or disorders that a child has (eg, absolute risk reduction, absolute risk increase, odds ratio, relative risk, number needed to treat, number needed to harm) and the "average" expected gain (eg, the effect size or the specific cutoff used to determine benefit or harm in the study for which the absolute risk reduction was calculated). Parents also need an explanation of an average means based on what we know about the patient and the participants in the study or studies with whom he or she is being compared. Focusing on this central clinical conversation in EBM pediatric psychopharmacology offsets a misleading view that we will find an absolute answer in our quantitative, logical positivist scientific view. Establishing realistic expectations based on the best available scientific evidence helps establish a strong therapeutic alliance and ensures good adherence to treatment. (Adherence is shown to be poor in pediatric pharmacology [23].)

These same issues apply to psychotherapy data and are even more important to address when combined with psychopharmacology. The combination of psychosocial treatments with drug treatments promises to bring a stronger dose effect, address multiple targets caused by comorbidities, and augment the treatment of partial responders [2] The pediatric EBM seminar at Duke includes child residents and faculty from psychology, social work, and psychiatry. The presence of a multidisciplinary group of faculty ensures the integration of evidence-based psychopharmacology and psychotherapy across the continuum of care from developing research questions to working with individual patients. This forum has the essence of "bench to bedside," and EBM is the lens that allows this vision to form clearly.

Bias is one of the main sources of overestimation of treatment effects and usually the result of a poor trial design. Being able to determine whether a treatment effect is clinically real requires that the scientific method be used and reported accurately. Although quality studies exist, there is certainly an impression in academia and private practice that these studies are frequently weighted unfairly in the interest of the sponsor. The use of EBM critical appraisal skills to review medication studies gives residents an opportunity to assess properly for biases and validity of trials. Examples of important questions to answer are as follows [24,25]:

Is the comparison valid?

Is an appropriate dose of the treatment drug being compared against an appropriate dose of a comparison drug and for an equivalent period of time?

If being compared against psychotherapy, is the psychotherapy gold standard well validated?

Are the patients of an appropriate clinical sample?

Are they only marginally ill, with the intent to show a large number of responders, even if the response is minimal?

How were they selected?

Is the outcome measure meaningful or chosen with the intent of giving the best chance show an effect, even if it has little clinical or ecologic validity?

Here is an example of our critical appraisal of a published pharmaceutical industry sponsored trial during one of our EBM seminars. Wagner and colleagues [26] presented at American Psychiatric Association in 2002 and in 2004 had published in *American Journal of Psychiatry* a randomized, controlled trial studying the use of citalopram in treating major depression in children and adolescents. The basic design of the study of this medication was an 8-week, randomized, double-blind, placebo-controlled study that compared the safety and efficacy of citalopram with placebo in the treatment of children (aged 7–11) and adolescents (aged 12–17) with major depressive disorder. The primary outcome measure was score on the Children's Depression Rating Scale-Revised; the response criterion was defined as a score less than or equal to 28.

The authors reported an effect size of 2.9 (which is considered immense in terms of Cohen's formulae) and concluded "citalopram reduced depressive symptoms to a significantly greater extent than placebo…" In a follow-up editorial, Tamminga [27] stated, "The importance of this well-designed large study for therapeutic strategies in children and adolescents cannot be overstated. It is important that the methodology of this study is solid and the numbers adequate to test the efficacy question asked. The result that citalopram reduced depression more than placebo in this child and adolescent population provides a clear answer for physicians that will (in combination with results from additional studies) guide treatment decisions." Taken at face, without a critical evidence-based analysis, an effect size of 2.9 definitely could be interpreted as significant (statistically and clinically). Our EBM group and several other authors had concerns that were addressed through a systematic review of the study, however. There were questions as to the proportion of subjects excluded after the initial single-blind period and the method of elicitation of suicidal ideation (not clearly defined in the study), but for this example we focus on the statistical conclusions. An effect size of 2.9 seemed anomalous enough to elicit a response from Martin and colleagues [28] to question whether it represented a calculation error or a calculation using a different formula. This second option seemed reasonable considering that the number needed to treat was 8 and the difference in percent responders between treatment and placebo was 36% to 24%, respectively. Mathews and colleagues [29] reported in their reanalysis an odds ratio of 1.75 (95% CI, 0.92–3.43), which straddles the value of no effect. In their response, Wagner and colleagues [30] gave the formula they used to calculate the effect size, which differed from the commonly used (and likely assumed) Cohen method. When they recalculated the effect size with Cohen's method, it was 0.32, a modest estimate and one that should temper the enthusiasm over the outcome of the study. What is important in terms of EBM is that critical questions were raised regarding methodology, an understanding of the specific statistics used and more appropriate alternatives were considered, and a critical evaluation of the outcome and conclusions to be drawn was performed independent of the original authors. Without the application of these EBM tools, the child psychiatrist is left to accept the assertions of the primary researchers based on their authority. It is this responsibility of the child psychiatrist to critically interpret and apply the results of such studies of medications to the care of patients. This is a central theme in our pediatric psychopharmacology curriculum.

To further promote evidence-based practice in pediatric psychopharmacology we also participate in the Child and Adolescent Simple Trials Network (CAPTN) [31]. The training director is the principal investigator and each resident is a co-principal investigator, which establishes their individual role as a future principal investigator during training. The CAPTN experience includes each resident formulating clinical and research questions for consideration by John March, MD, as the principal investigator of CAPTN and the application of EBM critical appraisal skills during reviews of the protocols in the pediatric psychopharmacology seminar.

In this era of genomics the definitions of disease and schema for diagnosis and taxonomy are being re-examined in adult and pediatric psychiatry [32]. It is increasingly clear that treatment response is likely to be one of the criterion used in defining disease, which has tremendous implications for the importance of knowing EBM principles in pediatric psychopharmacology. The measurement of treatment response (ie, clinically meaningful reduction of symptoms and improved functionality with the use of rating scales) is a current standard. Having an EBM-informed understanding of how these tools are used to measure independent variables is critical to the appraisal of present and future studies about the effect of medications.

EBM serves us as useful steering tool in teaching pediatric psychopharmacology. Integration across fields related to pediatric psychiatry and through the spectrum of basic research to individual patient care is the unifying concept with EBM as the common language. This approach allows residents to learn a set of strategies and tactics to navigate the ever-expanding volume of clinical research in a systematic, critical manner and have an appreciation of the larger context in which pediatric psychiatric care takes place.

## Curriculum design

The classical model for teaching child and adolescent psychopharmacology (as in all of medicine) has been an apprenticeship model whereby the experiences and accumulated knowledge of multiple individuals has been passed down through anecdotes, individual relationships, and somewhat arbitrary experiences [33]. Although the role of mentors in medicine is critical in helping individuals develop skills in diagnosis and critical thinking, it has had limitations because of great variability in what is learned and taught between training programs and between trainees within their programs. The current trend in all of medicine has been to make decisions based on concrete clinical evidence where available (ie, to review the research literature and faithfully apply data from studies of populations to individual patients based on multiple variables, such as symptoms and diagnoses, response to treatment and harm, and demographics of the studied population). In the clinical encounter, decisions about individual patients are dichotomous: treat or don't treat.

A serious limitation for EBM psychopharmacology is paucity of data on medications being used to treat children and adolescents. There has been a lack of incentives for the pharmaceutical industry to study medications in children until recently. Consequently, the use of most medications for pediatric psychiatric disorders has been off label and extrapolated from adult studies. It was not "until the late 1990's the National Institute of Mental Health (NIMH) funded most of the research in pediatric psychopharmacology, including almost all of the placebo-controlled trials of tricyclic antidepressants and most studies of stimulant medications in ADHD" and "the first placebo-controlled trial of fluoxetine that showed efficacy in pediatric depression" [5].

There has been a lot of discussion in the literature about what specific topics and information should be covered in a pediatric psychopharmacology-training program, yet there is no specific delineation in the Accreditation Council of Graduated Medical Education requirements. It has been noted that the Psychiatry Residency Review Committee mandates that the didactic curriculum should include presentations on the treatment and prevention of all major psychiatric disorders and "adequate and systematic instruction in psychopharmacology and other clinical sciences relevant to psychiatry." Teaching EBM pediatric psychopharmacology addresses several issues in the presentation of these materials. First, whatever is taught must have the evidence well delineated in the hierarchy of evidence. Second, the material must be relevant and generalizable to the clinical practice. This requirement follows the adult learning principle that the information be deemed relevant and practical to enhance retention of information [14]. Third, the curriculum should be comprehensive enough to provide a solid general background for the purpose of allowing the trainee to perform well on standardized testing and have a foundation for independent study. On the certification and recertification examinations of the American Board of Psychiatry and Neurology, a significant number of the core competencies involved psychopharmacology, and most individuals who failed the patient section of the oral examination had inadequate performance in the area of drug treatment, which indicated that trainees may need additional experience with applying psychopharmacologic knowledge in the context of patient cases [34].

We have been designing and using a case-based approach to facilitate learning. This approach to the teaching of EBM psychopharmacology integrates it into the context of clinical practice discussions to reinforce practice behaviors [35]. The use of cases is designed to approximate this experience. Combining this method of learning with a team approach gives residents various experiences through the active processes of (1) discussion, (2) practice by doing, and (3) teaching others, which have been suggested to be the most successful techniques in building retention of materials [14]. These cumulative experiences of learning the scientific facts with the Socratic method and their application to clinical practice serve as the foundation for future life-long learning as a model of "practice sessions that are distributed over time produce greater and longer lasting skill acquisition than practice sessions of a long duration conducted over a shorter time period" [36].

An initial survey was conducted through review of texts, discussion with faculty and trainees as to the type of clinical cases, diagnoses, and general topics that are more commonly encountered, essential for the treatment of patients, and should be addressed throughout training. Although this list of topics is subject to revision, ours includes various clinically relevant and frequently encountered topics:

Normal development
Attention deficit hyperactivity disorder
Pediatric "bipolar disorder"
Learning disorders
Oppositional defiant disorder/externalizing disorders
Obsessive-compulsive disorder
Depression
Posttraumatic stress disorder
Separation anxiety, social phobia, generalized anxiety disorder
Eating disorders
Forensic topics and custody evaluations
Emergency topics/suicidality
Pervasive developmental delays/autism

Cultural competency
Tics/movement disorders

Each module contains several elements: (1) A pretest to prime individuals, engage them in learning, and help them to assess their initial fund of knowledge. (2) Background readings, which are chosen to cover specific elements. Readings are chosen from literature searches, systematic reviews (eg, Cochrane database), or current tests. The background readings should cover the epidemiology, etiology, and diagnosis (often including American Academy of Child and Adolescent Psychiatry practice parameters and available clinically validated instruments to track symptoms).

The modules are created (or updated with the newest literature) by persons who will be using them, thus engaging trainees to conduct their own literature searches and seek exemplar cases from their own or colleagues' clinical experiences. A flow diagram for creating the module may be conceptualized (Fig. 1).

In addition to the specific disorders covered, certain essential core topics are covered, such as neurophysiology, pharmacokinetics, and pharmacodynamics, which are also systematically reviewed in a separate seminar that uses an evidence-based text on pediatric psychopharmacology [37]. These topics are worthy of review in a pharmacology course specific to child and adolescent psychiatry because of the unique biologic and developmental needs of children. Future plans include a detailed review by a pediatric pharmacist on drug-drug interactions, with clinically relevant material from consultations and practice.

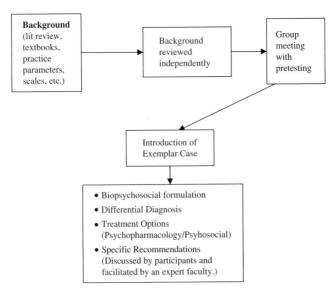

Fig. 1. Process model of case-bound learning method.

Overall pediatric psychopharmacology is best learned when integrated with the rest of the curriculum. To accomplish this goal it is necessary to have a block of protected time, which we have achieved by using an academic half-day 1 day per week. The half-day starts at 8AM with a specific module and topic on which to focus for 1 to 1.5 hours. It is sometimes necessary to continue the module sessions from one week to the next given their pith. This module is followed that morning by our EBM seminar in which up-to-date articles on diagnosis, therapy, prognosis, systematic reviews, and pediatric treatment guidelines are reviewed to address clinical questions specifically related to the topic. A critical appraisal is done of the papers reviewed, and the findings are discussed. The crowning element to this half-day of study is the psychopharmacology seminar, in which we use our comprehensive text and articles while reviewing the specific medications appropriate to the clinical case. Given the context and repetition of some material from the module groups and EBM seminar, it is easier to form a more cohesive and comprehensive picture about how and where psychopharmacology fits in to the treatment of the whole patient. This also allows the child residents to discuss the properties, mechanism of action, adverse effects, and pediatric pharmacokinetics of specific agents in an integrated way with the rest of the material. The most gratifying aspect occurs when a resident takes his or her knowledge into the faculty supervised clinic to improve the lives of patients and their families through treatment and education.

**Summary**

Psychopharmacology is taught in the DUHCAP training program within the context of an EBM model. The curriculum design has incorporated adult learning theory into an integrated format that starts with a case-based learning module followed by the pediatric EBM seminar and then the pediatric psychopharmacology seminar. In a case-based module, first- and second-year child residents work together to develop a differential diagnosis and treatment plan for a patient described in a detailed clinical vignette. A clinical expert who uses the Socratic method to draw information from the fellows and delineate gaps in their knowledge informs this process, which presses fellows to sharpen their analytic skills and stimulates new patient-centered EBM questions. Medication studies, practice guidelines, and treatment algorithms relevant to the case are then critically appraised in the EBM seminar. Finally the pediatric psychopharmacology seminar reviews in-depth details regarding pharmacokinetics, pharmacodynamics, safety issues, and treatment resistance. This hub of academic activity is linked with spokes of clinical practice in various settings, populations, and modalities. Collaborative care and combined treatments are also reviewed and applied in a seminar on empirically based psychosocial treatments shared with psychology interns as part of the outpatient teaching clinic. Taken together, these threads of teaching methods combined with the goals and objectives of DUHCAP pediatric psychopharmacology create the clinical care experience for the child psychiatry residents.

## References

[1] Barondes S. Drugs, DNA and the analyst's couch. In: Brockman J, editor. The next fifty years: science in the first half of the twenty-first century. New York: Vintage Books; 2002. p. 267–76.

[2] March JS, Wells K. Coordinating pharmacotherapy with psychotherapy: an evidence-based approach. In: Andrés Martin LS, Charney DS, Leckman JF, editors. Pediatric psychopharmacology: principles and practice. New York: Oxford University Press; 2003. p. 426–43.

[3] Green ML. Evidence-based medicine training in graduate medical education: past, present and future. J Eval Clin Pract 2000;6(2):121–38.

[4] Goldner EM, Abbass A, Leverette JS, et al. Evidence-based psychiatric practice: implications for education and continuing professional development. Canadian Psychiatric Association position paper. Can J Psychiatry 2001;46(5):15.

[5] DeVeaugh-Geiss J, March J, Shapiro M, et al. Child and adolescent psychopharmacology in the new millennium: a workshop for academia, industry, and government. J Am Acad Child Adolesc Psychiatry 2006;45(3):261–70.

[6] Costello EJ, Mustillo S, Erkanli A, et al. Prevalence and development of psychiatric disorders in childhood and adolescence. Arch Gen Psychiatry 2003;60(8):837–44.

[7] Osser DN, Patterson RD, Levitt JJ. Guidelines, algorithms, and evidence-based psychopharmacology training for psychiatric residents. Acad Psychiatry 2005;29(2):180–6.

[8] Klein DF. Comments on psychiatric education. Acad Psychiatry 2005;29(2):128–33.

[9] March JS, Chrisman A, Breland-Noble A, et al. Using and teaching evidence-based medicine: the Duke University child and adolescent psychiatry model. Child Adolesc Psychiatr Clin N Am 2005;14(2):273–96.

[10] Green ML, Ruff TR. Why do residents fail to answer their clinical questions? A qualitative study of barriers to practicing evidence-based medicine. Acad Med 2005;80(2):176–82.

[11] Ellison JM. Teaching collaboration between pharmacotherapist and psychotherapist. Acad Psychiatry 2005;29(2):195–202.

[12] Ying P, Hadge L, Elliot A, et al. Teaching effective collaboration between psychology interns and psychiatry residents in the outpatient clinic. New York: New York University; 2006.

[13] Carraccio C, Wolfsthal SD, Englander R, et al. Shifting paradigms: from Flexner to competencies. Acad Med 2002;77(5):361–7.

[14] Zisook S, Benjamin S, Balon R, et al. Alternate methods of teaching psychopharmacology. Acad Psychiatry 2005;29(2):141–54.

[15] Kern DA, Thomas PA, Howard DM, et al. Curriculum development for medical education: a six step approach. Baltimore (MD): The John Hopkins University Press; 1998.

[16] Georgiopoulos AM, Huffman JC. Teaching psychopharmacology: two trainees' perspectives. Acad Psychiatry 2005;29(2):167–75.

[17] Group TMC. A 14-month randomized clinical trial of treatment strategies for attention-deficit/hyperactivity disorder: the MTA Cooperative Group. Multimodal Treatment Study of Children with ADHD. Arch Gen Psychiatry 1999;56(12):1073–86.

[18] March J, Silva S, Petrycki S, et al. Fluoxetine, cognitive-behavioral therapy, and their combination for adolescents with depression: treatment for adolescents with depression study (TADS) randomized controlled trial. JAMA 2004;292(7):807–20.

[19] Group POTS. Cognitive-behavior therapy, sertraline, and their combination for children and adolescents with obsessive-compulsive disorder: the Pediatric OCD Treatment Study (POTS) randomized controlled trial. JAMA 2004;292(16):1969–76.

[20] March J. Child and adolescent anxiety multisite study (CAMS). Grant Number: 5U01MH064107–04. 2002.
[21] March J. Treatment in pediatric obsessive-compulsive disorder. Grant Number: 5R01MH055121–08. 2003. Available at: http://crisp.cit.nih.gov/. Accessed September 14, 2006.
[22] Emslie G. Treatment of adolescent suicide attempters in Dallas. 2002. Available at: http://crisp.cit.nih.gov/. Accessed September 14, 2006.
[23] Haynes RB, Yao X, Degani A, et al. Interventions to enhance medication adherence. Cochrane Database Syst Rev 2005;(4):CD000011.
[24] Gray G. Evidence-based psychiatry. Washington, DC: American Psychiatric Publishing; 2004.
[25] Guyatt GH, Sackett DL, Cook DJ. Users' guides to the medical literature. II. How to use an article about therapy or prevention. B. What were the results and will they help me in caring for my patients? Evidence-Based Medicine Working Group. JAMA 1994;271(1):59–63.
[26] Wagner KD, Robb AS, Findling RL, et al. A randomized, placebo-controlled trial of citalopram for the treatment of major depression in children and adolescents. Am J Psychiatry 2004;161(6):1079–83.
[27] Tamminga CA. Demonstrating drug action. Am J Psychiatry 2004;161(6):943–5.
[28] Martin A, Gilliam WS, Bostic JQ, et al. Child psychopharmacology, effect sizes, and the big bang. Am J Psychiatry 2005;162(4):817 [author reply: 818–9].
[29] Mathews M, Adetunji B, Mathews J, et al. Child psychopharmacology, effect sizes, and the big bang. Am J Psychiatry 2005;162(4):818 [author reply: 818–9].
[30] Wagner KD, Robb AS, Findling RL, et al. Dr. Wagner and colleagues reply. Am J Psychiatry 2005;162(4):818–9.
[31] March J. Child and adolescent psychiatry trials network (CAPTN). Grant Number: 5P30MH066386–03. 2003. Available at: http://crisp.cit.nih.gov/. Accessed September 14, 2006.
[32] Krishnan KR. Psychiatric disease in the genomic era: rational approach. Mol Psychiatry 2005;10(11):978–84.
[33] Glick ID, Zisook S. The challenge of teaching psychopharmacology in the new millennium: the role of curricula. Acad Psychiatry 2005;29(2):134–40.
[34] Juul D, Winstead DK, Sheiber SC. Assessment of psychopharmacology on the American Board of Psychiatry and Neurology examinations. Acad Psychiatry 2005;29(2):211–4.
[35] Coomarasamy A, Khan KS. What is the evidence that postgraduate teaching in evidence based medicine changes anything? A systematic review. BMJ 2004;329(7473):1017.
[36] Blanco C, Lujan JJ, Nunes EV. Education and training in psychopharmacology. Acad Psychiatry 2005;29(2):124–7.
[37] Andrés Martin LS, Charney DS, Leckman JF, editors. Pediatric psychopharmacology: principles and practice. New York: Oxford University Press; 2003.

ELSEVIER
SAUNDERS

Child Adolesc Psychiatric Clin N Am
16 (2007) 183–206

CHILD AND
ADOLESCENT
PSYCHIATRIC CLINICS
OF NORTH AMERICA

# Teaching Evidence-Based Psychotherapies

Margo Thienemann, MD*, Shashank V. Joshi, MD

*Psychiatry and Behavioral Sciences, Division of Child and Adolescent Psychiatry,
Stanford University School of Medicine, 401 Quarry Road, Stanford, CA 94305-5719, USA*

"I swear to fulfill, to the best of my ability and judgment, this covenant: I will respect the hard-won scientific gains of those physicians in whose steps I walk, and gladly share such knowledge as is mine with those who are to follow..." *A Modern Hippocratic Oath*, Louis Lasagna

As scientist-clinicians, psychiatric physicians seek to and are bound to practice in a manner informed by evidence about causality, classification, and treatment for the troubles causing suffering in our patients. Over time, physicians have attributed the causes of psychiatric conditions to diverse factors: circulating emotion-regulating humors, pressure points that induce hysterical fits, disequilibrium of psychic energies, and genetic neurotransmitter promoter region variation. As the fields of general psychiatry and child psychiatry have developed, causal theories and observations have suggested various therapeutic interventions: effective and ineffective, ethical and unethical, examined and unexamined, acceptable and unacceptable to patients. What is the process by which ethical, effective, and acceptable practice and teaching evolve?

Over time, basic science and clinician researchers gather knowledge about factors that influence children's and adolescents' mental health. As that knowledge accumulates, we bootstrap our diagnostic paradigms, treatments, and teachings into more helpful interventions by integrating scientific findings and clinical evidence into practices aimed at improving symptoms and addressing dysfunction in psychiatrically ill youth and their families. Persons who train child and adolescent psychiatrists are charged, as are those teaching any branch of medicine, with teaching students that knowledge evolves continuously and that fellowship training only begins a career-long process of integrating new information into one's

---

* Corresponding author.
*E-mail address:* mthiene@stanford.edu (M. Thienemann).

understanding and practice. (Note: For the remainder of this paper, "child psychiatry and child & adolescent psychiatry" will be used interchangeably.) As teachers, we must help trainees appreciate the growth of the knowledge base in child psychiatry and acquire competence in evaluating and integrating new information. A substantial amount of current diagnostic, prognostic and treatment evidence likely will be obsolete during the lifetime of the child psychiatry fellow's practice.

Currently our field is actively involved in developing new ways to characterize and treat children and adolescents with psychiatric disorders and in evaluating the effects of our therapies. We also are beginning to examine the effectiveness of our teaching methods. This article aims to present evidence for, ideas about, and a philosophy to guide those who are privileged to train child psychiatrists in psychotherapies. Specifically, it discusses the issues of the evidence base for diagnosis and for nonspecific and specific active elements of child psychotherapy. Evidence for methods of training is presented. The article addresses the need for supervising psychiatrists to keep abreast of developments in teaching methods so that we can best train competent, curious, and compassionate child psychiatrists.

## Evidence base for child and adolescent psychiatry

A well-trained child and adolescent psychiatrist confronting a new patient thoughtfully addresses and as accurately as possible answers these questions: Why has this family or child sought treatment now? What are my patient's problems? On what basis have I made the diagnostic impression? What evidence do I have for proposing treatment for these problems? What other options are available? Am I skilled to deliver this therapy? Does this intervention fit my patient's needs? Will the patient and family accept this treatment? To answer these questions, the child psychiatrist draws from the reservoir of experiences with other patients whose presentations vary in degrees of similarity.

As clinicians, we use our own patient assessment and others' experiences to inform our medical decisions. We access these experiences by reviewing the best information available: from well-designed research studies to preliminary pilot investigations, case reports, recall of cases supervised and presented during training, and examples from our own clinical experience. We compare information about the patient at hand with information about other patients, noting similarities and differences. In this process we integrate scientific evidence with knowledge of current patient characteristics to determine patient diagnosis and then choose and recommend a course of action. To practice evidence-based child psychiatry, we (ideally) adhere to "the conscientious, explicit and judicious use of current evidence in making decisions about the care of individual patients...integrating individual clinical expertise with the best available external clinical evidence from systematic research" [1].

## Making evidence-based diagnoses

This article aims to address evidence-based therapy. For one to treat using an evidence-based approach, the intervention should target the problem for which the treatment was actually designed. Using an evidence-based method to define patients' problems is desirable. The Diagnostic Schedule for Mental Disorders (DSM) [2] has improved our ability to communicate to each other by labeling different symptom clusters based on expert consensus. Unlike the situation in other medical disciplines, in which laboratory findings inform diagnosis, in child psychiatry, subjective reports from young patients and others who are not the patient comprise much of the data available for consideration by the diagnostician. Making an accurate, evidence-based diagnosis would be a good first step toward considering an evidence-based treatment.

Unfortunately, the literature on this approach suggests that most psychiatric diagnosticians do not make diagnostic and treatment decisions predictably or scientifically. In child psychiatry, diagnostic agreement between clinicians and evaluators using standard research interviews ranges from poor to moderate [3,4]. For example, a study that compared reliability of clinician diagnoses of 393 adolescents found poor agreement between clinicians when making affective, anxiety disorder, and adjustment disorder diagnoses [5]. Clinician-generated diagnoses agreed poorly with standardized research diagnoses generated by the Diagnostic Interview Schedule for Children (DISC-P-2.3) for 245 referred youths [6]. In another investigation, outpatient physicians' clinical diagnoses were less similar to those made by bachelor-level investigators administering a standardized assessment package than inpatient physicians' diagnoses were. Another group found that even with the information available to inpatient child psychiatrists, research evaluations using a structured diagnostic interview during admission were more diagnostically sensitive than were the psychiatrists' evaluations [7]. The research diagnoses had low agreement with clinician admission and discharge diagnoses. Our trainees should appreciate that different methods, each designed to clarify psychiatric diagnosis, may yield different diagnoses.

Not only are diagnoses made by clinical interview different than those made using structured interviews but also consistent differences are found in which diagnoses are likely to be established by a clinical interview. In Jensen's study of 245 subjects, agreement between structured and clinical interviews was higher for externalizing categories than for internalizing disorders [6]. Similarly, interrater reliability was best for attention deficit and substance abuse disorders in a study by Hughes and colleagues [8]. Ezpeleta and colleagues [9] examined the diagnostic agreement between clinicians and the Diagnostic Interview for Children and Adolescents in 137 outpatient children and adolescents. Except for conduct disorder, the agreement between clinicians and DICA-R was low to moderate. The authors attributed sources of disagreement to choice of informant, whether information was observed or reported, differences in which conditions were focused upon, strictness of criteria application, and time span consideration. Including information from the child and parents improved diagnostic accuracy [9]. Children who have internalizing disorders (who are less often brought to clinics than children who have externalizing disorders) are less often detected even in the clinic.

In addition to understanding these diagnostic discrepancies, child psychiatry trainees must understand that research has consistently found that information elicited from children and parents differs. Parents report more behavioral and externalizing symptoms than children, and children report more internalizing and subjective symptoms than parents [10,11]. Parents report more observable symptoms and fewer school-related symptoms than do children [12]. Comparing diagnoses made using the semi-structured Anxiety Disorders Interview Schedule for Children, when interviewing parents alone, children alone, and children and parents together, Rapee and colleagues [13] found poor agreement between children and parents. In reviewing answers to questions about specific symptoms, Herjanic and Reich [10] found that parents and their children agreed more about symptoms that were concrete, severe, and unambiguous. These studies point out the necessity for using multiple informants in performing diagnostic assessments and identify some characteristics of discrepancies between reporters.

Why does this gap between clinical and structured interview diagnoses exist? Some researchers suggest that structured diagnostic interviews improve the diagnostic process by organizing clinical data collection and eliminating biases when applying diagnostic criteria [14]. Researchers who study medical decision making agree and have worked to identify sources of diagnostic inaccuracy [3]. Cognitive errors and bias errors may result in clinicians taking cognitive short cuts and making irrational decisions in assessment and treatment planning. Awareness of this possibility is important for child psychiatry trainees and educators as they monitor students' evolving diagnostic and treatment decisions and practices.

Disorders that are in the news (eg, disorders getting publicity because of new drug indications) may be more frequently diagnosed. Diagnoses may be made with inadequate consideration of their prevalence rate. Especially for beginning and intermediate clinicians, generating a diagnostic hypothesis prematurely in the interview may lead to neglecting consideration of the actual diagnosis. The order in which information is presented, time spent in discussing particular symptoms, and recent or emotional clinician experiences are factors that can lead to errors. The level of clinical experience of the physician correlates with different types of errors. Experienced clinicians are more likely to make errors by omitting diagnostic consideration and basing decisions on clinical experience. Less experienced clinicians make errors in including excessive diagnoses and, lacking practice, tend to rely on available scientific evidence. Intermediate clinicians perform most poorly [3].

Teachers and students benefit from knowledge of these potential sources of bias and differences in the process of making diagnoses.

Supervisors will benefit from understanding the extent of trainees' knowledge of normal child development. Some childhood internal reactions and behaviors are considered pathologic based on developmental level. Examples include separation anxiety, tantrums, and bedwetting. The most recent child experience for many trainees in child and adolescent psychiatry is their own experience of childhood. Trainees may or may not have studied developmental psychology, have their own children, have had exposure to younger children, have babysat, or have had much experience in pediatrics. Their lack of knowledge and exposure handicaps them in considering age appropriateness, temperamental variation, or pathology of children's and adolescents' symptoms and behaviors. Teachers should be aware of their trainees' level of awareness of normal development and aid trainees in filling the gaps in this area.

### Teaching trainees to make diagnoses to choose therapeutic interventions

The more a clinician can access and apply knowledge about accurately characterizing patients' problems, the firmer the ground on which he or she stands in making treatment recommendations. In our field, there is no one gold standard method of diagnostic evaluation or of teaching diagnostic skills. The following suggestions are designed to teach diagnostic skills and trainee appreciation of issues involved in making diagnoses.

- Familiarizing students with the existence and use of structured interviews in child psychiatry. The interviews developed for research paradigms are varied and evolving, with improving validity and reliability. To accomplish this, trainees either view a tape of an interview or watch a supervisor perform the interview before doing one themselves. Trainees should perform a clinical interview and a structured interview on the same clinical patient and compare findings. The trainee should be observed either live or via videotape to ascertain his or her reliability on the interview. Administering the interview separately to parent and child informs the student about differences in reporting between these sources. In our anxiety disorders clinic, we have integrated the use of the Anxiety Disorders Interview Schedule for Children into clinical practice [15]. We have found that experiencing the discrepancy between the interviews by doing them is more informative than simply describing the differences using passive didactics.
- In supervision, trainees should be queried on the methods by which they came to make the diagnoses. What were the sources of information? How reliable does the trainee consider each informant? Are there other ways to gather the information, such as psychometric measures or a structured interview? What information is missing? How could that be secured? The supervising child psychiatrist can help trainees identify

the most salient questions and ensure that trainees investigate to get an answer. Assigning trainees to search the literature for these questions reinforces the importance of continual evaluation and integration of evidence in making clinical decisions. This skill has been captured by Sackett and colleagues in the book "Evidence Based Medicine: How to Practice and Teach EBM." March and colleagues describe applicability of this method to child psychiatry training [1,16]. First, the team defines a specific question. Then, using the method called critical appraisal of a topic, clinicians research the question in a systematic fashion, which entails defining a cogent question, performing a literature search, evaluating the data, and then presenting findings to the treatment team. Software for creating critical appraisal of a topic and assisting with calculations is available for free from the Center for Evidence Based Medicine at http://www.cebm.net/catmaker.asp. Authors attribute the use and success of this method of teaching to learning skills for evaluating available information in a clinically salient context and sharing work between trainees and faculty in keeping up with current research.

- Participation in research as part of training also helps trainees to make diagnoses in several ways. First, by performing diagnostic evaluations using structured interviews, they become familiar with DSM criteria. They also may come to appreciate limitations of these interviews, such as the quality of informant recall, restrictions involved in scripted questioning, and subjective patient and interviewer reactions within the structured interview situation. Our fellows often have noted that subjects' families felt especially pleased at feeling they have had a thorough evaluation.

### Accreditation Council on Graduate Medical Education's psychotherapy competency requirements for child psychiatry fellows

"Opportunities for the development of both conceptual understanding of and beginning clinical skills in the major treatment modalities with children and adolescents, which include brief and long-term individual therapy, family therapy, group therapy, crisis intervention, supportive therapy, psychodynamic psychotherapy, cognitive-behavioral therapy, and pharmacotherapy must be provided." (http://www.acgme.org/acWebsite/downloads/RRC_progReq/405pr1104.pdf)

Mellman and Beresin [17] noted that psychotherapy training typically follows an "apprenticeship" model. The adage of "see one, do one, teach one" included undertaking one's own psychotherapy and observing faculty interviews and therapy sessions with patients (seeing), spending hours treating patients and receiving supervision (doing), and passing on the craft to others during the final years of training and afterwards (teaching). Until the recent establishment of the Accreditation Council on Graduate Medical Education core competencies, residency review committee requirements for psychiatry could be met by "passively completing rotations, showing up for sessions with patients, and attending classes and supervision." The lack of uniform standards for exposure to psychotherapy modalities led to much interprogram variability. Many programs continue to determine their rotation sites based primarily on sources of funding, and with some sites more focused on clinical service than education, psychotherapy opportunities have diminished even further. The authors write that "psychotherapeutic foods were sampled by residents, but a balanced diet and attention to comprehensive nutrition was not necessarily guaranteed." To address this, several national work groups have been formed to assist the field in establishing, implementing, and assessing the core competencies in psychiatry training to include five specific competencies for general psychotherapy training: supportive, brief, cognitive-behavioral, psychodynamic, and combined pharmacotherapy and psychotherapy [18–21].

For child and adolescent training directors, Dingle and Beresin [22] have written a highly practical paper on the topic of competencies in this issue that includes samples of general competency-based evaluation forms and a master list of evaluation methods.

## Researched methods for teaching psychotherapies

Just as measuring the outcome of psychotherapy interventions is required for establishing evidence for its utility, individuals desiring to teach evidence-based therapies perform best if they follow suit and determine the results of their teaching interventions. We must determine whether the material taught was learned and used effectively in patient care. We must monitor and measure our teaching behavior to improve and optimize training outcome. The following section addresses the topics of teaching the evidence-based psychotherapies, measuring trainee competency in these therapies, and measuring supervisor competence in teaching.

## Evidence for psychotherapy

Although a single diagnostic gold standard child psychiatry diagnostic evaluation has not been established, evidence-supported diagnostic measures for particular diagnostic entities, such as anxiety or mood disorders, do exist. Similarly, several specific psychotherapies developed to target specific disorders have been researched sufficiently to receive the label "well established." To qualify as well established as designated by the American Psychological Association guidelines, the treatment must be manualized and tested in at least two sites and must be a randomized, controlled study of a nonselected subject population, with outcomes measured by raters blind to treatment group [23]. The studies must include sufficient numbers of subjects to demonstrate differences between the tested treatment and some other nonspecific active intervention in light of many uncontrolled differences between subjects, such as differences in intelligence, education, talents, medical health, social support, socioeconomic situation, clinical and subclinical emotional disorders, life experiences, and differences between local environments, treatment sites, treatment providers, and their therapeutic skills.

As helpful as this evidence base is, it does not have automatic applicability to practice or teaching. Possible pitfalls include choice of specific treatments for specific patients, adequacy of therapist training and supervision, knowledge about which problem to address in what order, and failure of specified treatments to describe and direct many nonspecific elements of therapy. Within the field of psychiatry exist controversies about and resistances to adopting evidence-based psychotherapies, as illustrated in this tale in a controversial article [24,25].

> Once upon a time, psychotherapists practiced without adequate empirical guidance, assuming that the therapies of their own persuasion were the best. Many of their practices were probably helpful to many of their patients, but knowing which were helpful and which were inert or iatrogenic was a matter of opinion and anecdote. Then a group of clinical scientists developed a set of procedures that became the gold standard for assessing the validity of psychotherapies. Their goal was a valorous one that required tremendous courage in the face of the vast resources of the Drug Lords and the nonempirical bent of mind of many clinician-dragons, who tended to breathe some admixture of hot air, fire, and wisdom.
>
> In their quest, the Knights identified interventions for several disorders that showed substantial promise. The treatments upon which they bestowed Empirical Support helped many people feel better—some considerably so, and some completely. In the excitement, however, some important details seemed to get overlooked. Many of the assumptions underlying the methods used to test psychotherapies were themselves empirically untested, disconfirmed, or appropriate only for a range of treatments and disorders. Although many patients improved, most did not recover, or they initially recovered but then relapsed or sought additional treatment within the next 2 years. Equally troubling, the Scientific Method (Excalibur) seemed to pledge its allegiance to whomsoever had the time and funding to wield it. Most of the time, psychotherapy outcome studies supported the preferred position of the gallant knight who happened to conduct them (Sir Grantsalot).
>
> Nevertheless, clinical lore and anecdotal alchemy provided no alternative to experimental rigor, and as word of the Knights' crusade became legendary, their tales set the agenda for clinical work, training, and research throughout the land. Many graduate programs began teaching new professionals only those treatments that had the imprimatur of Empirical Validation, clinicians seeking licensure had to memorize the tales told by the Knights and pledge allegiance to them on the national licensing examination, and insurance companies used the results of controlled clinical trials to curtail the treatment of patients who did not improve in 6 to 16 sessions, invoking the name of Empirical Validation [26].

Despite controversy about particular issues in developing and using substantiated treatments, evidence-supported psychotherapies have credible evidence that treatment-as-usual does not. Meta-analyses of controlled studies of psychotherapy of children and adolescents in unconstrained treatment have demonstrated no additional benefit of treatment over no treatment [25,27]. Over time, we as a field will learn more about how evidence-supported therapies work among various patients, settings, and therapists, more about "doses of therapy" required, and about therapist training methods. Successful therapies that target specific problems will become increasingly accessible to practitioners, who may pick and choose as is clinically relevant. Familiarizing trainees with methods of accessing and learning evidence-supported therapies primes them for evaluating and integrating therapies as they evolve.

### Where to start in teaching evidence-based psychotherapy

For each particular provisional diagnosis or clinical problem, the child psychiatry trainee must become aware of available relevant evidence-based treatments. Because the body of work accomplished is substantial and because the internet and literature search engines are accessible, child psychiatrists have a great experience pool from which to glean information. Text books such as "Evidence-Based Psychotherapies for Children and Adolescents," edited by Alan E. Kazdin and John R. Weisz, are currently a good starting reference [28]. Up-to-date information about evidence-based therapies for children and adolescents is available at the Center for Evidence Based Health Care, a center developed to promote the teaching and practice of evidence-based interventions (with special emphasis on evidence-based mental health) and to develop, evaluate, and disseminate improved methods of using research in practice and incorporate these in the teaching methods of the Centre for Evidence-Based Medicine Healthcare (CEBMH) (http://cebmh.com). The Department of Health's Child and Adolescent Mental Health Division of the State of Hawaii maintains a resource guide in evidence-based psychosocial and pharmacologic interventions for children (http://www.hawaii.gov/health/mental-health/camhd/library/pdf/ebs/ ebs016.pdf). Pub Med's Clinical Queries site runs specialized Medline searches (for topic choices: etiology, diagnosis, therapy, prognosis, and clinical prediction guides) for clinicians (www.pubmed.gov). Searches using this site may be performed as narrow and specific or broad and sensitive. Using the critical appraisal of a topic format in teaching about choice of therapy is an active, hands-on method for organizing the research literature that engages trainees in addressing questions about available treatments.

### Applicability of empirically supported therapies to clinical patients

Empirical studies must include sufficient numbers of subjects to control for myriad differences. These differences highlight the need for judgment about applicability of treatment for a particular patient. Because children who present to a mental health provider often have more than one diagnosis and unique biologic and family predispositions, environments, strengths, weaknesses, and desires for treatment, we have imperfect evidence to guide us as to where and how to first intervene. Clinicians in training must consider the patient and family's chief complaints, values and belief systems, the diagnostic assessment tool, the applicability of evidence-based treatments to the patient's problems (considering differences between the patient and documented study populations), and the family's reaction to and feasibility of recommendations. Sackett and colleagues [1] in "Evidence Based Medicine" suggest that unless patients' characteristics are so different from those of the study population as to be considered useless, one may accept a treatment's efficacy in the study population as a good starting point for estimating treatment efficacy in one's patient.

Current psychotherapies in child and adolescent psychiatry have well-established efficacy. Because this article focuses more on the process of teaching trainees to learn to select and administer appropriate treatments and because the evidence base is constantly changing, we refer readers to current texts and literature for specifics. At the time of this writing, some (but not all) evidence-based nonpharmacologic treatments include discrete trial training and pivotal response training for autism, participant modeling and cognitive behavioral therapy for childhood anxiety disorders, cognitive behavioral and interpersonal therapies for adolescent depression, family-based therapy for anorexia nervosa, parent-child interactive therapy for oppositional children, parent training for attention deficit hyperactivity disorder, parent, teacher, and child multi-faceted treatment for young children with conduct disorders, problem-solving skills training and parent management for youth with conduct disorders, and multidimensional treatment foster care for antisocial youth [29].

It seems safe to say that most instructors of child psychiatry trainees are not trained and competent in each of these interventions. A survey of general psychiatry residents at one institution reported that they were overwhelmingly enthusiastic about learning cognitive behavioral therapy, but two thirds of them had difficulty accessing adequate supervision [30]. Having determined an appropriate treatment using the available evidence, how might the instructor and trainee proceed to help a particular patient? How do teacher and trainee learn these psychotherapies? Current research on child psychotherapies is heavily weighted toward the substantiation of interventions' benefits in select populations when administered by specially trained, supervised practitioners. Evidence on translation of these therapies into the community lags far behind, as does actual training. To teach these psychotherapies, we must (1) learn to do them and (2) attempt to teach them in a manner that has evidence for success.

## Words about manualized treatments

Therapies cannot be tested without explicitly defining the intervention in a way that many individuals may use. To individuals unfamiliar with administering treatment guided by a manual, the prospect can seem mechanistic and stifling. Manualized treatments are not cookbooks for robotic psychotherapists, however. Most manualized treatments assume that one has therapeutic skills for building an alliance, dealing with emergent events, prioritizing issues, and maintaining confidentiality. In addition to requiring these basic psychotherapeutic skills, most treatments require therapist flexibility and creativity to implement them successfully [31,32]. Despite their use, treatment manuals have some built-in limitations. Usually they are written early in process of treatment development and testing, without opportunity for bootstrapping into improved versions. Manualized treatments are tested as a whole package rather than element by element, so determining the active ingredients often requires cumbersome "dismantling studies." Manuals are designed typically to address one diagnosis only and do not directly address comorbid and non-DSM issues. Because the research design is for brief interventions, follow-up and maintenance interventions may not be tested or included. Finally, manualized treatments are designed (as are most scientific developments) by the efforts of interested and motivated researchers. If one is to accept manualized treatment as a necessary and useful improvement for our field, one also might wish for a systematic plan development and testing of needed interventions.

## Teaching nonspecific elements of psychotherapy

Manualized therapies on the whole do not directly address all mediators of therapeutic change. Treatment alliance, therapist and patient attention, support, empathy, treatment acceptability, and barriers to treatment are among these factors, and are issues that raise objections with some therapists uncomfortable with manualized treatments. Children are not usually and adolescents are often not the ones seeking therapy. For that reason, establishing a collaborative relationship within which to address goals and therapy tasks (establishing a therapeutic alliance) may be more challenging in the child psychiatric population. Learning to establish this connection is important, because the strength of the therapeutic alliance between therapist and child predicts change across diverse types and modes of child treatment [33].

Patient-perceived therapist empathy and warmth also mediate treatment outcome. Research has shown that after a session together, patients and therapists may rate therapist empathy differently [34]. Across therapeutic modalities, technical interventions require an adequate relationship (minimally) or a strong working alliance (ideally). The working alliance has been researched extensively [18,35–41] and can be defined as a mutual collaboration against the common foe of the patient's presenting problems

[42]. Also termed "therapeutic alliance," this construct has proved to be a strongly independent predictor of clinical outcomes across the major schools of psychotherapy [43].

A strong alliance requires a shared understanding and agreement about goals for change and about the necessary tasks to achieve these goals [37,38]. This collaboration between therapist and patient involves three essential components: tasks, goals, and bonds. Tasks refer to in-therapy cognitions and behaviors that form the core of the therapeutic process. If the therapeutic relationship is strong, the patient and therapist perceive the tasks in therapy as relevant and potentially beneficial, and each party accepts responsibility to take part in this process. A good working alliance requires a common endorsement of the goals (clinical outcomes), which are the targets of an intervention. The term "bonds" refers to the attachment status of the patient-therapist relationship and includes mutual trust, acceptance, and confidence [18,35,36,40,44].

Research on the therapeutic alliance in psychotherapy with children and teens has concentrated largely on interpersonal processes, one of which considers a developmental perspective [45–47]. Recent investigators also have paid attention to the dual alliance with caregivers, who must play an important role in treatment while not impeding the therapeutic activity between doctor and patient [35,46,48–50]. Although research on the working alliance in adult therapy suggests that the alliance is usually established early (by sessions 3–5) [39,51,52], a recent meta-analysis on alliance formation in children by Shirk and Karver [33] found that relationship measures obtained later in therapy were more strongly associated with clinical outcomes compared with measures taken early, perhaps because of relationship formation evolving more slowly with younger patients. With regard to the dual alliance, we propose that although a strong first session alliance may not always be possible with patient and parent, a good enough alliance is crucial for the family to return for the second session.

Aspects of interpersonal technical activity are teachable in psychiatry residencies, often through modeling opportunities [53–62]. Among these are active skills of expressed responsiveness and the ability to generate a sense of hope, an open, clear, and empathic communication style, and minimization of negative therapist behaviors (irritability or impatience with patient/family efforts, premature insight or interpretation, perceived coldness of the therapist by the patient/family, and a take-charge attitude that may lead to patient dependency in the early phases of treatment) [35,40,63–66]. Training programs may foster the ability to develop therapeutic alliance-building skills through attention to accumulated clinical hours (eg, a strong alliance is correlated with cumulative numbers of patient hours) [55], complex case formulation, and attention to specific factors, such as patient and therapist nonverbal communication. A qualitative study by Kurcias [58] links the evolution in trainee abilities with supervisor assistance in conceptualization and the clinical "seasoning" that occurs with time and experience. As training progressed, psychology trainees in this study became more clinically sophisticated, more comfortable with discussing patient-therapist relationship issues, more patient with the slow pace of change, and more adept at managing relationship and alliance ruptures. Finally, Summers and Barber [61] concluded that (1) certain concrete aspects of the working alliance, such as goal setting and task recognition, may be more teachable (and learnable) than other aspects, such as bond development and (2) pre-existing factors that affect the therapist's ability to build and maintain an alliance must be attended to in didactic form and individual supervision.

Because of its central importance to all forms of psychotherapy, development of the therapeutic alliance is being examined as a potentially measurable skill in psychiatry residency training programs [61]. For a detailed discussion of effect sizes for specific modalities, please see the discussion by Horvath [39,52]. The quality of the alliance may be measured. For therapy with children, therapeutic alliance instruments include the Modified Therapeutic Alliance Questionnaire for Children and Parents (HAq-CP) [67], Therapeutic Alliance Scale for Children, revised (TASC-R) [33], and the Therapeutic Alliance in Pediatric Pharmacotherapy Scale (TAPPs; in development) [35]. Direct observations of trainee, patient, and caregiver interactions also inform supervisors in assessing and addressing this issue.

Empathy is another nonspecific therapy element. Although some clinicians have cautioned that empathy could, in situations of excessive dependency, lead to temporary mood elevation (decreasing motivation to do therapeutic work) or inadvertent reinforcement of patients' self-defeating behaviors or detract from progress, warmth and empathy generally improve clinical outcome. Burns and Nolen-Hoeksema [34] suggested that the feedback obtained by having patients fill out empathy rating forms at the end of sessions helps therapists learn empathy. Summers and Barber [61] have recommended that the alliance be rated at sessions 2, 5, and 10, followed by 3-month intervals for longer term therapies in adult patients. Validated scales in adults include the Working Alliance Inventory (WAI), Penn Helping Alliance (HAq), the California Psychotherapy Alliance Scales (CALPAS) and the California Pharmacotherapy Alliance Scale (patient and pharmacotherapist versions) [68–71].

## Combined psychotherapy and pharmacotherapy

Beitman and colleagues [36] developed a manual for teaching combined psychotherapy and pharmacotherapy that may be used as one tool to fulfill this Accreditation Council on Graduate Medical Education competency requirement. Goals of the ten-session program include (1) becoming familiar with the research findings and limitations of combined treatments, (2) learning to use pharmacotherapy during psychotherapy, (3) learning to use psychotherapy during pharmacotherapy, (4) learning and addressing the issues involved during "split" treatment, (5) understanding the sequencing of pharmacotherapy and psychotherapy, and (6) conceptualizing the neurobiology of psychotherapy. Three other examples of curricula include Mintz's psychology of psychopharmacology/therapeutic role of the prescriber [72], Weiden and Rao's medication compliance curriculum [73], and the medication alliance training program by Byrne and colleagues [74]. Riba and Balon [75] also have written a guide for training directors in this competency as part of the core competencies in psychotherapy series. (This series, edited by Glen O. Gabbard, includes a basic text on each of the five basic competencies and is available through American Psychiatric Publishing, Inc. [http://www.appi.org].) Although these guides were written for general psychiatry training programs, the material is applicable and adaptable for child and adolescent training programs.

## Psychotherapy for psychotherapists

This article summarizes some of the empirical research in psychotherapy demonstrating that nonspecific factors account for a significant amount of the variance of outcome in treatment studies. To this end, Norcross [76] has written in support of the therapist's participation in his or her own psychotherapy as part of psychotherapy training. In a 2005 article, he reported that approximately 75% of psychotherapists (versus 25% of all Americans who have received specialized health care) have undergone at least one episode of psychotherapy, including therapists with analytic, psychodynamic, cognitive behavioral, or systems orientations. Although well-designed studies of the effects of therapists' participation in personal psychotherapy and patient outcome are few, some studies do suggest that therapists' personal therapy is correlated with rater-observed warmth, empathy, genuineness, awareness of countertransference, and an increased emphasis on the therapeutic relationship. In a retrospective study of training elements found most helpful to psychotherapists, personal therapy placed in the top three (after direct patient contact and formal supervision) and outranked didactic experiences [76].

## Translating researched therapy protocols into clinical use

Although the following study is not an example of teaching child psychiatry trainees to do an evidence-based therapy, this translational study by Mufson [77] and colleagues describes the process used when university-based clinical researchers train other mental health professionals (frontline staff in public treatment settings) to perform interpersonal therapy for depressed adolescents (IPT-A). The group created new training materials that describe how to use specific techniques (eg, communication analysis and the interpersonal inventory), which provide guidelines for introducing the treatment to the adolescents. Therapists were required to read the treatment manual before attending the didactic sessions. The trainees then attended training that lasted 2.5 days. The researchers suggested scripts for use by the therapists. Therapists began treating their first case using IPT-A under weekly supervision of an IPT-A expert clinician. Clinicians did not record sessions because of concerns about confidentiality but filled out adherence checklists after each session. Supervisors completed an assessment based on their impressions for 6 of the 12 sessions and rated the therapists' overall competence as IPT-A therapists for each IPT-A treatment case. The training was reported to be effective when outcomes of IPT-A were compared with clinic treatment-as-usual for treating adolescent depression in school-based health clinics in impoverished urban communities in New York City [78].

### Translation of multisystem family therapy

Another translational study is presented to highlight the development of tools to measure adherence to treatment protocol, a behavior necessary for learning and training in manual-based therapies for supervisor and therapist. A study of translation of multisystem family therapy from a research to a clinical setting aimed to validate measures of therapist adherence and supervisory practices [79]. Clinicians received 40 hours of training in the form of didactic instruction and practicing opportunities in multisystem family therapy. During the study, clinicians also participated in weekly 90-minute group supervision, 60-minute group telephone consultations, and quarterly topical updates. The measures of therapist and supervisor adherence demonstrated good psychometric properties. This type of measure may be useful in monitoring psychiatric trainees' adherence to evidence-based therapies and their supervisors' adherence to a supervisory protocol.

### The Coping with Depression Program at the University of California San Francisco

The following discussion illustrates a successful integration of two evidence-based therapies into a training clinic. In the general psychiatry clinic at the University of California San Francisco, a faculty task force developed a program that aimed to improve clinical care and resident training in evidence-based psychotherapy [80]. Previously at this site, all depressed patients were treated with long-term psychotherapy. In the Coping with Depression Program, residents treat depressed adult patients using cognitive therapy and interpersonal therapy. Components of the intervention include (1) patient/family psychoeducational classes, (2) patient access to a psychoeducational website (http://www.ucsf.edu/psych/cwd.htm), (3) 12 weeks of group cognitive therapy co-led by a resident and faculty member, (4) 16 weeks of individual interpersonal therapy, (5) booster sessions of each therapy, (6) evidence-based medication management, and (7) initial and follow-up Beck Depression Inventories.

Residents participate in didactic cognitive therapy and interpersonal therapy seminars and may participate in weekly case conferences about cognitive therapy. Two faculty members meet weekly with groups of three residents to supervise interpersonal therapy using videotapes of sessions. Most psychiatry residents in the training program completed a supervised empirically based treatment. Residents also learned to use objective outcome information to supplement their clinical assessments.

## The McMaster psychotherapy program

More than 10 years ago, McMaster University in Hamilton, Ontario, implemented an empirically oriented psychotherapy training program aimed at standardizing an approach to the training and assessment of trainee competence [81]. This program teaches seven therapies, most of which are manualized (except long-term psychodynamic psychotherapy, which is taught but not manualized). Trainees audiotape or videotape each therapy session. Tapes are reviewed weekly by the trainee's primary supervisor. An alternate supervisor reviews selected tapes blindly using an empirically validated therapist competency rating scale. The faculty is assessed on supervisory and formal didactic skills.

Psychotherapy training begins with client-centered supportive therapy, on which nonspecific therapeutic alliance skills and empathy are focused. Seminars use the active learning tools of videotape and role play. Trainee skills are assessed using evaluation forms to record supervisors' ratings of empathic attunement, support, and alliance. Cognitive-behavioral therapies for depression and anxiety, family therapy, and interpersonal therapy are evaluated similarly. Couples therapy is supervised live. Group therapies are taught by involving trainees as co-therapists. The authors note that this successful program is not possible without funding for (at least) a psychotherapy coordinator and an administrative assistant.

## Assessing trainee competence in psychotherapy

How do we evaluate trainee competence in psychotherapy? Paralleling the situation that trainees are rarely offered an opportunity to observe examples of specific therapies, few faculty watch trainees' therapies or review taped sessions of an entire therapy. Supervisors also rarely have a defined standard by which to judge residents' competence at therapy [82]. Competence in psychotherapy is hard to ascertain because of the overwhelming number of choice points and microprocedures involved in the complex interaction between patient and therapist [83]. Assessing competence re-quires multiple observations of multiple performances, the demonstration of acquisition of a knowledge base of evidence and theories, and trainee experience of conducting each kind of therapy under qualified supervision. To be competent, therapists must be able to perform the work and demonstrate that they know why they are doing what they are doing.

Yager and Kay [83] and Yager and Bienenfeld [82] recommended some assessment methods to assess trainees' proficiencies in psychotherapies. Among these methods are (1) development of knowledge-base examinations; (2) development of tape libraries demonstrating complete examples of specific therapies performed by experts (which could form the basis of seminars); (3) meetings between supervisors and trainees' psychotherapy patients to assess progress; (4) routine monitoring of therapy by auditing taped therapy sessions; (5) trainee production of a "process folio" for training cases that would contain a case write-up and formulation, essays addressing indications for the form of psychotherapy chosen, goals for the treatment, training goals for the resident as applicable to the case, possible problems, and probable outcomes (the portfolio could be augmented with taped sessions, regularly scheduled follow-up entries, selected references and notes about the references' influence on the therapeutic process, and a termination note, which would enable trainees to document knowledge of a case and issues involved in the treatment); (6) development of simulated cases, either on computer or paper, with situations designed to address particular competencies.

### The psychodynamic psychotherapy competency test

Researchers at Columbia University developed a multiple-choice, written test of psychodynamic psychotherapy skills to objectively test trainee's therapeutic competencies [84]. Developers generated selected vignettes describing situations in psychodynamic therapy. Multiple-choice questions were generated to assess core areas of psychodynamic psychotherapy knowledge and skills: (1) establishing a therapeutic framework and alliance, (2) recognizing and managing transference, countertransference, and resistance, (3) recognizing defensive organization and therapeutic change, and (4) assessing and recommending several psychodynamic interventions. The test was designed to take approximately 2 hours to administer. Initial testing with psychoanalytic experts and general psychiatry residents supported the validity and feasibility of testing this knowledge and these skills. The test may be accessed at http://psychotherapy.columbia.cursum.net. This endeavor is another example of progress in documenting resident competency in a standardized manner.

### A Canadian way

In 2004, Ravitz and Silver [85] accomplished a survey of postgraduate training programs for the Canadian Psychiatric Association Psychotherapy

Task Force to find out how psychiatry trainees learn to do psychotherapies. In the article, the authors noted that to be effective, training should be relevant to trainees, take place over an extended period of time, facilitate active participation, and integrate new learning actively into clinical work. Quoting psychotherapy researchers Henry and Strupp, the authors sought teaching methods that relied on specific learning tasks and specific feedback about the interventions. They suggested "Evaluation of expertise assesses educational effectiveness and can also serve as an impetus to consolidate learning...Evaluating competencies represents a change from documenting what is taught to documenting the residents have actually learned" [85].

Goals of education for trainees in psychotherapy include theoretical knowledge, which is easily tested in traditional ways, technical therapy skills (eg, using treatment manuals), which can be assessed using adherence measures, and clinical competence in applying the knowledge skillfully within therapeutic relationships. Innovations reported in the survey include the following:

- Clinical supervision guidelines
- Computerized patient logs
- Sequencing psychotherapy training to begin with training in the basics of psychotherapy
- Intensive small group learning that incorporates videotape review of faculty and trainees
- Psychotherapy supervisor groups
- Faculty training in psychotherapy adherence and competency rating scales
- Delay of supervisory privileges until after 1 year of participation in supervisory training

Other teaching suggestions included using standardized simulated psychotherapy patients, role-plays, creation of benchmark psychotherapy practice videos and completion of 360° evaluations (in which patients, parents, and teachers participate in evaluating trainee competence).

**Training supervisors**

*Lessons from the one-minute preceptor*

In an attempt to improve and evaluate the results of teaching in the clinical setting, a teaching model called the one-minute preceptor was developed [86]. Using this method, when confronted with a clinical question, the teacher (1) encourages trainees to commit to an answer, (2) provides supporting evidence, (3) teaches general rules, (4) provides positive reinforcement, and (5) corrects mistakes. The method takes approximately 5 minutes and provides the teacher with feedback about the trainees' knowledge. The method is powerful. A study of teaching this method to attendings illustrated other important facts about learning clinical and teaching skills:

(1) learners tend to avoid role playing, (2) those who participated by role playing learned better, and (3) providing scripted cases and small group experiences as starters loosened up trainees to more actively (instead of passively) learn this teaching method.

In general, supervisors have not been trained to supervise. To test a method of training supervisors to use more effective, experiential learning, Milne and James [87] designed a study in which supervisors were taped and given feedback on supervision. The training aimed to increase supervisors' balanced uses of all four modes of experiential learning: (1) reflection (having trainees reflect on their actions), (2) conceptualization (leading trainees to become aware of the knowledge base that might guide them), (3) planning (having reflected on actions and thought about it, motivating trainees to determine what to do next time), and (4) practical experience (encouraging trainees to engage in modeling/demonstrating correct performance, role play exercises, learning tasks, and behavioral exercises). In this study, supervision of the supervisors resulted in improved supervisory competence. The authors concluded that supervision seems to require training and that training supervisors can improve their capacity to train.

*Challenges for training programs*

As noted by Mellman and Beresin [17], the announcement of the residency review committee essentials for psychotherapy competencies generated much anxiety among training directors, who felt a sense of urgency and difficulty in meeting these challenges. Programs must specify how they will systematically teach these competencies in writing while attending to knowledge, skills, and attitudes for each competency. Valid assessment measures also must be developed for these activities and outcomes demonstrated to the residency review committee at the time of site visits. Although training directors may have newfound leverage to secure resources from their departments, department chairs/division chiefs still must find the dollars to fulfill these new requirements. Teaching time in the curriculum is already stretched to the maximum in most programs, which requires an artful balance of scheduling required, important, and competing topics [17].

## Summary

This article presented an overview and description of recent work regarding training in evidence-based therapies. It highlighted the need for training directors to help trainees understand the complex issues that affect diagnostic evaluations, a starting point for choosing an evidence-based therapy. Sources of information and methods helpful in helping trainees (and their trainers) assess the current knowledge regarding a clinical diagnostic or therapy issue were discussed. The article also provided examples of methods to teach nonspecific therapy skills by designing the curriculum's sequence to teach basic psychotherapy skills first, reviewing recorded (video/audiotaped) sessions, and providing personal psychotherapy for trainees. Evidence for methods of training specific psychotherapies by translating manualized and other research-based psychotherapies from the research and university setting to the community was presented. Finally, ideas about assessing residency competence and assessing and training supervisors were reviewed. For individuals who train child and adolescent psychiatrists, this is a time during which ideas for improved teaching are developing, with a focus on making the learning process more active and more planful and the results more measured. As therapies develop to be evidence supported, so too must our diagnostic and teaching methods.

## References

[1] Sackett DL, Straus SE, Richardson WS, et al. Evidence based medicine: how to practice and teach EBM. 2nd Edition. Philadelphia(PA); Churchill Livingstone; 2000.
[2] APA. Diagnostic and statistical manual of mental disorders. 4th Edition. Washington, DC: American Psychiatric Association; 2000.
[3] Galanter CA, Patel VL. Medical decision making: a selective review for child psychiatrists and psychologists. J Child Psychol Psychiatry 2005;46(7):675–89.
[4] Piacentini J, Shaffer D, Fisher P, et al. The diagnostic interview schedule for children-revised version (DISC-R): III. Concurrent criterion validity. J Am Acad Child Adolesc Psychiatry 1993;32(3):658–65.
[5] Rey JM, Plapp JM, Stewart GW. Reliability of psychiatric diagnosis in referred adolescents. J Child Psychol Psychiatry 1989;30(6):879–88.
[6] Jensen AL, Weisz JR. Assessing match and mismatch between practitioner-generated and standardized interview-generated diagnoses for clinic-referred children and adolescents. J Consult Clin Psychol 2002;70(1):158–68.
[7] Aronen ET, Noam GG, Weinstein SR. Structured diagnostic interviews and clinicians' discharge diagnoses in hospitalized adolescents. J Am Acad Child Adolesc Psychiatry 1993; 32(3):674–81.
[8] Hughes CW, Rintelmann J, Mayes T, et al. Structured interview and uniform assessment improves diagnostic reliability. J Child Adolesc Psychopharmacol 2000;10(2):119–31.
[9] Ezpeleta L, de la Osa N, Domenech JM, et al. Diagnostic agreement between clinicians and the Diagnostic Interview for Children and Adolescents—DICA-R—in an outpatient sample. J Child Psychol Psychiatry 1997;38(4):431–40.
[10] Herjanic B, Reich W. Development of a structured psychiatric interview for children: agreement between child and parent on individual symptoms. J Abnorm Child Psychol 1997; 25(1):21–31.
[11] Rubio-Stipec M, Canino GJ, Shrout P, et al. Psychometric properties of parents and children as informants in child psychiatry epidemiology with the Spanish Diagnostic Interview Schedule for Children (DISC.2). J Abnorm Child Psychol 1994;22(6):703–20.
[12] Comer JS, Kendall PC. A symptom-level examination of parent-child agreement in the diagnosis of anxious youths. J Am Acad Child Adolesc Psychiatry 2004;43(7):878–86.
[13] Rapee RM, Barrett PM, Dadds MR, et al. Reliability of the DSM-III-R childhood anxiety disorders using structured interview: interrater and parent-child agreement. J Am Acad Child Adolesc Psychiatry 1994;33(7):984–92.
[14] Calinoiu I, McClellan J. Diagnostic interviews. Curr Psychiatry Rep 2004;6(2):88–95.
[15] Thienemann M. Introducing a structured interview into a clinical setting. J Am Acad Child Adolesc Psychiatry 2004;43(8):1057–60.

[16] March JS, Chrisman A, Breland-Noble A, et al. Using and teaching evidence-based medicine: the Duke University child and adolescent psychiatry model. Child Adolesc Psychiatr Clin N Am 2005;14(2):273–96.

[17] Mellman L, Beresin E. Psychotherapy competencies: development and implementation. Acad Psychiatry 2003;27(3):149–53.

[18] Beitman BD, Yue D. A new psychotherapy training program: description and preliminary results. Acad Psychiatry 1999;23(2):95–102.

[19] Goin M, Kline F. Supervision observed. J Nerv Ment Dis 1974;158(3):208–13.

[20] Goldberg D. Structuring training goals for psychodynamic training. J Psychother Pract Res 1998;7:10–22.

[21] Wright J, Beck A. Cognitive therapy. In: Hales R, Yudofsky S, Talbott J, editors. Textbook of psychiatry. 3$^{rd}$ edition. Washington, DC: American Psychiatric Press; 1999.

[22] Dingle A, Beresin E. Competencies. Child Adolesc Psychiatr Clin N Am 2007;16(1):225–47.

[23] Chambless DL, Ollendick TH. Empirically supported psychological interventions: controversies and evidence. Annu Rev Psychol 2001;52:685–716.

[24] Crits-Christoph P, Wilson GT, Hollon SD. Empirically supported psychotherapies: comment on Westen, Novotny, and Thompson-Brenner (2004). Psychol Bull 2005;131(3):412–7 [discussion: 427–33].

[25] Weisz JR, Weersing VR, Henggeler SW. Jousting with straw men: comment on Westen, Novotny, and Thompson-Brenner (2004). Psychol Bull 2005;131(3):418–26 [discussion: 427–33].

[26] Westen D, Novotny CM, Thompson-Brenner H. The empirical status of empirically supported psychotherapies: assumptions, findings, and reporting in controlled clinical trials. Psychol Bull 2004;130(4):631–63.

[27] Weisz JR, Weiss B, Han SS, et al. Effects of psychotherapy with children and adolescents revisited: a meta-analysis of treatment outcome studies. Psychol Bull 1995;117(3):450–68.

[28] Kadzin AE, Weisz JR, editors. Evidence-based psychotherapies for children and adolescents. New York; Guilford Press; 2003.

[29] Kazdin AE, Nock MK. Delineating mechanisms of change in child and adolescent therapy: methodological issues and research recommendations. J Child Psychol Psychiatry 2003; 44(8):1116–29.

[30] Cassidy KL. The adult learner rediscovered: psychiatry residents' push for cognitive-behavioral therapy training and a learner-driven model of educational change. Acad Psychiatry 2004;28(3):215–20.

[31] Kendall PC. Flexibility within fidelity. Clinical Child and Adolescent Psychology Newsletter 2001;16(2).

[32] Kendall PC. Pros and cons of manual-based treatments. Clinical Child and Adolescent Psychology Newsletter 2001;16(1).

[33] Shirk S, Karver M. Prediction of treatment outcome from relationship variables in child and adolescent therapy: a meta-analytic review. J Consult Clin Psychol 2003;71(3):452–64.

[34] Burns DD, Nolen-Hoeksema S. Therapeutic empathy and recovery from depression in cognitive-behavioral therapy: a structural equation model. J Consult Clin Psychol 1992; 60(3):441–9.

[35] Joshi S. Teamwork: the therapeutic alliance in pediatric pharmacotherapy. Child Adolesc Psychiatr Clin N Am 2006;15:239–62.

[36] Beitman BD, Blinder BJ, Thase ME, et al. Integrating Psychotherapy and pharmacotherapy: dissolving the mind-brain barrier. New York: WW Norton; 2003.

[37] Bordin E. The generalizability of the psychoanalytic concept of the working alliance. Psychotherapy, Theory, Research, and Practice 1979;16:252–60.

[38] Bordin E. Theory and research on the therapeutic working alliance: new directions. In: Horvath A, Greenberg L, editors. The working alliance: theory, research, and practice. New York: John Wiley & Sons; 1994. p. 304.

[39] Horvath A. Research on the alliance. In: Horvath A, Greenberg L, editors. The working alliance: theory, research, and practice. New York: John Wiley & Sons; 1994. p. 314.

[40] Horvath A, Bedi R. The alliance. In: Norcross JC, editor. Psychotherapy relationships that work. New York: Oxford University Press; 2002. p. 37–69.
[41] Horvath A, Symonds B. Relation between working alliance and outcome in psychotherapy: a meta-analysis. J Couns Psychol 1991;38:139–49.
[42] Morgan R, Luborsky L, Crits-Cristoph P, et al. Predicting the outcomes of psychotherapy by the Penn Helping Alliance Rating Method. Arch Gen Psychiatry 1982;39: 397–402.
[43] Plakun E, Sudak D, Beitman BD. Psychotherapists CoPb: teaching the alliance across schools of therapy. Presented at the 35th Annual Meeting of the American Association of Directors of Psychiatry Residency Training (AADPRT). San Diego, 2006.
[44] Horvath A, Greenberg L. Development of the working alliance inventory. In: Greenberg L, Pinsof W, editors. The psychotherapeutic process: a research handbook. New York: Guilford Press; 1987.
[45] Castonguay L, Constantino M. Engagement in psychotherapy: factors contributing to the facilitation, demise, and restoration of the working alliance. In: Castro-Blanco D, editor. Treatment engagement with adolescents. Washington, DC: American Psychological Association; 2005.
[46] Morrisey-Kane E, Prinz R. Engagement in child and adolescent treatment: the role of parental cognitions and attributions. Clin Child Fam Psychol Rev 1999;2(3):183–97.
[47] Oetzel K, Scere D. Therapeutic engagement with adolescents in psychotherapy. Psychotherapy: Theory, Research, and Practice 2003;40(3):215–25.
[48] Hawley KM, Weisz JR. Child, parent, and therapist (dis)agreement on target problems in outpatient therapy: the therapist's dilemma and its implications. J Consult Clin Psychol 2003;71(1):62–70.
[49] Hawley KM, Weisz JR. Youth versus parent working alliance in usual clinical care: distinctive associations with retention, satisfaction, and treatment outcome. J Clin Child Adolesc Psychol 2005;34(1):117–28.
[50] Nevas D, Farber B. Parents' attitudes toward their child's therapist and therapy. Prof Psychol Res Pr 2001;32(2):165–70.
[51] Alexander L, Dore M. Making the parents as partners principle a reality: the role of the alliance. J Child Fam Stud 1999;8(3):255–70.
[52] Horvath A, Greenberg L. Introduction. In: Horvath A, Greenberg L, editors. The working alliance: theory, research, and practice. New York: John Wiley & Sons; 1994. p. 304.
[53] Beitman BD, Yue D. Learning psychotherapy. New York: WW Norton; 1999.
[54] Crits-Christoph P, Barber J, Kurcias J. The accuracy of therapists' interpretations and the development of the therapeutic alliance. Psychother Res 1993;3:25–35.
[55] Davenport B, Ratliff D. Alliance ratings as a part of trainee evaluations within family therapy training. Contemporary Family Therapy 2001;23(4):441–54.
[56] Dunkle J, Friedlander M. Contribution of therapist experience and personal characteristics to the working alliance. J Couns Psychol 1996;43:456–60.
[57] Grace M, Kivlighan JD, Kunce J. The effect of nonverbal skills training on counselor trainee nonverbal sensitivity and responsiveness and on session impact and working alliance ratings. J Couns Dev 1995;73:547–52.
[58] Kurcias J. Therapy trainees and developmental changes in the alliance. Sciences and Engineering 2000;60(11-B):5779.
[59] Mallinckrodt B, Nelson M. Counselor training level and the formation of the psychotherapeutic working alliance. J Couns Psychol 1991;38(2):133–8.
[60] Safran J, McMain S. Therapeutic alliance rupture as a therapy even for empirical investigation. Psychotherapy 1990;27(2):154–65.
[61] Summers R, Barber J. Therapeutic alliance as a measurable psychotherapy skill. Acad Psychiatry 2003;27(3):160–5.
[62] Weiden P, Havens L. Psychotherapeutic management techniques in the treatment of outpatients with schizophrenia. Hosp Community Psychiatry 1994;45(6):549–55.

[63] Henry W, Strupp H. The therapeutic alliance as interpersonal process. In: Horvath A, Greenberg L, editors. The working alliance: theory, research and practice. New York: John Wiley & Sons; 1994.

[64] Hersoug A, Monsen J, Havik O, et al. Prediction of early working alliance: diagnoses, relationship, and intrapsychic variables as predictors. Presented at the Society for Psychotherapy Research. Chicago, 2000.

[65] Lichenberg J, Wettersten K, Mull H, et al. Relationship and control as correlates of psychotherapy quality and outcome. J Consult Clin Psychol 1988;45:322–37.

[66] Sexton H. Process, life events, and symptomatic change in brief, eclectic psychotherapy. J Consult Clin Psychol 1996;64:1358–65.

[67] Kabuth B, Remy C, Saxena K, et al. The modified therapeutic alliance questionnaire for children and parents (HAq-CP). Presented at the Scientific Proceedings of the 49th American Academy of Child and Adolescent Psychiatry Meeting. San Francisco, 2002.

[68] Horvath AO, Greenberg L. Development and validation of the working alliance inventory. J Couns Psychol 1989;36(2):223–33.

[69] Luborsky L, Barber J, Siqueland L, et al. The revised helping alliance questionnaire (HAq II). J Psychother Pract Res 1996;5:260–71.

[70] Marmar C, Gaston L, Gallagher D, et al. Towards the validation of the California Therapeutic Alliance Rating System psychological assessment. J Consult Clin Psychol 1989;1:46–52.

[71] Weiss M, Gaston L, Propst A, et al. The role of the alliance in the pharmacologic treatment of depression. J Clin Psychiatry 1997;58(5):196–204.

[72] Mintz D. Teaching the prescriber's role: the psychology of psychopharmacology. Acad Psychiatry 2005;29(2):187–94.

[73] Weiden P, Rao N. Teaching medication compliance to psychiatric residents: placing an orphan topic into a training curriculum. Acad Psychiatry 2005;29(2):203–10.

[74] Byrne M, Deane F, Lambert G, et al. Enhancing medication adherence: clinician outcomes from the Medication Alliance Training Program. Aust N Z J Psychiatry 2004;38:246–53.

[75] Riba M, Balon R, editors. Competency in combining pharmacotherapy and psychotherapy. Washington, DC: American Psychiatric Publishing; 2005.

[76] Norcross JC. The psychotherapist's own psychotherapy: educating and developing psychologists. Am Psychol 2005;60(8):840–50.

[77] Mufson LH, Dorta KP, Olfson M, et al. Effectiveness research: transporting interpersonal psychotherapy for depressed adolescents (IPT-A) from the lab to school-based health clinics. Clin Child Fam Psychol Rev 2004;7(4):251–61.

[78] Mufson L, Dorta K, Wickramaratne P, et al. A randomized effectiveness trial of interpersonal psychotherapy for depressed adolescents. Arch Gen Psychiatry 2004;61:577–84.

[79] Henggeler SW, Schoenwald SK, Liao JG, et al. Transporting efficacious treatments to field settings: the link between supervisory practices and therapist fidelity in MST programs. J Clin Child Adolesc Psychol 2002;31(2):155–67.

[80] Eisendrath SJ, Lichtmacher JE, Haller E, et al. Training psychiatry residents in evidence-based treatments for major depression. Psychother Psychosom 2003;72(2):108–9 [author reply: 109].

[81] Weerasekera P, Antony MM, Bellissimo A, et al. Competency assessment in the McMaster Psychotherapy Program. Acad Psychiatry 2003;27(3):166–73.

[82] Yager J, Bienenfeld D. How competent are we to assess psychotherapeutic competence in psychiatric residents? Acad Psychiatry 2003;27(3):174–81.

[83] Yager J, Kay J. Assessing psychotherapy competence in psychiatric residents: getting real. Harv Rev Psychiatry 2003;11(2):109–12.

[84] Mullen LS, Rieder RO, Glick RA, et al. Testing psychodynamic psychotherapy skills among psychiatric residents: the psychodynamic psychotherapy competency test. Am J Psychiatry 2004;161(9):1658–64.

[85] Ravitz P, Silver I. Advances in psychotherapy education. Can J Psychiatry 2004;49(4):230–7.

[86] Bowen JL, Eckstrom E, Muller M, et al. Enhancing the effectiveness of one-minute preceptor faculty development workshops. Teach Learn Med 2006;18(1):35–41.

[87] Milne DL, James IA. The observed impact of training on competence in clinical supervision. Br J Clin Psychol 2002;41(Pt 1):55–72.

ELSEVIER
SAUNDERS

Child Adolesc Psychiatric Clin N Am
16 (2007) 207–224

CHILD AND
ADOLESCENT
PSYCHIATRIC CLINICS
OF NORTH AMERICA

# The Impending and Perhaps Inevitable Collapse of Psychodynamic Psychotherapy as Performed by Psychiatrists

## Martin J. Drell, MD[a,b],*

[a]*Department of Infant, Child, and Adolescent Psychiatry, Louisiana State University Health Sciences Center, 2020 Gravier, 7th Floor, New Orleans, LA 70112, USA*
[b]*New Orleans Adolescent Hospital and Community System of Care, 210 State Street, New Orleans, LA 70118, USA*

"There were no facts, only interpretations." Nietzche

During my training in Boston in the 1970s, described by one of my supervisors as the tail end of the "golden age" of psychodynamic psychotherapy training, psychodynamic psychotherapy was king. It was the main focus of my residencies in child and general psychiatry. In my child training, I had five psychotherapy supervisors, one of whom was a child-training analyst. One supervisor focused on counter-transference issues specifically. I carried approximately 15 hours of therapy cases, most of whom came at least weekly. Many came twice weekly; some even came three times per week. On my inpatient rotation, I had psychotherapy sessions daily with all my caseload. Process notes were expected on all cases [1]. The long stay inpatient unit on which I trained had a therapeutic/administrative split so that I could focus on the therapeutic issues of my cases and preserve neutrality from the exigencies of having to administer the ward's milieu and my case's behavior. Others managed the administration. I did the psychodynamic therapy. Likewise, the parent work was done by the social workers, again to allow me to focus solely on the therapy.

There was an active debate at the time as to what constituted a "proper" evaluation, with the senior supervisors saying that eight session evaluations were better than the six session model set forth by the "young bucks," as they called the less senior supervisors.

---

* New Orleans Adolescent Hospital and Community System of Care, 210 State Street, New Orleans, LA 70118.
*E-mail address:* mdrell@lsuhsc.edu

1056-4993/07/$ - see front matter © 2006 Elsevier Inc. All rights reserved.
doi:10.1016/j.chc.2006.09.002
*childpsych.theclinics.com*

During my 2 years in my child residency (it was not yet a child and adolescent psychiatry residency), I gave one patient medications—tricyclic antidepressants to be exact. The severely depressed 16-year-old patient who had anorexia responded well. For this psychopharmacologic act, I was roundly chastised by my supervisor, who attributed my problematic act to the chief resident on the unit who had trained at Massachusetts General Hospital, where they were "ruining the field" with in their interest in biologic issues.

I read the psychodynamic literature extensively, including Freud (Sigmund and Anna), Donald Winnicott, Melanie Klein, and Heinz Kohut. There was a superb family therapy seminar with world-class faculty, to which I paid almost no attention because it was not the reigning favorite, which was individual psychodynamic psychotherapy. Most residents were expected to have their own analysis. Many considered applying to one of the institutes. I seriously wondered if my failure to have done the first and my lack of interest in doing the latter would harm my career and my desire to be a therapist, a vocation that at that point seemed the totality of my profession. My goal was to be the best child therapist in the world!

Contrast this approach with the current situation, in which dynamic psychotherapy is not king and currently vies with numerous other treatment modalities (biologic and psychotherapeutic), many of which are distinguished by having more available and better publicized "evidence" as to their effectiveness. The chairs of most departments are seldom analysts or therapists, as they were when I trained, and are increasingly chosen for their abilities to generate lucrative and prestigious federal and pharma grants.

Inpatient units currently focus on short stays and crisis stabilization as dictated by insurance and other funding imperatives. There is little time for psychodynamic therapy, much less longer term psychotherapy. Supportive, strength-based, and cognitive behavioral therapies predominate and are often conducted by social workers and other "therapy extenders." The medical staff models a managerial style that emphasizes diagnosis, putting together measurable and objective treatment plans, and psychopharmacologic treatments. The therapeutic/administrative split divides along disciplinary lines, with the administration and management handled by the physicians who are still in charge and the other, poorer paid disciplines handling the therapeutic half of the equation.

I recall two incidents that highlight what is happening. In the first incident, I came out of my office at 10:30 AM and found an excellent postgraduate year 2 resident signing out for the day. I asked him why he was leaving so soon. He remarked that "he was done" because rounds were over and he had written his notes. In the second incident, another excellent resident on her inpatient rotation asked me if she could do more therapy. When I suggested that she could talk daily to the patients on the unit, she responded "Can I do that?" It should be noted that on that resident's unit, the attending happens to be psychoanalytically trained [2] yet chooses, in keeping with the culture of the hospital, to do mainly administrative and psychopharma-cologic duties on the unit. When I suggested to the supervisor that there were absolutely no prohibitions as to his doing psychotherapy or psychody-namic psychotherapy supervision with the residents on the unit, he replied, "When I talk to the residents about psychodynamic issues, they treat me ei-ther like I'm an idiot or a magician. When the residents ask me for psycho-dynamic formulations, which is usually after they hear that formulations are back as part of the board exams, I have to tell them that I can't do a formu-lation as they had not provided me enough data. They think I can pull for-mulations out of thin air."

In outpatient training clinics, the time spent doing psychodynamic thera-pies is dwindling. A modal evaluation seems to be approximating one ses-sion. Training directors are obligated by the last iteration of the Residency Review Committee (RRC) regulations to teach numerous therapies, includ-ing cognitive behavioral therapy, psychotherapy with psychopharmacology, psychodynamic psychotherapy, brief therapy, and supportive psychother-apy. I remember thinking at the time the regulations were changed: "If the training programs are having trouble teaching one type of therapy, does it make sense to deal with this issue by making programs teach five types?" This admirable and well-meaning prescription to teach five types of therapy is thought by many to have further diluted psychodynamic therapy training and to have lessened the overall training end product by turning out residents that are "Jacks of all therapies" and masters of/competent at none.

As for supervision and seminar time, they need to be shared with other therapies. Process notes are seemingly a thing of the past. Many residents I have encountered have no idea what they actually are. More and more residents are choosing not to have personal therapies, and membership in psychoanalytic institutes has dwindled. Biologic therapies and the neurosciences are currently the king. Long live the king?

In this article, I try to explain what has happened over the last 30 years. It is my hope that this discussion will clarify some of the current challenges to teaching and practicing psychodynamic psychotherapy and point to some ways to preserve it as a skill for psychiatrists. My personal belief is that psy-chotherapy as a general skill for psychiatrists is an endangered species that will all but disappear within our field without thoughtful and effective inter-vention. I have come sadly to this conclusion after seeing what has happened over time to my psychotherapy practice and those of my colleagues. The general response to my question to my colleagues as to whether they still conduct psychodynamic therapy is inevitably a "yes, but..." answer. "Yes, I do psychodynamic therapy, but not like in the old days." When pressed for details as to what they mean, they respond that almost all their patients are on medication and that they use their dynamic skills "all the time." When further pressed, most say that they are not conducting formal psychodynamic therapy per se. Many seem upset by this shift in their prac-tice and invariably lament that something important is being lost. They especially lament that residents do not really learn psychodynamic psycho-therapy in their residencies anymore.

Other child and adolescent psychiatrists remark that we are in the midst of a paradigm shift to the neurosciences and that psychotherapy should be seen as an antiquated vestige of the past. These child and adolescent psychiatrists tend to wonder why pediatric psychopharmacology and the neurosciences are not specified as mandatory competences to be taught like the psychotherapies. Still other child and adolescent psychiatrists take the middle road of advocating for a biopsychosocial approach in which residents are taught psychotherapies and the biologically based therapies.

From my perspective as a long time training director, I believe that the fundamental "holding environment" for psychodynamic psychotherapy has been so compromised that it is not "good enough" to support its survival. It is hard for me to conceive that the training environment in most residency programs could possibly assist residents through the difficult process of becoming therapists described by Salman Akhtar, MD in his March 10, 2006 American Association of Directors of Psychiatric Residency Training (AADPRT) Shein Lecture entitled "From Hesitation through Borrowed Faith to Conviction." In his presentation, Dr. Akhtar suggested a process that sounds conspicuously like the training I had years ago. He did not, however, mention the impact and importance of not having psychodynamics as the supraordinant organizing theory in our field. His suggestions included the following:

Having more than one faculty member who believes in therapy
Reading psychotherapy books and successful case histories
Reading studies that show therapeutic efficacy
Seeing faculty members conduct psychodynamic interviews and construct
    formulations
Seeing faculty members present their own cases over time
Being a member of a psychotherapy group
Being in one's own therapy
Having ongoing and effective supervision

I am concerned that many training programs do not provide their trainees with this host of opportunities.

It should be noted that predicting the demise of psychodynamic psychotherapy as a general skill in our field does not mean I think that psychodynamic psychotherapy will die. On the contrary, I believe that psychodynamic psychotherapy as a skill and treatment modality will continue and may flourish in the future under the leadership of other disciplines. I might add that I will continue to enjoy this form of therapy and continue to practice it, unfortunately more as an avocation than a vocation.

My way of conceptualizing and organizing my response to the question of what has happened over the last 30 years regarding psychodynamic psychotherapy has been influenced and guided greatly by the works of Jared

Diamond, a professor of geography at University of California, Los Angeles, whose interests in evolutionary biology and biogeography led to his 1997 Pulitzer Prize–winning book "Guns, Germs, and Steel: The Fate of Human Societies" [1] and the related 2004 book "Collapse: How Societies Choose to Fail or Succeed" [2]. In the first book, Diamond attempts to answer the complicated question of why certain cultures prosper economically and others do not. Throughout his award-winning book, he speaks of the importance of geography and climate and the impact they have on farming, the domestication of animals, isolation from other cultures, intellectual and commercial trade, communication, innovation, and productivity. He speaks of the advantages of certain climates and geography yet always points to the power of individuals and groups to enhance or nullify these advantages, however great.

Diamond focuses more directly on the decline and fall of specific societies in his second book, "Collapse: How Societies Choose to Fail or Succeed." In this book, he details the demise of past societies, such as those on Easter Island and Pitcairn Island, the Anasazi, the Mayan Empire, and the Norse in Greenland, and discusses the dilemmas threatening modern societies, such as those in Somalia, Rwanda, Haiti, China, Australia, and parts of the United States, such as Montana.

> "Past people were neither ignorant bad managers who deserved to be exterminated or dispossessed, nor all-knowing conscientious environmentalists who solved problems broadly similar to those we face today. They were people like us, facing problems broadly similar to those we now face. They were prone either to succeed or to fail, depending on circumstances similar to those making us prone to succeed or fail today. Yes, there are differences between the situation we face today and that faced by past peoples, but there are still enough similarities for us to be able to learn from the past." [2]

The lessons learned and premises set forth by Diamond will guide the rest of this article.

Diamond formulated a five-point framework of possible contributing factors that he believes helps to understand societal collapses. The first four of these systemically interconnecting factors are listed here:

1. Environmental damage, which refers to "damage that people do inadvertently to the environment. The extent and reversibility of that damage depends partly on properties of people...and partly on properties of the environment...Those properties are referred to either as fragility...or as resilience."
2. Climate change, which refers to "climate change, a term that today we tend to associate with global warning caused by humans...Natural climate changes may make conditions either better or worst...and may benefit one society while hurting another."
3. Hostile neighbors, which refers to other societies (or societal forces) that endanger the society. "A society may be able to hold off its enemies as

long as it is strong, only to succumb when it becomes weakened for any reason."

4. Friendly trade partners, which refers to decreased support by friendly neighbors. Societies depend on friendly neighbors and are impacted negatively if these neighbors should—for whatever reason—become weakened themselves.

The fifth set of factors involves societies' responses to its problems. Diamond stresses continually that these responses may forestall or alleviate collapse.

For the purposes of this article, I ask the forbearance of the reader to make the large conceptual leap of considering the endeavor to support, maintain, and train others in therapy as a culture or society (psychoanalytic societies) mired in problems and in danger of collapse similar to those societies Diamond refers to in his book. If this leap is made, then Diamond's five factors can be used to provide an organizational framework for my discussion. In the interests of time, I condense the five factors into two main groupings. The first group includes Diamond's factors one to four, which I term "Societal Responses Contributing to Collapse in the Training of Psychodynamic Psychotherapy." The second group includes factor five, which I term "Societal Responses That Might Forestall the Threat of Collapse in the Training of Psychodynamic Psychotherapy."

## Societal factors that contribute to the collapse in the training of psychodynamic psychotherapy

Numerous factors come to mind that complicate and impede the training of psychodynamic psychotherapy. I list them to be comprehensive, although the factors are interrelated and potentiate one another. I believe that the totality of these factors leads to a vicious downward cycle. One wonders if the entire endeavor has reached its tipping point and that psychodynamic psychiatry as performed by psychiatrists is careening down the proverbial slippery slope that inevitably comes after one reaches the peak of one's success.

### Our field focuses on different patients

It could be argued that our field has refocused on more seriously mentally ill patients. This shift, having been made, focuses on a population that is less responsive to psychodynamic psychotherapy. Because of this, the training programs have redesigned their training curriculum toward treatment modalities that better suit more seriously mentally ill patients. This redefinition of our clinical population has been in progress for decades. I first became aware of this in a seminar with Larry Silver, MD (in the early 1980s), who set forth the case that psychiatry was the only specialty in which its practitioners saw easier and less ill patients as they became more senior, that we were the only specialty that stuck so intensely to one treatment modality, and that we needed to become proficient at a wider range of treatment modalities to adapt to changing circumstances. These sentiments paralleled those set forth in the American Academy of Child Psychiatry's "Project Future" [3], which predicted and suggested forcefully that child and adolescent psychiatry as a discipline would, over time, switch to more severe and emotionally ill populations. This report greatly influenced the field and seems to have been prescient. Whether the report merely reflected the early stages of a trend that already had started or influenced professional behaviors or both is unclear. The fact that child and adolescent psychiatrists are seeing more complex and complicated cases is absolutely clear.

*Therapeutic movements have developmental lifespans of their own*

*Psychodynamic psychotherapy has run its course*

There seems to be a natural course of therapeutic movements. History shows that these various movements come and go, either being proven ineffective, less effective than other modalities that surpass them, being integrated into other modalities, or being absorbed into general practice and society. At the time of their success, these movements are all exciting and fascinating, have charismatic leaders, have no problems attracting converts and recruits, and seem to be destined for eternal life. As a matter of course, the movements demean, devalue, denigrate, and upset their competitors, which are portrayed as having been made of "baser metals." Having seen the rise and decline in popularity and predominance of many popular therapies (eg, behavioral therapy and family therapy) in my professional lifetime, one wonders if psychodynamic therapy is not succumbing to its inevitable self-limited course as new modalities, such as cognitive behavioral therapy, dialectical behavior therapy, and psychopharmacology, which are destined for the same fate, ascend in popularity.

*No coherent and effective group is entrusted with the maintenance of psychodynamic psychotherapy*

My initial thoughts concerning this factor focused on what I believed to be a failure on the part of the psychoanalytic establishment to recognize and deal with challenges to the practice of psychodynamic psychotherapy. My first drafts bemoaned the analysts' love of the status quo and their defensive "circle the wagons" isolation. Upon further thought, however, I realized that it is unfair to put the burden on "saving" psychodynamic psychotherapy on the analysts and that this was an artifact of their long-standing and admirable involvement in teaching psychodynamic principles and practices. This realization led to the larger question as to who is entrusted to ensure the viability of psychodynamic psychotherapy. Should it be the analysts, the RRC, the AADPRT, the American Psychiatric Association, the

American Academy of Child and Adolescent Psychiatry, or specific training programs? I could not answer my own question and suspect that the lack of a coordinated and effective organization or group of organizations to champion psychodynamic psychotherapy has endangered its viability. The reality, I suspect, is that many "isolated" individuals, groups, and constituencies are dearly interested in the survival of psychodynamic therapy and that each "in their isolation" is ultimately ineffective. I suspect that the dominance of psychodynamics and psychodynamic psychotherapy in the past may have led to a feeling that organization and action were not needed. After all, there used to be no need to champion this area. It was the king!

Diamond notes that "isolated groups are at a disadvantage" because "most groups get most of their ideas and innovations from the outside." I believe that individuals who are interested in psychodynamic psychotherapy have by tradition isolated themselves, circled their wagons, and spent more time demonizing and belittling their competitors than proactively responding to them.

When asked how a society could fail to recognize the dangers to their existence that seem so clear in retrospect, Diamond offers four reasons:

1. The group may fail to anticipate a problem before it actually arrives because of having no prior experiences to help it recognize the problem or having false assumptions that precluded seeing the problem.
2. When the problem arrives the group may fail to perceive it either because the change is imperceptive or is covered by up-and-down shifts that obscure its detection.
3. When dangers are perceived, the group fails to solve them because of failure to be systemic or because of selfishness and perceived self-interest on its part.
4. The group tries to solve the problem but fails because of clashes of interest in various parties, denial, group irrationality, or false hopes.

*Analytic societies are attracting fewer physicians*

Having let the analytic societies "off the hook," I do not wish to neglect their importance in this endeavor and lament the recent trend of psychoanalytic societies to attract fewer physicians. This translates into a smaller pool of supervisors and role models for future general psychiatry and child and adolescent psychiatry training. A correlated reality is that the physicians currently involved are growing older and will be less available for training should residency programs wish training to occur. In New Orleans over the last 3 years, two of the senior child analyst supervisors have died, one has retired, and one left the city after Hurricane Katrina. Only one physician analyst remains, and he is in his seventies. There are few child and adolescent psychiatrists (ie, physicians) to replenish this supervisory pool. There are several psychologist candidates that we will enlist, but the same discipline role modeling will have been greatly reduced.

*The trend toward the neurosciences*

The push toward studying the brain (Decade of the Brain) and the neurosciences has made the study of the mind and psychosocial issues seem outdated along with the psychosocial modalities that accompany them.

*The trend toward evidence-based medicine*

The trend toward the increased rise of research as an arbiter of what practitioners should be doing has been long-standing and necessary but seems to have intensified in the past decade with a more trenchant gatekeeping function called evidence-based medicine. Many practitioners feel that evidence-based medicine, in the full flush of its ascendancy, is being overinterpreted to mean that a modality cannot be used if there is no evidence of its efficacy or that presence of evidence for another modality mandates that it be used instead. A recent example of this approach came during a workshop at the 2006 AADPRT meeting, in which a training program described its evidence-based psychotherapy seminar that focused overwhelmingly on cognitive behavioral therapies as if they were the therapies with the best research. There was a brief discussion of psychodynamic psychotherapy that highlighted its meager research base. The presenters specifically mentioned a treatment manual created for psychodynamic work with children with conduct disorder. This manual was quickly dismissed as not having been researched appropriately, however. The presenters did their best to qualify what they were saying by pointing out that certain therapies, often coincidentally those that were more researched, were easier to research than others. Despite these efforts, the general tone that pervaded the presentation seemed to favor therapies with better databases. The low-lying research fruits were being enjoyed at this feast.

The vehemence of the evidence-based medicine movement seems at times to outstrip its database, which leads to conclusions that may not stand the test of time or more rigorous research. The sentiments of evidence-based medicine are worthy and understandable, but its implementation must be moderated. If not, many modalities, such as psychodynamic therapy, that are complex and difficult to research or whose impact demands a lengthy timeline that dissuades research will be relegated to a lesser status. As Einstein said, "That which can be counted may not count and that which counts may not be countable." (I would add "hard to count.") It is my firm belief that psychoanalytic therapy can be researched, should be researched, and will be researched in the future as our field figures out what it needs to count and how better to count it.

*Researchers beget researchers*

Once medical schools identify research as the most prestigious leg of the three-legged stool of research, training, and clinical service, the entire system is subtly and not so subtly configured to perform research. This priority status impacts who is recruited into medical schools via the biases of admissions' committees, who are chosen as department chairs, who are chosen for faculty, who are chosen for residencies, and who are chosen as training directors. The confluence of these choices and the lure of research grants and their overheads cannot but impact the priorities set in the curricula. Recent research initiatives, such as those spawned by the Institute of Medicine, that try to develop more researchers only further complicate the already complicated training mission. They especially harm the training efforts in psychotherapy if they specify that the preferred research is biologic. This provides still another shift away from the psychosocial aspects of our biopsychosocial mission.

### Research begets research articles

Similarly, an emphasis on research skews what articles are accepted into journals. Over the years, the *Journal of the American Academy of Child and Adolescent Psychiatry* has focused on empirical articles. This focus favors subjects that are easiest to research, such as psychopharmacologic/drug studies. There are psychotherapy research articles, but they seem to favor modalities such as short-term therapies and cognitive behavioral therapy, which are easier to research. The editors of the journals correctly state that the bar is set the same for all submitted articles and that psychodynamic therapy articles, when written to these standards, are happily accepted. Therapy articles and other articles that fall below these standards are rejected or placed in specially designated sections that relegate the work to a different—perhaps secondary—status. The complexity and rigors of psychodynamic therapy research limit its visibility in the benchmark journals for our field.

### Diagnostic and Statistical Manual-IV

The Diagnostic and Statistical Manual of Mental Disorders (DSM) was created as a research tool to ensure that varying researchers were performing research on similar and standardized populations. Its focus on phenomenology (things that can be perceived objectively) is by definition antithetical to psychodynamic approaches, which focus more on the subjective. The DSM's popularity and user-friendly cookbook quality have undermined the way our field has looked at diagnosis and how disorders are formulated. Likewise, the use of DSM for reimbursement is a powerful reinforcer of the phenomenologic approach. What is paid for becomes what is deemed important.

### There is little support for psychodynamic research

It is not by mistake that the journals are filled with psychopharmacology articles as big pharma funds research to market and license their medications. Similarly, the research into cognitive-behavioral therapy and its related therapies is provided by thousands of eager PhD candidates in clinical psychology training programs that currently favor cognitive-behavioral approaches and have a research requirement as part of their training curricula. Few psychiatry programs have ever had such a requirement. This fact means that little research was performed on psychodynamic therapy during its heyday in our field and that little research on it will occur now that other therapies—perhaps those easier to research—predominate interest in our field.

## Competing disciplines

General psychiatry and child and adolescent psychiatry are dwarfed when compared with the total number of psychologists, social workers, licensed professional counselors, marriage and family counselors, and nurse practitioners. These disciplines understandably seek to serve their own interests, enhance their scopes of practice, and increase their market share of the psychotherapy business. They do so by marketing, advertising, price concessions, general advocacy, and legislative advocacy. Their competition, in concert with managed care practices, has moderated and prevented the increase in charges for psychodynamic psychotherapy to the point at which many psychiatrists, serving their own economic interests, have switched their valuable billable hours to the more lucrative practice of medication management. Some individuals in the competing disciplines, especially psychologists and nurse practitioners, recently have attempted to extend their scopes of practice to psychopharmacology to compete with psychiatrists for market share in this arena also.

## The looming health care budget, managed care, and insurance companies

This list would not be complete without formally mentioning the complicated and complex world of health care financing. Over the past decades the percentage of the gross national product (GNP) dedicated to health care has increased steadily to the point at which society has become concerned. The response has been a panoply of decisions and legislation that have been named by many "managed care." This process has led to redefining who gets care, the types of care rendered, where this care is delivered, and how this care is financed. The results have proved a challenge for all of health care, especially mental health care. It has constrained the provision of psychodynamic psychotherapy by physicians in various ways. Some of the most well-known practices include determining that some patients' conditions, which were formerly paid for by insurance companies and other funders, will not be paid for because they are not "medically necessary," reducing monetary payments for services, providing incentives for psychopharmacologic services so that practitioners who deliver those services will be paid more per hour than for psychodynamic psychotherapy, limiting the number of sessions paid for per year, having patients pay increasing percentages of the cost (deductibles and co-pays), and limiting access via such procedures as selection panels, credentialing processes, and precertification procedures. Regardless of the necessity of these measures to ensure the economic strength of our nation, they have added many barriers to the delivery of psychodynamic psychotherapy by physicians. Many psychiatrists and child psychiatrists have shifted their practices accordingly and are delivering more psychopharmacologic services and fewer psychotherapy services. This shift has been accordingly reinforced by "big pharma," and its knowledge that there is a direct correlation between the numbers of physicians prescribing the numbers of scripts written and corporate profits.

*Stigma*

Stigma, with its subtle and not so subtle discrimination against individuals with mental disorders, must be mentioned on any list of barriers to psychotherapy conducted by physicians. Stigma and the cognitive biases that reinforce it lead to secrecy and a lack of advocacy at the levels of the individual, family, and larger society. Stigma decreases the use of all treatment services and the amount of services available, including psychodynamic psychotherapy.

## Societal responses that might forestall the threat of collapse in the training of psychodynamic psychotherapy

This section is needed only if one has come to the conclusion that there is a problem in the training of psychiatrists to conduct psychodynamic therapy. Inevitably some individuals will believe that there is no problem in the training of psychodynamic psychotherapy to physicians and that the status quo should and can be maintained. Likewise, some individuals believe that there is no problem because psychiatrists do not currently need this skill or will not need it in the future and that that there is no need to forestall its demise. In this case, individuals who believe such will either press for the elimination of therapy training from the RRC requirements and training curriculums or, if they believe that therapy training is on the slippery slope to demise as I have suggested, they need only to opt for the continuation of what is currently occurring.

Even if one does believe that there is a problem, Diamond makes it clear that there are, in certain situations, no viable solutions because the factors leading to collapse are so thoroughly in play as to be unstoppable or that forces such as conflicts of interest or group irrationality will contribute to a lack of success. Assuming that the pessimistic scenarios just mentioned do not dominate and that one feels there is a problem, then what responses can be made to ensure the viability of psychodynamic psychotherapy for psychiatrists?

*We need data on the scope of the current problem*

My sense that psychodynamic psychotherapy as an endeavor for psychiatrists is waning is based on anecdotal evidence. Ongoing research must be conducted to see what is exactly the current state of psychotherapy during the residency period and afterwards. Questions regarding the impact of the RRC regulations on therapy must be asked and answered in a sophisticated manner. Questions abound. Can we effectively teach numerous types of therapy? What is the impact of having to teach numerous types of therapy? What has been the cost of this endeavor for the teaching of psychodynamic psychotherapy? Are psychiatrists doing psychodynamic psychotherapy in their practices? If so, with which patients, how often, for how long per session, and for what duration? Research of this nature over time will help clarify whether a problem exists, what its extent is, and whether it is getting worse. Such data are necessary to mount a measured and thoughtful response.

*More research on psychodynamic psychotherapy must occur*

In this age of evidence-based medicine and empiricism, there must be a concerted effort to find the will and the funds to perform psychodynamic psychotherapy research, against "no treatment" conditions and other psychosocial treatments, and against biologic treatments. This effort may necessitate advocacy and new forms of fundraising and training. I often have advocated that psychoanalytic institutes pool their resources to create a fund to support research in psychoanalytic and psychodynamic psychotherapy. Other fundraising initiatives should be considered with this goal in mind.

*The psychotherapy research that is present must be better disseminated*

Approximately a decade ago I was asked to participate in what I thought to be "a fool's mission": to present on the research database for infant psychotherapy on a head-to-head basis against the databases for psychopharmacology and family therapy. When I performed my literature search I was pleased to find that elegant and well-designed studies on infant therapy clearly showed its effectiveness. It was interesting that the various infant therapies were proved effective for different aspects of the clinical problems and that certain therapies sustained their effectiveness or proved superior to other therapies only after the passage of time. I was even more pleased to find that the quality of the modest number of studies conducted held up well in comparison to psychopharmacology and family therapy research.

Efforts must be made to communicate better the psychodynamic psychotherapy research that has been done. Strategies for the dissemination of this research should be created, which would include the creation of review articles for the "gold standard" journals in our field and initiatives to have empirical research articles preferentially submitted to these journals. Having such articles in "guild" psychoanalytic and psychodynamic journals, where they are adoringly read by true believers, is not as helpful.

Such strategies would include an analysis of barriers to the dissemination of this information. A recent example of such a barrier was identified by the psychotherapy committee of the American Academy of Child and Adolescent Psychiatry, which noticed that the literature reviews done in preparation for the Academy's practice parameters did not include many of the psychodynamic articles of which the members of the committee were aware. A brief investigation led to the finding that this was partly because of the lack of use of DSM-IV TR diagnoses in psychoanalytic articles. When the authors of the practice parameters used DSM diagnoses as key words in their literature searches for the parameters, no psychoanalytic articles showed up. It is hoped that meetings between the committee and their psychoanalytical counterparts will lead to a solution in which DSM-IV TR diagnoses are added to the key words indices of psychoanalytic articles. I believe that similar efforts, including meeting with journal editors, will assist in disseminating the research that is available.

*Support research on all psychosocial therapies*

Although it often seems that other psychotherapies, such as cognitive behavioral therapy or dialectical behavior therapy, are the enemies, it is my contention that a larger mega-battle is going on between individuals who espouse a biologic vision of the future and those who espouse a psychosocial vision. If a biologic model predominates in our field, then all psychosocial treatments may be in danger of collapse for psychiatrists. Winning the head-to-head battles between one psychosocial therapy and another and not the biologic versus psychosocial battle may be short sighted and ultimately lead to the weakening of training for all of the psychosocial interventions. Implicit in this strategy is advocacy for a model that supports biologic and psychosocial conceptions of reality and truth.

*Individuals interested in psychodynamic therapies should unite to become an advocacy group*

To remedy factor four from the list of factors that contribute to the potential collapse of psychodynamic therapies as performed by psychiatrists, I would urge that the considerable number of groups interested in the survival of psychodynamic therapy for physicians find ways to unite into a larger advocacy group. This larger group hypothetically would be better able to define and analyze the problem and design complex and multi-pronged solutions. These solutions would include vigorous advocacy with key organizations involved in deciding the course of mental health and health care. To be effective, these efforts would necessitate subjugating the current and long-standing focus on differences in techniques, skills, underlying theories, and lengths of treatment to focus on similarities and the threat of survival for the entire field.

Once united, this new, larger consortium should ensure that it does not become a large, more articulate "circle the wagon" quorum for detailing the threats to their field and the woes that beset it. Although "misery does indeed love company," the larger group should be careful to eschew the tendency toward larger scale isolation. It is important for psychodynamic therapies to not take a "bunker mentality" stance that reinforces and rationalizes the superiority of their position as the resources and support for it dwindle. They should open themselves to dialogues with other groups and disciplines, especially groups that are skeptical of their positions. Recent cross-disciplinary efforts to identify the neuroscience and neuroanatomic underpinnings of "talk therapy" would serve as examples.

In a recent interview in which he focused on the field of psychoanalysis specifically, Dr. Eric Kandel, a Columbia University Professor and a 2000 Nobel Prize winner, summarized points two through five this way:

> "The problem with psychoanalysis, and it's a deep problem, is not with Freud. Subsequent generations have failed to make it a rigorous, biological based science. Psychoanalysis as a therapy has declined in popularity because it is time consuming and expensive. Most importantly, people have lost confidence in whether or not it works. I think its going to go down the tubes if the psychoanalytic community doesn't make a serious effort to verify its concepts and show which aspects of the therapy work, under what conditions, for what patients, and with which therapists. We need to look for the biological effectiveness of all kinds of therapy in the same way we do for drugs. I think that's the leitmotif of the next 15 years. If we can do it, we can revolutionize the field. After all, Freud said that one day in the future we will need to bring psychoanalysis and the biology of the mind together."[4]

## Go the subspecialty route

This strategy involves conceptualizing psychodynamic therapy as an "elite therapy" and creating specialty tracks and fellowships to teach it. This strategy, which has been embraced by all other specialties (eg, those that deal with substance abuse, consultation-liaison, geriatrics), assumes the need for special knowledge, experiences, and skills that are above and beyond what is expected for a trainee, in general, psychiatry or child and adolescent psychiatry. Although some say that the psychoanalytic institutes already provide such training, I contend that that route may be less effective than via mainstream training efforts and the creation of approved subspecialties for psychotherapies. It would be an added bonus if this subspecialty had a research requirement.

## Go the special track/enhanced focus route

This strategy is similar to the subspecialty track except that it would embed enhanced psychotherapy training in the regular training curriculum. Such tracks have been implemented in programs to focus interested

residents on various areas in the programs. Research tracks are being advocated as some of the ways to address the current lack of clinicians-re-
searchers in the fields of psychiatry and child and adolescent psychiatry.

Psychoanalytic institutes could assist in this strategy by offering their faculty to teach seminars and provide supervision. A model for such activities
would be the relationship between the Houston-Galveston Family Institute
and Baylor College of Medicine's child psychiatry division in the 1980s. In
that case, the Institute offered to do whatever was needed to promote interest
in family therapy, including consultation concerning the curriculum, actually
designing the family therapy curriculum, and providing supervisors and seminar participants. This collaboration facilitated Baylor's increased focus on
family therapy in its child residency and was a win-win situation for both sides.

### The Center of Excellence approach: the haves get richer while the have nots do not

In a related strategy, it has been suggested that such a specialty training
focus as mentioned in points six and seven be maintained in the programs
already strong in training psychodynamic psychotherapy. This strategy is
appealing because these programs have the necessary resources. It is less
popular with the "have nots," whose resources might not match their aspirations for teaching psychotherapy. Diamond adds an overall precautionary
note to this strategy when he states that if a society is in the process of col-
lapsing, the "haves" (ie, the chiefs and the rich) often find themselves pursuing short-term objectives, which in the longer term only obtain for them
the "privilege of being the last to starve."

### Boutique practices

A result of strategies six, seven, and eight inevitably would lead to bou-
tique practices in psychodynamic psychotherapy after one's training. These
practices undoubtedly would be "cash and carry" practices like many analysts currently have and would carry on the psychodynamic tradition, albeit
in a downsized manner. I remind my trainees that nothing keeps them from
having a psychodynamic psychotherapy practice at this point other than
financial constraints. "If you are willing to take what the insurance companies pay then you, too, can have a therapy practice." Few students see the
attractiveness of my proposition.

### Advocacy: attempt to influence the Accreditation Council for Graduate Medical Education, Residency Review Committee and the boards

This approach, which is invoked on a regular basis by organizations, is
a worthwhile one but is prone to responses that often reflect and favor
the prevailing forces, which currently are not necessarily in favor of the
training of psychodynamic psychotherapists. These organizations are

generally the agents of the "haves" and are not prone to massive innovations, which can threaten their perceptions of their power, prestige, and interests. Many organizations, perhaps because of the paradigm shifts in our field, are having trouble defining the future and subsequently their missions for themselves and are divided on what specifically to advocate for.

### Take a different tack and go generic

When faced with the swelter of more than 400 types of psychotherapy, all of which are vying for attention, there is a tendency to accentuate the differences or the similarities between them. If one takes the latter approach, one seeks to identify generic psychotherapeutic skills that all psychiatrists and perhaps all doctors need to know, including skills such as engaging patients, listening actively, being empathic, increasing motivation, and practicing countertransference. When one talks to psychodynamic therapists about the demise of therapy in psychiatric training, they often say that it would be a shame and then claim regret that the above mentioned skills would be lost if psychodynamic therapy training diminishes. One wonders if they are not making the false assumption that because training in psychodynamic therapy teaches these valuable skills, that these skills will not or cannot be taught through other methods. Are not these core skills more important than the therapeutic modalities used to teach them? Leading advocates for the teaching of core skills are Bernard Beitman and Dongmei Yue [5], who have authored a book in which they describe a curriculum that teaches a toolbox of therapeutic skills, such as verbal response modes and intentions, working alliance, inductive reasoning to determine patterns, strategies of change, resistance, transference, and countertransference. Their goal is to provide a standardized, time-efficient program that teaches the basics of psychotherapy.

### Await the demise of one's enemies

Individuals interested in psychodynamic psychotherapy could revel in the spate of bad press lately given to big pharma and medications in general. These articles about the overprescribing of medications, noxious side effects (including death and diabetes), and black box warnings might trigger a backlash that might re-enervate interest and use of psychodynamic psychotherapy. This is a possibility; however, it would, in my estimation, be better to take a proactive stance that does not leave one's fate in the hands of individuals who do not have one's best interests at heart.

## Summary

In this article I have attempted to set forth factors that I believe are conspiring to end the practice of psychodynamic psychotherapy by physicians. The list is a daunting one whose factors are certainly additive and most likely end up as more than the sum of its parts via their interrelatedness. They have been in play for years and do not show signs of major diminution, despite wishes by some practitioners that they might. They have already impacted the performance of psychodynamic psychotherapy by physicians and probably will continue to do so. There are arguments that this process is inevitable and part of a major paradigm shift for the field of psychiatry in response to exciting and revolutionizing discoveries in the neurosciences, including brain imaging, the human gene project, and psychopharmacology. Science, people would say, is inexorably moving us from a focus on the mind to that of the brain. This paradigm shift seems to have taken its toll on the practice of psychodynamic psychotherapy, although to be fair, the same focus on the neurosciences has made it clear that therapies have the ability to change brains as do the medications.

There are just as cogent arguments that psychodynamic therapy is a victim of its high costs, questionable results, and societal wishes for quick fixes and streamlined health care costs. Why pay a physician higher fees when other disciplines can do the same work for less money? There is scant evidence that psychodynamic psychotherapy as performed by medical doctors is any better than that performed by psychologists or social workers. Why pay psychiatrists more to deliver the same product just because of their increased years of education or stature?

This broad-ranging scientific/economic "one-two punch" has sent the psychodynamic psychotherapies for a loop. When science—or the illusion of such—and money saving come together, quick changes are likely to occur. Whether we, as a field, have passed the tipping point and are on the downward slippery slope is unclear. What seems clear, however, is that this situation probably will not slow or reverse without concerted efforts to address these factors. I have provided a list of strategies that might be used to counteract the factors leading to a decline in the practice of psychodynamic psychotherapy by psychiatrists. The list is certainly not exhaustive. It is up to us as a field to decide whether psychodynamic psychotherapy is worth saving and why. If the decision is made that it is valuable, then effective strategies must be used to support its continued existence. As Diamond says, "The future is up for grabs" and lies "in our hands."

## References

[1] Diamond J. Guns, germs, and steel: the fate of human societies. New York: WW Norton and Company; 1997.
[2] Diamond J. Collapse: how societies choose to fail or succeed. New York: Penquin Books; 2005.
[3] American Academy of Child Psychiatry. Project future. Washington, DC: American Academy of Child Psychiatry; 1983.
[4] Adler J. Freud in our midst. Newsweek. March 27, 2006; 47.
[5] Beitman B, Yue D. Learning psychotherapy: a time-efficient, research-based, and outcome-measured psychotherapy training program. 2nd edition. New York: WW Norton and Company; 2004.

ELSEVIER
SAUNDERS

Child Adolesc Psychiatric Clin N Am
16 (2007) 225–247

CHILD AND
ADOLESCENT
PSYCHIATRIC CLINICS
OF NORTH AMERICA

# Competencies

## Arden D. Dingle, MD[a,*], Eugene Beresin, MD[b,c]

[a]*Department of Child and Adolescent Psychiatry, Emory University School of Medicine,*
*1256 Briarcliff Road, #317 South, Atlanta, GA 30306, USA*
[b]*Department of Psychiatry, Harvard Medical School, Cambridge, MA*
[c]*Department of Child and Adolescent Psychiatry, Massachusetts General Hospital and*
*McLean Hospital, Wang 812, Parkman Street, Boston, MA 02114, USA*

Essential characteristics of good education systems include regularly evaluating the standards of teaching, monitoring the progress and development of students, and ensuring the quality of the graduates. Over the last 25 years, increasing interest developed in documenting the competency of professionals in a wide range of fields. Naturally, the education of physicians—undergraduate, graduate and postgraduate—became a focus of attention. Various organizations took the lead in concentrating on the different levels of medical education, with all groups focusing on the identification, description, and implementation of the basic areas of knowledge, skills, and attitudes considered essential for the practice of medicine: the core competencies. The competency movement promotes a model in which a defined outcome drives the educational process, unlike the present system, which is generally structure and process oriented. Within the competency framework, child and adolescent psychiatry trainees would do inpatient care until they achieved and demonstrated competence. In our current educational structure, they do inpatient work for a specified amount of time and ideally reach competence. Ultimately, the competence model will define a continuum of competencies with benchmarks for each level of medical education: medical students, residents, and practicing physicians [1,2].

## Undergraduate medical education

The accreditation standards of the Liaison Committee of Medical Education require medical schools to have learning objectives for their medical

---

Bonus material pertaining to this article is available online at www.childpsych.theclinics.com. See notations, within this article for details.

\* Corresponding author.

*E-mail address:* adingle@emory.edu (A.D. Dingle).

degree programs. The American Association Medical Council's Medical School Objectives Project was created to help the medical schools with this aim. It identified four necessary attributes of physicians: altruistic, knowledgeable, skillful, and dutiful. It recommended that medical schools use these criteria to define the undergraduate medical educational experience [3]. Brown Medical School has developed a competency model that defines nine abilities that must be achieved by graduation. These abilities were defined by observable behaviors and assessed at three levels of competence: beginning, intermediate, and advanced. New evaluation techniques were created based on identified performance standards. Students were required to achieve intermediate competence in all abilities except problem solving, which required advanced competence [4–6]. The University of Washington has implemented an integrated developmental curriculum that uses competency domains and uses a new administrative structure that emphasizes mentors and core clinical teachers [7]. Indiana University has a formal curriculum based on nine competencies and a program to implement an informal curriculum to foster professionalism [8]. Currently, medical schools are being encouraged to incorporate the competencies into their curriculum [9]. There is increasing interest in developing evaluation methods to assess students during medical school and as they transition into residency [10–12].

## Graduate medical education

In the United States, the American Council on Graduate Medical Education (ACGME) and the American Board of Medical Specialties (ABMS) took the lead in developing and determining the core competencies for all medical specialties and then ensured their use by mandating their incorporation into residency training programs by including them in the Residency Review Committee (RRC) program requirements for each specialty [2]. The ACGME oversees issues related to graduate medical education, including the accreditation of medical educational institutions and residency programs. Every medical specialty has its own RRC, which oversees residency training for that specialty. Each RRC is required to define the training requirements for the specialty and ensure adherence by regular reviews of residency programs, including site visits. The RRC program requirements for any particular program must be approved by the ACGME that oversees each of the component RRCs. The ACGME also has common program requirements for all specialties and institutional requirements for all institutions that sponsor residencies. ABMS is the organization that oversees specialty certification for physicians. Each specialty has a board that determines the criteria to be eligible for certification, the certification process, the certification standards, and the procedure by which certification is maintained. This article describes the core competencies as defined by the ACGME Outcome Project and some of the approaches that child and adolescent residency programs have taken to implement and use these competencies to enhance their educational curricula and be in compliance with the RRC requirements.

## Background

Because of growing demands for accountability from the public and health care delivery funding sources, the ACGME initiated its Outcomes Project to define the core qualities of a competent physician. The mission of this endeavor was to keep apace with other fields, such as business, aviation, and education, which had long attempted to define and assess the minimal expected standards of professional behavior. The ACGME believes that physicians have a social contract to perform certain duties as professionals and an obligation to ensure that there are ongoing means to evaluate the performance of practitioners with a mandate to maintain certain defined minimal standards. In 2000, the ACGME published the results of the project, defining the core competencies.

Six core competencies were identified for medicine; by definition, these proficiencies are considered to define the knowledge, skills, and attitudes that are essential for the practice of medicine and represent the minimal standard that physicians are expected to attain for clinical practice. The core competencies adopted by the ACGME are medical knowledge, patient care, interpersonal and communication skills, practice-based learning and improvement, professionalism, and systems-based practice. The ACGME developed basic descriptions of the expected content area for each competency with the requirement that each competency address expected knowledge, skills, and attitude and have identified associated assessment methods. The idea was that this information would be used as a structure and stimulus for the medical specialties to develop first a national consensus about the essential content in each competency for their field and ultimately to have reliable and valid methods of assessing the acquisition of these competencies during residencies and afterward [13–15]. To help with this process, in 2001 the RRC program requirements included a mandate that each program implement the core competencies in their curricula. Although national standards are highly desirable, the actual definition of each competency and its assessment was left to the individual programs.

The ACGME core competences are defined as follows (ACGME Outcomes Project):

1. Patient care that is compassionate, appropriate, and effective for the treatment of health problems and the promotion of health
2. Medical knowledge about established and evolving biomedical, clinical, and cognate (eg, epidemiologic and social-behavioral) sciences and the application of this knowledge to patient care
3. Practice-based learning and improvement that involves investigation and evaluation of their own patient care, appraisal and assimilation of scientific evidence, and improvements in patient care

4. Interpersonal and communication skills that result in effective information exchange and teaming with patients, their families, and other health
   care professionals
5. Professionalism, as manifested through a commitment to carrying out
   professional responsibilities, adherence to ethical principles, and sensitivity to a diverse patient population
6. Systems-based practice, as manifested by actions that demonstrate an
   awareness of and responsiveness to the larger context and system of
   health care and the ability to effectively call on system resources to provide care that is of optimal value

One way to understand the core competencies is to view patient care and
medical knowledge as unique to each particular medical specialty. The other
core competencies are generic and share many features across fields; there
are discussions among the ACGME and other organizations about incorporating these competencies into the common program requirements, with
patient care and medical knowledge remaining in each specialty's requirements. Currently, each specialty and program is required to define the
core competencies independently.

The psychiatry RRC included the ACGME categories in their program
requirements though medical knowledge was replaced by clinical science.
Child and adolescent psychiatry was one of the first specialties that had to
demonstrate incorporation and use of the core competencies with the
2001 program requirements, including an expectation that there be at least
one written core competency for each main competency area [16]. The next
set of program requirements, effective January 2007, will require an integration of the core competencies into the education plan with identified
methods of assessment that produce an accurate assessment of a resident's
competence in the six core competencies [17].

Implementing new mandated educational initiatives at the local level
generally tends not to be viewed by program personnel with enthusiasm
because of the reluctance to accept externally imposed directives and the
difficulties of integrating new requirements into existing curricula. The
core competencies provide some exciting possibilities for enhancing medical education, however. They provide a common structure and language
across medical specialties to define and discuss the essential aspects of capable physicians, those that all physicians share and those that are unique
to each specialty. This framework promotes the development of defined,
observable endpoints that describe the desired product of residency education: ethical, responsible physicians who provide excellent patient care.
Ultimately, this project will result in reliable and accurate strategies and
techniques to measure these qualities of physicians. Understanding how
to define and assess the knowledge, skills, and attitudes of effective, competent physicians will enhance further insight into how to refine and improve educational practices.

Traditionally, programs and individuals in medicine were evaluated and monitored by separate models and systems. Program content and quality were reviewed by the RRC and physician abilities by the American Board of Psychiatry and Neurology, a board of the ABMS. The RRC and the ACGME accredited programs; the ABPN certified individuals. The competency movement offers an alternative model—an integration of program evaluation and improvement with an ongoing assessment of its constituents, the residents. This model is in concert with what training programs had long been expected to do, namely, to certify that their graduates were clinicians who were capable of practicing competently and independently. The competencies, as an organizing structure, encourage an integrated perspective in which the program and participants are viewed as interdependent and are considered in the decisions about the desired outcome, the methods used, and the quality of the end product. Although programs continue to be accredited by the ACGME/RRC system and individual physicians are certified by the ABMS, both organizations have adopted the core competencies as an organizing framework promoting a more coherent structure for individuals as they progress through training and graduate and become practitioners.

## Resources

Over the last few years, there has been increasing data available on suggested content and approach to the competencies, in general and for specific competencies and on strategies for and types of evaluation. The ACGME website (www.acgme.org) offers descriptions of the Outcomes Project and competencies, strategies and methods of assessment, and implementation and possible resources for training programs. The website (www.aadprt.com) of the American Association of Directors of Psychiatric Training also has recommended resources and sample documentation from several programs. The ABPN also has information on the core competencies on its website (www.abpn.com). Although still limited, there has been increasing literature related to the competencies in psychiatry [2,18–24], including suggestions about how to produce an optimal learning environment for residents [25]. The Work Group on Training and Education of the American Academy of Child and Adolescent Psychiatry developed potential templates for the various core competencies [26]. Literature on how to assess various aspects of the competencies in psychiatry [24,27–31] has been growing, including information specifically for child and adolescent psychiatry [32]. Investigators also have started looking at residents' opinions about the competencies, program implementation, evaluation methods, and effectiveness and exploring methods to engage the residents actively in the competency process [33–35]. Literature from other specialties also can be helpful for discussing the issues, developing programs, and designing assessment methods, including methods to evaluate competencies across specialties [36–66].

## Using the core competencies

### Development

The most helpful approach for a residency program is to consider the core competencies for child and adolescent psychiatry residency as a general template that covers the essential aspects of a child and adolescent psychiatrist. In other words, the competencies address the traits of an individual professional, whereas the RRC program requirements specify the educational mandates for the system of training. Because the psychiatry RRC defines national standards in general terms and does not delineate specific individual methods of developing and assessing the competencies, it does mean more work at the local level. Each program has to develop its own competencies within the ACGME format, which means that there is the flexibility to develop a competency-based curriculum in a way that best fits each individual program. Unfortunately, the core competencies are an unfunded mandate, although their development and implementation are required. Early in the process of developing and using the core competencies, it is essential to review the residency program resources to determine if they are adequate. Important elements include having people who are available and willing to devote the time and energy to this project, have adequate expertise in the residency's program and structure, are knowledgeable about expected minimal standards for child and adolescent psychiatrists, and are informed about psychiatric educational practices and assessments. Personnel also are necessary for the implementation and monitoring of the core competencies curriculum, in terms of resident performance and program development and maintenance. Assessing the available resources can be helpful in determining if additional support must be obtained from the child and adolescent psychiatry division, psychiatric department, participating hospitals, or graduate medical education. For example, requests can be made for the reorganization of faculty schedules to free up time, assignment of administrative or secretarial support or funds to attend workshops, or hire consultants.

A key to successful implementation and maintenance is to consider the core competencies as a tool to enhance the program's strengths and improve areas of weaknesses, because residency administrators, faculty, and residents usually view change to improve educational activities and outcomes more positively than change to comply with the rules. Programs have used various approaches to incorporating the core competencies, and it can be helpful to get examples from several different other programs to learn about various strategies and ideas that may be appropriate or adaptable. In general, several areas should be considered when incorporating the core competencies into a child and adolescent psychiatry program (Box 1).

---

**Box 1. Initial considerations**

Program organization
- Major institutions
- Key personnel
- Decision-making structure
- Decision-making process
- Timelines
- Products

Goals

Decisions
- Personnel involved
- Review/approval process
- Approach to the competencies

---

### Documentation organization

One of the major difficulties in implementing any type of change for residency programs is that most programs exist in established, sometimes entrenched systems that can be resistant to innovations and often fail to appreciate the need for revisions and different approaches. Before starting the process and initiating any changes, it is important to understand the existing program structure to determine the best strategy to enlist support for the successful development and implementation of the core competencies and explore the possible implications of implementing the core competencies on the involved systems and individuals. It is essential to identify early the major institutions and personnel involved in the program and appreciate who is likely to be supportive or resistant and for what underlying reasons. In the interest of garnering general support, key personnel and institutions should be involved early in the process so that the core competencies can be developed and implemented in a manner that accommodates their needs and standards and minimizes disruption. For many programs, instituting the core competency approach involves a significant amount of work and developing a different way of organizing and describing the program activities and resident progress. For many academic and clinical faculty, this change may generate wariness at the least, or at worst, outright resistance and resentment. It is essential for training directors to emphasize how the core competencies can help with any current concerns and with the required accreditation process. With this new challenge comes a unique opportunity—to review what a program is doing to enhance residency training and re-evaluate its efficacy.

Having faculty and residents embrace the core competencies as a defining and organizing principle for residency training in child and adolescent psychiatry is still a work in progress for most programs. Some programs have found the following perspectives to be useful in facilitating the acceptance and actual use of this model. Framing these requirements as a new method of describing and documenting existing program and resident activities can be helpful for individuals who resent the implication that their program was not producing competent child and adolescent psychiatrists before the existence of the core competencies requirements. It can be effective to emphasize the usefulness of the competency language and framework in developing specific markers for resident performance levels that are tied to key aspects of good psychiatric practice. With clearer markers, it can be easier for faculty to give meaningful feedback—positive and negative—so that residents have a better idea of their strengths and areas that need improvement. It also can be less demanding to document poor resident performance because the format aids in describing specific deficits, often making the desired outcome and possible strategies for remediation more evident. Programs also have used the required aspect of this project to acquire additional support or resources.

Key personnel need to understand that the ACGME has mandated the implementation of competencies for the training institutions themselves. Each graduate medical education committee at hospitals and medical schools currently has common program requirements that are reviewed and legislated by the ACGME. Within these and the institutional requirements is the need for the sponsoring organization to support each of its RRC-approved residency programs and help in the establishment of the competencies. Institutions are required to supply necessary support for the mandates of the programs. The faculty should appreciate that the ACGME has provided a new means to appeal to a program's parent institution to help and maintain the systematic introduction of the competency model. Programs and faculty have a newfound authority to appeal for educational resources should they be required. Several institutions, through their graduate medical education departments, are providing support and resources by holding specific meetings for program directors and administrators about the core competencies, sharing competency documents across residency programs, offering information during internal reviews, having a resource person within GME, and providing information on and access to consultants. Some institutions even have provided personnel to help develop the competencies. Other forms of support have included sending program directors and administrators to meetings that have information on the core competencies (ie, American Association of Directors of Psychiatric Training). When asking for additional program support or resources, it is essential to be clear about why these specific requests are necessary.

Key individuals involved in the process of developing and implementing the competencies generally include representatives of the training director, division chief, department chair, institutions sponsoring major rotations, faculty with significant teaching responsibilities, and residents. After identifying which individuals should be involved in making the initial decisions about the process and the content, the next step is establishing how the process should work. Clarifying the usual decision-making structure and process in the program for various issues is helpful, and using that information to determine whether the existing structure is appropriate or if a new system for the competencies should be created. For example, a program may decide that its education committee should be responsible for the core competencies because all of the key personnel participate in the group. Another program may create a task force with designated individuals that work on the project and report back to the education committee. Whatever system is chosen, it is important to be clear about the timelines, expected products, and the approval process. Regardless of the process chosen, having informative discussions near the beginning to orient and inform the faculty and residents of the issues and plans and ask for their input can prevent later feelings of being ambushed and the spread of misinformation.

## Goals

Once it has been determined who is going to work on the core competencies, the goals for the process should be decided. A major aim is for the program to be in compliance with the RRC accreditation standards. Other possible objectives can include identifying the essential components (ie, clinical areas) of child and adolescent psychiatry, defining competency for particular stages of professional development, defining the essentials in terms of the competencies, having a competency-based curriculum that enhances residency education, describing the curriculum in a manner that fits with the nature of the program, detailing the competencies in measurable ways, designing and implementing an effective system of ongoing feedback and evaluation, identifying methods of assessment, developing appropriate documentation, maintaining consistency with national and local standards, incorporating the competencies into the current program structure and systems, and establishing methods of educating faculty, residents, and others. In general, the goal should be to preserve the character and integrity of the department and program, tailoring the competencies to existing structures, reinforcing current strengths and improving existing weaknesses, and, above all, engaging and inspiring the faculty and administration to join in the process—to become active participants in this process of cultural change.

## Approaches to the competencies

The ACGME requires that programs have all six competencies and that certain minimal language be used. Each competency must include expectations in terms of knowledge, skills, and attitudes and assessment methods. By the end of training, residents must reach the level of a new practitioner [13]. Generally, it is suggested that for each competency, certain areas be covered (Box 2). Some programs adopted the ACGME terms and language systematically, whereas others were more selective and continued to use their own terminology. Defining the various criteria and standards during the initial stages of this process can help inform subsequent activities. For example, setting down the basic principles that define competency and the level of a new practitioner can identify the essential components for the content of each core competency description and the necessary types of evaluation and documentation.

There is considerable variation among programs as to how the competencies are described and integrated into the curricula. For the competencies to be an effective and useful tool in residency education and physician development, however, they must have some meaningful connection to the priorities and aims of the program and its participants; otherwise they inevitably are viewed as more bureaucratic paperwork that irritates individuals who must read and complete new forms. Typically, the core competencies cover content and behavior that has been previously identified by the program as essential, although the format and structure may be different. For example, the various aspects of professionalism are

---

**Box 2. Competencies content**

*Core competencies*
- Patient care
- Clinical science (ACGME, medical knowledge)
- Interpersonal and communication skills
- Practice-based learning and improvement
- Professionalism
- Systems-based practice

*Content*
- Definition
- Outcome
- Expectations
- Knowledge
- Skills
- Attitudes
- Assessment
  Objective methods
  Supervision
  Independent learning
- Needs for improvement/deficiency remediation

a program requirement for the residents but may not be grouped together and labeled as such. Competency descriptions can be general or specific. These examples are from the child and adolescent psychiatry programs at Emory University School of Medicine and Massachusetts General Hospital and McLean Hospitals. A general approach is to have one general patient care competency, which includes all aspects of care that a competent child and adolescent psychiatrist should provide (Appendix 1—available online) with various experiences and evaluation methods identified as being relevant. Having more specific patient care competencies could include several separate ones for different types of psychotherapy and psychopharmacology and ones for other services (Appendix 2—available online). Some programs have revised all of their paperwork (ie, goals and objectives, evaluation forms) to use the competency framework and language; other programs only have certain key forms, such as certain assessment paperwork with competency language. Many programs do not have the resources to develop and maintain separate evaluation forms for each rotation or course. An intermediate method is to have one master form that could be modified for specific experiences if the supervising faculty were interested in doing so (Appendices 3–5—available online). Generally, it is advisable to choose the approach that makes the most practical sense, because one of the major sources of resistance to the use of the core competencies framework tends to be the amount of work necessary for its development and ongoing use. Many programs have designed the core competencies work to be created and implemented in stages (eg, doing one core competency at a time, completing one aspect of the curriculum first, or developing the descriptions 1 year with the evaluation standards and methods completed subsequently).

During the development of the competencies, it is essential to consider simultaneously what evaluation methods will be used for assessment (Table 1). Often with careful review, programs realize that many of their existing assessment strategies can be used, sometimes with minor revisions. For example, adding a brief faculty form to already occurring observations of resident-patient interactions makes this activity a type of clinical skill evaluation. New styles of evaluation can seem appealing, but carefully reviewing whether they are achievable during the initial stages of implementing the competencies is crucial. For example, portfolios are impressive, but someone must monitor them and—more importantly—read and evaluate the contents. Developing and implementing different and innovative evaluation methods and forms take significant time and energy and may be better actualized and received if done after the core competencies have been introduced and accepted. A gradual approach of using existing methods with at least one assessment technique for each type of evaluation method (objective measures, supervision, clinical skills evaluation, and independent learning) initially and then adding additional ones with time can be more manageable and effective. It is

Table 1
Sample master list of evaluation methods

| Evaluation method | Description |
| --- | --- |
| Faculty evaluations (Global rating of live/recorded performance - GR) | All rotations and major didactic series; specific for each rotation and seminar |
| | Organized by core competencies; includes new practitioner status |
| | Definitions of rating points and new practitioner |
| | Done at the end of the rotation/every 6 months; faculty review with resident |
| Faculty chart review (record review) | Occurs on several rotations; requirements vary with rotation |
| | Use review process during one rotation |
| Patient observation form (checklist) | Targets skills necessary for patient engagement and treatment alliance |
| | Required annually; can be done on any rotation |
| Faculty observation (GR) | Occurs on most rotations |
| | Videotaping of patients required for some rotations/classes |
| Case presentations (GR) | Required for most rotations and some didactic seminars |
| Patient log (case log) | Master patient list with demographic, diagnostic and treatment data |
| | Reviewed by faculty and training director |
| | Data graphed by resident and rotation to track trends/content; all rotations |
| Resident checklist (portfolio - P) | Key elements of each rotation identified; covers all rotations |
| | Resident responsible for performing; reviewed by responsible faculty |
| | Monitored during training director reviews |
| CHILD PRITE (Written examination) | Modeled on written portion of the ABPN examination |
| | Given nationally, percentile scores compared with peer group |
| | Performance monitored; done annually |
| | Test content/group performance summary, reviewed with residents, faculty |
| Child clinical examination (standardized oral examination) | Replicates the oral portion of the ABPN examination; done annually |
| | Adolescent interview/presentation and video/vignette presentation |
| | Verbal and written feedback on performance |
| Presentations (P, GR) | Required presentations on various topics in several seminars and rotations |
| | Second-year residents present in child/adolescent psychiatry grand rounds |
| Second-year project (P) | Case presentation, literature review, or research project |
| | Presented during child/adolescent psychiatry grand rounds |
| | Written paper turned into training office |

(*continued on next page*)

Table 1 (*continued*)

| Evaluation method | Description |
|---|---|
| Submitted/published work (P) | Journal articles, book chapters |
| | Posters at local and national psychiatric/scientific meetings |
| | Some residents |
| Resident goals and objectives (P) | Every 6 months by each resident; at least three goals with specific measures |
| Modified 360° evaluation | Survey on resident performance/attitudes |
| (360° evaluation, patient survey) | • Completed by various individuals; during different rotations |
| | • Over the 2 years of training; tailored for each group of respondents |
| Co-worker survey | • During two first-year and one second-year rotations |
| | • By receptionist, nurses, and social workers |
| Consultant survey | • During first- and second-year rotations |
| | • Pediatric (MD) and school (teacher) |
| Patient survey | • Adolescent in intensive treatment—second-year rotation |
| Parent survey | • Parent of developmentally disabled child—second-year rotation |
| Peer (resident) survey | • Other child and adolescent psychiatry residents |

important to include all methods that are required, however. For example, the proposed program requirements dictate the use of assessment of resident performance by multiple other individuals (eg, a 360° evaluation) [17]. It is essential to develop forms that best fit the program and are appropriate for individuals using them. Some programs developed 360° evaluation forms, which are general and with similar formats (Appendices 6, 7—available online), whereas other programs have forms that use the competencies and vary depending on the informant (Appendices 8, 9—available online). During the process, it also can help to develop a master list of the assessment methods being used for each competency (Table 2).

Although general guidelines and content areas are specified by the ACGME [13] and the RRC [17] and there are recommendations from national organizations such as American Academy of Child and Adolescent Psychiatry and American Association of Directors of Psychiatric Training, most of the decisions and development are done at the local level, which allows considerable flexibility to create and shape something that explicitly fits each program. The potential drawback is that eventually a national standard format and criteria may be developed and imposed that do not match what particular programs have been using. The more that programs share information and strategies that can inform those organizations and institutions that determine the national standards, however (ie, RRC, ABPN), the greater the likelihood that the local and national versions of the core competencies will be compatible.

Table 2
Sample master list of assessment methods by competency

| General competencies | Evaluation methods |
|---|---|
| Clinical science (ACGME—medical knowledge) | Faculty evaluations, chart reviews, observation of clinical activities |
| | Patient observation form, case presentations, goals and objectives |
| | CHILD PRITE performance, child clinical examination performance |
| | Presentations, second-year project, submitted/published work |
| Interpersonal and communication skills | Faculty evaluations, observation of clinical activities |
| | Patient observation form, case presentations, goals and objectives |
| | Child clinical examination performance, modified 360° evaluation |
| | Presentations, second-year project, submitted/published work |
| Patient care | Faculty evaluations, chart reviews, observation of clinical activities |
| | Patient observation form, case presentations, modified 360° evaluation |
| | Patient log, resident checklist, goals and objectives |
| | CHILD PRITE performance, child clinical examination performance |
| Practice-based learning | Faculty evaluations, chart reviews, observation of clinical activities |
| | Patient observation form, case presentations, modified 360° evaluation |
| | Patient log, resident checklist, goals and objectives |
| | CHILD PRITE performance, child clinical examination performance |
| | Presentations, second-year project, submitted/published work |
| Professionalism | Faculty evaluations, chart reviews, observation of clinical activities |
| | Patient observation form, case presentations, goals and objectives |
| | Child clinical examination performance, presentations, modified 360° evaluation |
| Systems-based practice | Faculty evaluations, chart reviews, observation of clinical activities |
| | Patient observation form, case presentations, resident checklist |
| | CHILD PRITE performance, child clinical examination performance |
| | Presentations, second-year project, submitted/published work |
| | Goals and objectives, modified 360° evaluation |

## Documentation

Decisions about how a new procedure is going to be documented often are considered late in the process. Logically, it makes sense that determining the most appropriate methods of documentation is easier when one knows exactly what must be recorded. Given the typical structure of residency programs, however (ie, limited personnel with multiple demands on their time and often inadequate time or support for teaching), when designing curricula that require either additional or revised paperwork, considering the parameters of documentation in terms of what participants are willing or able to complete can be instrumental in facilitating acceptance. Some programs have done minimal revisions of their documentation, choosing to have the residency director complete a summary competency document on each resident. Others have kept the same number of forms but altered them to include the various elements of the competencies. Some programs have added additional competency-related documents to their existing paperwork.

## Implementation

When implementing the core competencies, it is suggested that every member of the residency program who might have an opinion about the process or outcome be invited to participate at some level and be periodically informed about how it is going. At the very least, individuals responsible for evaluating the competencies of the residents should provide the training director with ongoing feedback and a sense of possible problems or issues. When the competency-based model is going to be introduced, it should be clear to faculty and residents what the minimal expectations are about its use and what the timeline is for further modification. Having an identified individual (eg, the training director, associate director, or service chief) who is available for questions and takes the initiative to check on the participants' initial reaction and adjustment can assist acceptance and effective use. Depending on the situation, initial individual or group orientation/explanation sessions can be useful with ongoing monitoring. Activities that can be useful include faculty and resident retreats or focus groups, or designating part of a regular meeting and scheduling special meetings to focus on the status of the competency-based curriculum. Sending regular (brief) communications such as e-mail also can keep participants informed in a nonintrusive way.

## Maintenance

After the implementation of the core competencies in a training program, some plan for maintenance should be instituted to inform the new participants (ie, residents and faculty) and provide a framework for ongoing monitoring (quality control) and continued revision and improvement. Incorporating maintenance activities into existing systems is usually more manageable than developing new required events. An effective approach can be defining the core competencies as a mechanism to define and measure the program's and individual resident's achievement and progress. Program manuals that describe and explain the core competencies and their applications within the context of the residency program's educational mission can be provided to faculty and residents during their initial orientation. The manual can be updated yearly. On a regular basis, a portion of the education committee, faculty, and resident meetings can be devoted to the core competencies, with an emphasis on examining which aspects are effective, which are not, and what must be eliminated altered or added. Alternatively, a designated task force can meet periodically. Regardless of the system, however, involved faculty and the residents should be asked consistently and repeatedly for their perspectives and input on what needs improvement and should be changed, especially in terms of the evaluation methods and documentation. Faculty and residents should review the core competencies and associated documentation formally (paper or electronic versions) at least once a year. The core competencies should not be a static entity but should develop and improve as the program's curriculum does. Ideally, the program's participants will view the core competencies as a valuable component of the educational program and will take on some level of responsibility for ensuring that the competencies are useful and fulfill their expected role.

## Postgraduate medical education

The ABPN, along with other member boards of the ABMS, have begun to use the competency model. Because physicians should have to maintain the same competencies that they had to acquire for initial competency, the ABMS adopted the ACGME core competencies as the basic structure of their certification and maintenance of certification programs. One aspect of this integration has been the formal recognition that the ABPN cannot adequately assess all of the competencies in a written and oral examination format, which is the current organization of initial board certification. It has been suggested that some components of the ABPN board certification process be formally evaluated earlier in a physician's training. There are ongoing discussions between the ABPN and other educational organizations about which areas might be appropriate and possible mechanisms of evaluation. For example, one idea is that communication skills, specifically the ability to develop rapport with a patient and conduct a psychiatric interview, should be assessed during residency because it is a fundamental characteristic of a successful psychiatrist. Another realization has been that other competencies may be more appropriately assessed in the maintenance of certification program within which the written recertification examination has been included. The four parts of this program are evidence of professional standing, lifelong learning and periodic self-assessment, cognitive expertise, and evaluation of practice performance [67,68]. In addition to the written recertification, which is required every 10 years to measure cognitive expertise, the ABPN, in collaboration with several individuals and other organizations, is developing standards and assessment measures for the other parts of the program. The ABPN disseminates information about this program on its website (www.abpn. com) and in its newsletter, *ABPN Diplomate*. An increasing body of literature is devoted to discussing approaches for practicing physicians to maintain competence with an emphasis on promoting optimal adult learning opportunities [69–82].

**Future directions**

There has been a tendency to regard the competency model as a structure that will produce better child and adolescent psychiatrists, which it may. Currently, there are not enough data to comment on the impact of the core competencies on the field. Before the competency movement, however, programs were producing competent child and adolescent psychiatrists. A primary issue that is being addressed by the competency movement is that many residency programs did not have an adequate format to describe the specifics of a competent physician and how the program knew whether an individual resident met this standard. Another issue was the concern that there was an insufficient structure in some programs to ensure that residents had to achieve a minimal standard of performance to finish training. The most likely outcome of the core competencies is that programs will continue to produce good child and adolescent psychiatrists but will have the ability to systematically describe their specific characteristics and how they were measured and programs will be better at identifying individuals who are not meeting expected minimal standards and helping them meet those standards. Another advantage of the competencies is the benefit of continual, ongoing monitoring of outcomes, which enhances the process of clear, direct feedback. This format will improve the ability of residents and faculty to reflect on and examine their performances individually and together. This recognized, agreed-upon process was not formalized before the competency requirements, and many programs struggled with how to accomplish this practice effectively. Although the competency movement is geared toward assessing outcomes, it has resulted inadvertently in providing an integral forum for mindful, reflective practice that could have significant impact on our training and education.

Another potential outgrowth of the competency model is the reduction—perhaps ultimate elimination—of grade inflation and its replacement with a more honest, genuine, and accurate portrayal of what residents actually do. Significant progress has been made in using the core competencies framework to determine and describe what a competent child and adolescent psychiatrist should look and act like and what educational experiences are necessary and sufficient to ensure these attributes upon graduation. Several areas that need further exploration are related to assessment and measurement. There is a dearth of evaluation methods with documented reliability and validity [30]. Another issue for which the field must develop a strategy is the difficulty that individuals can have in accurately assessing their own performance, especially individuals who are doing poorly. This ability is essential for effective employment of the competency model, particularly once physicians are out of training [83–85]. As the field of child and adolescent psychiatry becomes more accustomed to and familiar with the core competencies model, it should be possible to use programs' experiences to develop various effective assessment techniques that can be shared among programs, with each choosing strategies that best fit their curricula, faculty, and residents. Improvement in evaluation methods also will promote the development of more systematic strategies to ascertain and correct deficits in educational activities, teaching methods, and performances of individuals. For example, programs might be encouraged to perform inter-rater reliability studies in their clinical assessment exercises.

Another challenge, perhaps even greater than the introduction of the competencies in residency programs, is to develop an effective, manageable system to assess the competency of practicing physicians. The literature is clear that it is far easier to measure knowledge than to assess clinical performance [86]. Clinical development occurs along a continuum from medical school through residency to postgraduate practice, with an expected increasing level of knowledge and skill as individuals progress. The only current assessments of postgraduate competence are the ABMS maintenance of certification examinations and the requirements for continuing medical education credits. The field must consider what outcomes should be used as the standards of clinical competence in addition to these and how to integrate the ABPN's developing maintenance of certification program with the requirements of other institutions, such as state licensing boards and hospitals. For example, many hospitals have annual performance reviews for quality assurance, improvement, and clinical credentialing.

Finally, the core competencies approach may have serious implications for our current medical education system, which is largely time-based for medical school and residency. Individuals must achieve a certain level of ability but also must put in a certain amount of time for required rotations (eg, clerkships in medical school and essential rotations in residency). Using the core competencies framework, trainees would only have to do a designated activity until competency was reached, meaning that they may finish in less than the time allotted or require additional time. Changing to primarily competency-based educational system from one that is somewhat based on time would profoundly alter the current medical educational system [2].

## Summary

The ultimate goal of the core competency project is to foster an educational and assessment system that can define the fundamental characteristics of a competent physician, describe what experiences are necessary to develop those attributes and abilities, and reliably evaluate whether a specific physician has and can use effectively the desired knowledge and skills. It is challenging to incorporate the core competencies into a child and adolescent psychiatry residency so that they enhance the education and promote the growth of individual residents without causing the residents and faculty major distress. The potential benefits of this integrative framework are considerable and worth pursuing, however. Being able to define and measure clearly the capabilities of a prospective child and adolescent psychiatrist allows residencies to refine and supplement their curricula using clear standards and criteria and identify and remediate deficiencies in individual residents. Finally, the competency movement, if implemented properly, may result in a true continuum of knowledge, skills, and attitudes through the life of the physician—from medical school through residency and postgraduate education.

## References

[1] Carraccio C, Wolfsthal SD, Englander R, et al. Shifting paradigms: from Flexner to competencies. Acad Med 2002;77(5):361–7.

[2] Schieber SC, Kramer TAM, Adamowski SE, editors. Core competencies for psychiatric practice: what clinicians need to know. Washington, DC: American Psychiatric Publishing; 2003.

[3] The Medical School Objectives Writing Group. Learning objectives for medical student education: guidelines for medical schools. Report I of the Medical School Objectives Project. Acad Med 1999;74:13–8.

[4] Smith SR, Dollase R. AMEE guide no. 14: outcome based education. Part 2: planning, implementing and evaluating a competency-based curriculum. Med Teach 1999;21(1): 15–22.

[5] Smith SR, Dollase RH, Boss JA. Assessing students' performance in a competency-based curriculum. Acad Med 2003;78(1):97–107.

[6] Smith SR, Fuller B. MD2000: a competency based curriculum for the Brown University School of Medicine. Med Health R I 1996;79(8):292–8.

[7] Goldstein EA, MacLaren CF, Smith S, et al. Promoting fundamental clinical skills: a competency-based college approach at the University of Washington. Acad Med 2005;80(5): 423–33.

[8] Suchman AL, Williamson PR, Litzelman DK, et al. Toward an informal curriculum that teaches professionalism: transforming the social environment of a medical school. J Gen Intern Med 2004;19:501–4.

[9] Whitcomb M. More on competency-based education. Acad Med 2004;79(6):493–4.

[10] Durning SJ, Pangaro LN, Lawrence LL, et al. The feasibility, reliability, and validity of a program director's (supervisor's) evaluation form for medical school graduates. Acad Med 2005;80(10):964–8.

[11] Lypson ML, Frohna JG, Gruppen LD, et al. Assessing residents' competencies at baseline: identifying the gaps. Acad Med 2004;79(6):564–70.

[12] Morgan PJ, Cleave-Hogg D. Comparison between medical students' experience, confidence and competence. Med Educ 2002;36:534–9.

[13] ACGME. Outcome project: ACGME general competencies version 1.3 (9.28.99). 2000. Available at: http://www.acgme.org. Accessed May 1, 2006.

[14] Batalden P, Leach D, Swing S, et al. General competencies and accreditation in graduate medical rducation. Health Aff 2002;21(5):103–11.

[15] Leach DC. Building and assessing competence: the potential for evidence-based graduate medical rducation. Qual Manag Health Care 2002;11(1):39–44.

[16] Accreditation Council for Graduate Medical Education. Program requirements for residency education in child and adolescent psychiatry: effective January 1, 2001. Available at: http://www.acgme. Accessed May 1, 2006.

[17] Accreditation Council for Graduate Medical Education. Program requirements for residency education in child and adolescent psychiatry. Available at: http://www.acgme. Accessed May 1, 2006.

[18] Beresin E, Mellman L. Competencies in psychiatry: the new outcomes-based approach to medical training and education. Harv Rev Psychiatry 2002;10:185–91.

[19] Berman EM, Heru AM, Grunebaum H, et al. Family skills for general psychiatry residents: meeting ACGME core competency requirements. Acad Psychiatry 2006;30(1):69–78.

[20] Martin L, Saperson K, Maddigan B. Residency training: challenges and opportunities in preparing trainees for the 21st century. Can J Psychiatry 2003;48(4):225–31.

[21] Mellman LA, Beresin E. Psychotherapy competencies: development and implementation. Acad Psychiatry 2003;27(3):149–53.

[22] Miller SI, Scully JH Jr, Winstead DK. The evolution of core competencies in psychiatry. Acad Psychiatry 2003;27(3):128–30.

[23] Scheiber SC, Kramer TA, Adamowski SE. The implications of core competencies for psychiatric education and practice in the US. Can J Psychiatry 2003;48(4):215–21.

[24] Sudak DM, Beck JS, Wright J. Cognitive behavioral therapy: a blueprint for attaining and assessing psychiatry resident competency. Acad Psychiatry 2003;27(3):154–9.

[25] Hoff TJ, Pohl H, Bartfield J. Creating a learning environment to produce competent residents: the roles of culture and context. Acad Med 2004;79(6):532–40.

[26] Sexson SB, Sargent J, Zima B, et al. Sample core competencies in child and adolescent psychiatry training: a starting point. Acad Psychiatry 2001;25(4):201–13.

[27] Bienenfeld D, Klykylo W, Lehrer D. Closing the loop: assessing the effectiveness of psychiatric competency measures. Acad Psychiatry 2003;27(3):131–5.

[28] Giordano FL, Briones DF. Assessing residents' competence in psychotherapy. Acad Psychiatry 2003;27(3):145–7.

[29] Mullen LS, Rieder RO, Glick RA, et al. Testing psychodynamic psychotherapy skills among psychiatric residents: the Psychodynamic Psychotherapy Competency Test. Am J Psychiatry 2004;161(9):1658–64.

[30] Swick SD, Hall S, Beresin E. Assessing the ACGME competencies in psychiatry training programs. Acad Psychiatry, in press.

[31] Yager J, Bienenfeld D. How competent are we to assess psychotherapeutic competence in psychiatric residents. Acad Psychiatry 2003;27(3):174–81.

[32] Sargent J, Sexson S, Cuffe S, et al. Assessment of competency in child and adolescent psychiatry training. Acad Psychiatry 2004;28(1):18–26.

[33] Coghill KK, O'Sullivan PS, Clardy J. Residents' perception of effectiveness of twelve evaluation methods for measuring competency. Acad Psychiatry 2005;29(1):76–81.

[34] Khurshid KA, Bennett JI, Vicari S, et al. Residency programs and psychotherapy competencies: a survey of chief residents. Acad Psychiatry 2005;29(5):452–8.

[35] Frey K, Edwards F, Altman K, et al. The collaborative care curriculum: an educational model addressing key ACGME core competencies in primary care residency training. Med Educ 2003;37(9):786–9.

[36] Brasel KJ, Bragg D, Simpson DE, et al. Meeting the Accreditation Council for Graduate Medical Education competencies using established residency training program assessment tools. Am J Surg 2004;188:9–12.

[37] Brown R, Doonan S, Shellenberger S. Using children as simulated patients in communication training for residents and medical students: a pilot program. Acad Med 2005;80(12):1114–20.

[38] Carraccio C, Englander R. Evaluating competence using a portfolio: a literature review and web-based application to the ACGME competencies. Teach Learn Med 2004;16(4):381–7.

[39] Carraccio C, Englander R, Wolfsthal S, et al. Educating the pediatrician of the 21st century: defining and implementing a competency-based system. Pediatrics 2004;113(2):252–8.

[40] Chapman DM, Hayden S, Sanders AB, et al. Integrating the Accreditation Council for Graduate Medical Education core competencies into the model of the clinical practice of emergency medicine. Ann Emerg Med 2004;43(6):756–69.

[41] Crain BJ, Alston SR, Bruch LA, et al. Accreditation Council for Graduate Medical Education (ACGME) competencies in neuropathology training. J Neuropathol Exp Neurol 2005;64(4):273–9.

[42] Duffy FD, Gordon GH, Whelan G, et al. Assessing competence in communication and interpersonal skills: the Kalamazoo II report. Acad Med 2004;79(6):495–507.

[43] Folberg R, Antonioli DA, Alexander CB. Competency-based residency training in pathology: challenges and opportunities. Hum Pathol 2002;33(1):3–6.

[44] Goroll AH, Sirio C, Duffy FD, et al. A new model for accreditation of residency programs in internal medicine. Ann Intern Med 2004;140(11):902–9.

[45] Higgins RSD, Bridges J, Burke JM, et al. Implementing the ACGME general competencies in a cardiothoracic surgery residency program using 360-degree feedback. Ann Thorac Surg 2004;77:12–7.

[46] Huddle TS. Teaching professionalism: is medical morality a competency? Acad Med 2005;80(10):885–91.

[47] Johnston KC. Responding to the ACGME's competency requirements: an innovative instrument from the University of Virginia's neurology residency. Acad Med 2003;78(12):1217–20.

[48] Joshi R, Ling FW, Jaeger J. Assessment of a 360-degree instrument to evaluate residents' competency in interpersonal and communication skills. Acad Med 2004;79(5):458–63.

[49] King RV, Murphy-Cullen CL, Krepcho M, et al. Tying it all together? A competency-based linkage model for family medicine. Fam Med 2003;35(9):632–6.

[50] Lockyer JM, Violato C. An examination of the appropriateness of using a common peer assessment instrument to assess physician skills across specialties. Acad Med 2004;79(Suppl)(10):S5–8.

[51] Long DM. Competency-based residency training: the next advance in graduate medical education. Acad Med 2000;75(12):1178–83.

[52] Reed VA, Jernstedt C, Ballow M, et al. Developing resources to teach and assess the core competencies: a collaborative approach. Acad Med 2004;79(11):1062–6.

[53] Rezet B, Risko W, Blaschke GS. Competency in community pediatrics: consensus statement of the Dyson Initiative Curriculum Committee. Pediatrics 2005;115(4):1172–83.

[54] Rogers J. Competency-based assessment and cultural compression in medical education: lessons from educational anthropology. Med Educ 2005;39:1110–7.

[55] Sectish TC, Zalneraitis EL, Carraccio C, et al. The state of pediatrics residency training: a period of transformation of graduate medical education. Pediatrics 2004;114(3):832–41.

[56] Sidhu RS, McIlroy JH, Regehr G. Using a comprehensive examination to assess multiple competencies in surgical residents: does the oral examination still have a role? J Am Coll Surg 2005;201(5):754–8.

[57] Silber CG, Nasca TJ, Paskin DL, et al. Do global rating forms enable program directors to assess ACGME competencies? Acad Med 2004;79(6):549–56.

[58] Talbot M. Monkey see, monkey do: a critique of the competency model in graduate medical education. Med Educ 2004;38:587–92.

[59] Torbeck L, Wrightson AS. A method for defining competency-based promotion criteria for family medicine residents. Acad Med 2005;80(9):832–9.

[60] Weiss BD. Are we competent to assess competence? Fam Med 2004;36(3):214–6.

[61] Whitcomb ME. Competency-based graduate medical education? Of course! But how should competency be assessed? Acad Med 2002;77(5):359–60.

[62] Reisdorff EJ, Hayes OW, Carlson DJ, et al. Assessing the new general competencies for resident education: a model from an emergency medicine program. Acad Med 2001;76(7): 753–7.

[63] Delzell JE, Ringdahl EN, Kruse RL. The ACGME core competencies: a national survey of family medicine program directors. Fam Med 2005;37(8):576–80.

[64] Britt LD. A major challenge for graduate medical education. Arch Surg 2005;140:250–3.

[65] Reich LM, David RA. Comprehensive educational performance improvement (CEPI): an innovative, competency-based assessment tool. Mt Sinai J Med 2005;72(5):300–6.

[66] Wang EE, Vozenilek JA. Addressing the systems-based practice core competency: a simulation-based curriculum. Acad Emerg Med 2005;12:1191–4.

[67] Miller SH. American Board of Medical Specialties and repositioning for excellence in lifelong learning: maintenance of certification. J Contin Educ Health Prof 2005;25: 151–6.

[68] Batmangelich S, Adamowski S. Maintenance of certification in the United States: a progress report. J Contin Educ Health Prof 2004;24:134–8.

[69] Armstrong E, Parsa-Parsi R. How can physicians' learning styles drive educational planning? Acad Med 2005;80(7):680–4.

[70] Burke D. A new model for postgraduate and continuing education in psychiatry. Australas Psychiatry 2001;9(3):215–8.

[71] Johnson DA, Austin DL, Thompson JN. Role of state medical boards in continuing medical education. J Contin Educ Health Prof 2005;25(3):183–9.

[72] Sachdeva AK. The new paradigm of continuing education in surgery. Arch Surg 2005;140: 264–9.

[73] Wann S. Determination of professional competency in a rapidly changing environment. J Am Coll Cardiol 2005;46(11):1996–8.

[74] Bellande BJ. The CME professional: challenges and opportunities in reforming CME. J Contin Educ Health Prof 2005;25:203–9.

[75] Melnick DE. Physician performance and assessment and their effect on continuing medical education and continuing professional development. J Contin Educ Health Prof 2004;24: S38–49.

[76] Spivey BE. Continuing medical education in the United States: why it needs reform and how we propose to accomplish it. J Contin Educ Health Prof 2005;25:6–15.

[77] Davis NL, Willis CE. A new metric for continuing medical education credit. J Contin Educ Health Prof 2004;24:139–44.

[78] Regnier K, Kopelow M, Lane D, et al. Accreditation for learning and change: quality and improvement as the outcome. J Contin Educ Health Prof 2005;25:174–82.

[79] Leach DC. In search of coherence: a view from the Accreditation Council for Graduate Medical Education. J Contin Educ Health Prof 2005;25:162–7.

[80] Nahrwold DL. Continuing medical education reform for competency-based education and assessment. J Contin Educ Health Prof 2005;25:168–73.

[81] Price D. Continuing medical education, quality improvement, and organizational change: implications of recent theories for twenty-first-century CME. Med Teach 2005;27(3):259–68.

[82] Hammond ME, Filling CM, Neumann AR, et al. Addressing the maintenance of certification challenge: the College of American Pathologists response. Arch Pathol Lab Med 2005;129:666–75.

[83] Hodges B, Regehr G, Martin D. Difficulties in recognizing one's own incompetence: novice physicians who are unskilled and unaware of it. Acad Medicine 2001;76(Suppl):S87–9.
[84] Kruger J, Dunning D. Unskilled and unaware of it: how difficulties in recognizing one's own incompetence lead to inflated self-assessments. J Pers Soc Psychol 1999;17(6):1121–34.
[85] Eva KW, Regehr G. Self-assessment in the health professions: a reformulation and research agenda. Acad Med 2005;80(Suppl):S46–54.
[86] Miller GE. Assessment of clinical skills/competence/performance. Acad Med 1990; 65(Suppl):S63–7.

Child Adolesc Psychiatric Clin N Am
16 (2007) 249–264

CHILD AND
ADOLESCENT
PSYCHIATRIC CLINICS
OF NORTH AMERICA

# A Stitch in Time Saves Nine: Intervention Strategies for the Remediation of Competency

Dorothy Stubbe, MD[a],*, Ellen Heyneman, MD[b],
Saundra Stock, MD[c]

[a] Yale University Child Study Center, Yale-New Haven Hospital Children's Psychiatric
Inpatient Service, 230 South Frontage Road, New Haven, CT 06520, USA
[b] Department of Psychiatry, University of California, San Diego, 3020 Children's Way,
San Diego, CA 92123, USA
[c] Department of Psychiatry and Behavioral Medicine, University of South Florida,
3515 East Fletcher Avenue, Tampa, FL 33613, USA

## The art and science of training competent practitioners

As with all of medicine, training and education in child and adolescent psychiatry are both art and science. A good training director serves as the conductor for the symphony—transmitting a serious and passionate commitment to the highest standards of comprehensive care for children, adolescents and families, a dedication to residents' personal and professional growth, and a vision of the field, where it is and where it needs to go. In each institution, the instrumentation and symphonic music varies, but the basic principles apply. Excellence in training requires coordinated and well-constructed training experiences that adhere to all training requirements within multiple systems (eg, medical school, hospital, clinics), are synchronized with the goals and structure of the broader administration (eg, dean, hospital administration, chair of department of psychiatry, division chair, directors of residency training), and are harmonized with the resources and needs of the division and department [1].

The enormous personal investment required of each resident to train and the institutional and national investment in each physician provide a crucial impetus to ensure that every resident competently completes training. The large number of underserved children and families in need of child and

---

* Corresponding author.
*E-mail address:* Dorothy.stubbe@yale.edu (D. Stubbe).

doi:10.1016/j.chc.2006.07.009

adolescent psychiatric care provides an added incentive to train competent child and adolescent psychiatrists to enter the workforce [2,3].

Each resident brings to the educational and training endeavor a unique set of personal assets and weaknesses. Some students easily master the cognitive and interpersonal challenges of training. Others may excel in the cognitive skills of didactics and struggle with the complex interpersonal and systems-based challenges of working in clinical settings. Residents may have ongoing difficulties passing the standardized cognitive examinations yet demonstrate superior and seemingly effortless skill in patient care and multidisciplinary collaboration.

In an effort to ensure that all medical practitioners have mastered the basic critical skills in six content areas determined to be essential to medical practice, the Accreditation Council for Graduate Medical Education (ACGME) identified six core areas in which a resident is required to obtain competence [4]. Programs must define the specific knowledge, skills, and attitudes required for competence in each of the six core competencies and provide educational experiences as needed in order for residents to demonstrate competence [5,6]. Elsewhere in this issue, Dingle and Beresin provide a comprehensive discussion of competency training in child and adolescent psychiatry [7]. Table 1 gives a summary of the core competencies in graduate medical education.

Training programs must document training experiences and resident achievement of the six core competencies. Supervisors assist residents with

Table 1
Core competencies in residency training

| Competency | Definition |
| --- | --- |
| Patient care | Compassionate, appropriate, and effective treatment of patients that serves to promote health and recovery |
| Medical knowledge | Established and evolving biomedical, clinical, and cognate sciences and the application of this knowledge to patient care |
| Practice-based learning and improvement | Investigation and evaluation of care for patients, the appraisal and assimilation of scientific evidence, and accessing of the evidence base for treatments to improve patient care |
| Interpersonal and communication skills | Effective exchange of information and collaboration with patients, their families, and other allied health professionals |
| Professionalism | Commitment to carrying out professional responsibilities, adherence to ethical principles, and sensitivity to patients of diverse backgrounds |
| Systems-based practice | Actions that demonstrate an awareness of and responsiveness to the larger context and system of health care and the ability to call effectively on other resources in the system to provide optimal health care for patients |

areas in which they are weak, and areas of strength are acknowledged. Situations in which the normal course of training is insufficient for an individual resident to master the knowledge, skills, and attitudinal challenges of the training program must be anticipated, however. In those instances, extra assistance and an individualized plan of attaining competence—remediation of competency—are required.

Surprisingly little has been written about the remediation of competency in medical education. Residents must meet competency criteria in knowledge, skills, and attitude for each of the competencies. Failure to meet the competency criteria in knowledge or skills can be described as a "deficiency" that must be made up, for example, through access to a missed learning opportunity or repetition of previously offered material [8–11]. In contrast, the "remediation" of attitudes is a more difficult definition, which suggests that a change is required in a resident's viewpoint or even personality style [12]. Health impairments caused by physical, psychiatric, or substance abuse problems are special challenges to remediation, and federal and state guidelines must be followed regarding the impaired physician and the safety of the public.

Remediation of competence is embedded within the overall philosophy of lifelong learning and improvement. At the start of any educational or training endeavor, the novice does not yet possess the knowledge, skills, and attitudes required for competence. Remediation is the act of identifying areas that are not yet performed competently and addressing them. Learners who are not making the progress expected of residents at their level of training require remediation to ensure that the skill level is consistent with the expertise needed to perform the tasks with competence.

## Competency evaluation and monitoring in residency training

"A stitch in time saves nine." This proverb is particularly relevant to the resident remediation process. Prevention of resident difficulties is multi-determined and begins with a carefully crafted interview and selection process to increase the probability of admitting residents who will adapt and be successful in the program. Unfortunately, selection criteria for residencies tend to be poorly correlated with predictions of which medical students may excel once they are in the residency [13,14]. Child and adolescent psychiatry training directors usually have the added advantage of possessing information about resident performance within the psychiatry residency program, which would be expected to correlate more highly with clinical performance. Several variables may obscure this correlation, however. First, letters of recommendation are often hard to "read between the lines" and may be glowing for even marginal residents. The shortage of child and adolescent psychiatry applicants may necessitate less stringent acceptance criteria at times. Evidence of the resident's dedication and motivation and a clear love of the work indicate that a resident will do well and respond positively to advice and assistance, if needed.

The competency training process includes the following crucial steps:

- Completing written competency goals and objectives for each rotation
- Using assessment measures of competency that are fair and using multiple evaluators (360° evaluations), including various formats (portfolio)
- Making, implementing, and monitoring a plan for remediation if competence is not attained

The training and evaluation process should be as transparent as possible [15]. Clear expectations, open and frequent communication with residents and their supervisors, and regular and ongoing feedback about areas of strength and areas of need do a great deal to prevent serious disciplinary problems. Experienced training directors have learned that setting clear expectations and reinforcing them early in training sets a professional pattern and standard of practice that may be maintained. Allowing tardiness or inconsiderate or low-level unprofessional behavior to go unnoticed can propagate bad habits quickly in an entire residency class [16].

**Productive feedback and the art of giving bad news**

Competency-based training, assessment, and remediation use a skills-attainment model rather than an apprentice model of training. For many faculty and supervisors, this method of teaching and supervision may be new or foreign, and faculty require a great deal of education to ensure that supervision is optimally interactive, with ongoing constructive feedback, monitoring, and engagement in the difficult task of gaining the skills needed for superior practice.

Except for the rare circumstance in which a trainee has such an egregious violation of ethics and practice that termination is required, residents should receive constructive feedback on strengths and relative weaknesses in their skill set and be engaged and motivated for self-improvement on an ongoing basis. From this theoretical stance, training and supervision may be conceptualized as ongoing remediation—or remediation may be conceptualized as ongoing improvement of medical practice. Remediation is not discipline. Only when a resident does not meet required expectations for improvement of practice should the process move forward into a more disciplinary procedure.

The supervisory process, when done in a respectful and nonjudgmental manner, allows for the open discussion of areas in which a resident may be struggling. Giving this feedback early and often and addressing concerning behavior or negative test scores promptly is helpful and frequently welcomed by residents. Hearing from the training director that there is a completely unexpected negative review at the end of a rotation tends to demoralize a resident, breed resentment, and increase anxiety [1].

Faculty seminars on providing constructive supervision may be helpful in assuring greater consistency in the supervisory process. The art and science of supervision are rarely taught to trainees, so after graduation when a junior faculty member is asked to supervise, he or she may lack the skill set. Supervisors frequently emulate individuals who supervised them. As the training endeavor becomes more complex, the effectiveness of supervision becomes more important. Resources are available to assist faculty in the process of effective supervision [17,18].

The steps in the training and evaluation process include

Engaging faculty and residents in the process of competency-based training
Providing open communication and supervision about strengths and weaknesses on an ongoing basis
Having a comprehensive evaluation system that allows residents to understand their areas of strength and weakness and identify any problem areas early (360° evaluations and a training portfolio are recommended)
Ensuring that the training program has a training atmosphere that promotes professionalism and does not tolerate exploitation of residents or unprofessional behavior of any faculty or staff
Implementing a transparent, fair, and uniformly applied process to address lack of competence or unprofessional behavior

## Remediation of competency

### Remediation versus discipline

A remediation process is not disciplinary. It is a written plan to assist a resident for whom areas of deficiency have been identified. Successful remediation avoids disciplinary interventions. It requires devotion to the resident and the dedication of departmental resources to the process to help the struggling resident become successful.

Within a training program, there are multiple levels of intervention that informally—or formally—address performance problems. It must be made clear as to whether a remediation process will enter into the formal record of the resident. It also is essential to articulate whether successful remediation will result in a recording of performance problems in a resident's permanent file. Some programs have remediation strategies that expunge from the resident's permanent record any perceived deficiencies that are fully remedied, a so-called "pencil probation."

The training director also must comply with the policies and procedures of the graduate medical education office of the institution in which the training program resides. Regulations vary from one institution to another, so it is essential to be aware of regulations at the local site. The training director must clarify when he or she must correspond, formally or informally, regarding performance problems of a resident with the graduate medical education office and with the chair of the department.

If a trainee displays deficiencies in competence that are severe, pose a danger to the public, or have not been modified by a concerted and comprehensive remediation plan, the remediation process may need to enter into a disciplinary phase. Each institution has a "due process" procedure in place for trainees, and the program director should be familiar with the process and ensure that all residents are informed.

Residents are interested in what information about their performance will be conveyed to external agencies. It must be specified to the resident and understood by the training director as to what information about the remediation process ultimately is included in a resident's permanent file or noted in subsequent requests for information about a resident's performance that are received after completion of training [19].

## Identification of the resident in need of remediation

Identifying, with as much specificity as possible, the knowledge, skills, and attitudes of a resident that require remediation is the first step in solving the difficulty. To do this, clear and objective data are required about resident performance. Effective training for weaker residents relies on faculty being comfortable identifying a trainee's areas of weakness, being willing to discuss this with the resident, and clearly documenting the resident's areas of difficulties and progress in addressing them.

It is all too common for training directors to receive written evaluations indicating that a resident is functioning at the expected level despite verbal reports indicating the resident is struggling. Dudek and colleagues [20] looked at supervisors in medicine and surgery departments to assess their perspective on impediments to giving failing marks to medical students or residents. They found that the supervisors felt confident in their ability to recognize trainees with problems but did not know what specific behaviors to document. Some supervisors also felt that there was no point to failing a trainee because they either anticipated an appeal of their evaluation or felt that no intervention would occur to help the trainee improve. Some faculty felt reluctant to be the first person to identify below-expected performance for a trainee and admitted to being more willing to reflect failure in their evaluation if other supervisors shared their concerns. Having faculty get together as a group on a regular basis to discuss all of the residents' performance may help faculty feel more comfortable documenting their own assessment of an individual resident. Clearly, addressing expectations regarding documentation and potential outcomes for below average performance with the faculty is important.

## Process and monitoring of a remediation plan

Once you have identified and clearly documented the area of weakness for a resident, a specific remediation plan should be created. In a recent article, Boiselle and Siewert [21] recommend that the following questions be addressed when devising a plan of remediation:

1. What is the nature of the problem? Is it knowledge, skills, or attitude/behaviors?
2. What is the resident's perception of the issue?
3. What is the faculty member's perception of the issue?
4. Are there other contributing factors (eg, health problems or relationship problems)? For instance, according to Friedman [22], 30% of residents suffer with significant depression and 40% have marital or relationship difficulties during their training.
5. What is the potential impact of the problem? Does it impact the resident's well-being? Does it impact patient care? Does it affect others on the team?

The training director is responsible for meeting with the resident and discussing the problem. It is important to foster and promote the core philosophy—that the goal of remediation is to provide a benefit for the trainee, not to serve as a punishment.

Understandably, residents are often defensive when first approached about remediation, and care should be taken to discuss the expected outcomes in a positive light of fostering professional development and growth. A remediation plan should be crafted to target the specific deficiencies for the resident. For example, cognitive deficits may be addressed through a structured review of core content. Difficulties with interpersonal and communication skills or professionalism require identification of specific measurable expectations, clear role definition, and regular meetings scheduled with a faculty mentor.

Engaging a resident in the process of improvement of practice is one of the key challenges facing a training director. Some helpful techniques for engaging a resident in the remediation process are as follows:

Meeting regularly with each resident at times other than evaluation feedback to discuss issues of training. Review strengths and areas of ongoing improvement in the resident's professional training as a matter of course. This atmosphere of reflecting upon performance, as well as the caring and objective discussion about strengths and weaknesses, sets the stage for frank discussions if there is a need for remediation.

Having as much objective data as possible. Generalities and nonspecific criticism of performance elicit defensiveness (eg, "The staff says that you are disrespectful to them"). Specificity allows for a more productive conversation (eg, "When you told the nurse that she should be able to handle that situation without calling you, she felt that you were not treating her in a respectful manner").

Referring to training goals and objectives (knowledge, skills and attitudes) of the rotation and overall training program to help base resident performance in the context of reaching these goals during training. The goals can be helpful in clarifying the aspects of training that have not yet been achieved and aspects that have.

Asking the resident to help you formulate the specifics of a remediation plan. The resident who can help craft the solution is an engaged resident.

The remediation plan should document the nature and extent of the problem, discussions between the training director and the resident, the plan for remediation, the time interval in which the remediation is to occur, how the remediation will be evaluated during this time period, and the person who will conduct the evaluation [16]. Typically, the frequency of evaluation and feedback to the resident is increased during the period of remediation. Common remediation methods include meeting with faculty advisors, assigned core content reviews, change in rotation schedules, videotaping patient interactions, modified clinic schedules, and extended training. In some circumstances, referrals for formal monitoring, counseling, or psychiatric assessment are warranted in addition to the formal education plan. The specific remediation plan should be put in writing and signed by the training director and the resident, including any change in status that accompanies the remediation (ie, formal warnings or placing the resident on probation).

The training director should be vigilant about the approach with a resident and how this fits with the overarching institutional policies regarding due process and resident expectations. Any time a remediation plan is being developed, it is wise to involve the graduate medical education office. It may be prudent to have the graduate medical education office review the resident's file regarding the documentation of the problem, especially if the resident's status is affected or if the program wants to consider nonrenewal of the resident for the following year. The graduate medical education office also may want the institution's legal consultants to review the file. The training director must know if there will be institutional support for recommendations coming from the faculty of their program. Clear and frequent documentation is the key to effective remediation and disciplinary procedure. Many training directors are concerned about potential liability of attesting to the competency of a resident, a requirement for the resident to graduate, for whom they had concerns. The legal implications of failing to terminate a resident whom the training director and institution deemed substandard in his or her clinical performance have yet to be determined.

*Remediation of attitudes*

Remediation of attitude problems, such as deficits in professionalism and interpersonal and communication skills, presents a particularly difficult but important task for the residency training director. Residents' attitudes may be difficult to assess in an objective manner and are far less straightforward to remediate than deficits in resident knowledge or skills. Attitudes within the core competencies include various categories, such as assuming responsibility for active and continuous learning, demonstrating flexibility by respecting others, working collaboratively and welcoming diverse opinions, placing the needs of the patient ahead of one's own needs, behaving ethically, and being willing to self-observe and confront personal biases and emotions. The evaluation of these attitudes is often subjective, which may lead to misunderstanding and conflict between the resident and the training director.

Professionalism is a complex competency that has been viewed as particularly important yet difficult to assess and remediate. Studies have suggested that attitude problems and unprofessional behavior in medical school have been associated with disciplinary action by state licensing board decades later. Three domains of unprofessional behavior that were related to later disciplinary outcome included poor reliability and responsibility, lack of self-improvement and adaptability, and poor initiative and motivation [23,24]. Medical students who displayed unprofessional behavior were three times more likely to be disciplined later by a medical board [23,25]. Training directors should screen applicants carefully for evidence of attitude problems or unprofessional behavior during medical school or other residencies to reduce the likelihood of future problems with unprofessional behavior. Once a resident is hired, however, it is the training director's responsibility to remediate attitudes and unprofessional behavior when observed. Can attitudes be taught, and how should these behaviors be addressed?

There has been considerable recent interest in developing professionalism curricula within various medical schools [26]. These curricula have emphasized the importance of professional responsibility, competence and self-improvement, respect for others and professional relationships, honesty, and social responsibility. The importance of these principles has been incorporated into medical student courses and clerkships throughout the 4 years of medical school. Several medical schools have emphasized use of a professionalism portfolio to document examples of professionalism. This portfolio may include the use of self-reflection exercises or vignettes, patient testimonials, faculty recommendations, ancillary staff observations, and peer ratings similar to the 360° evaluations used by residency programs. The professionalism portfolio has been used by the dean of student affairs in composing letters of recommendation for residency application and may be used by residency training directors as one means of documenting growth in professionalism. The professionalism portfolio sends a message that professionalism to the community is an important value that must be addressed as part of the education of physicians-in-training.

Vignettes that describe unprofessional behaviors also may be used as a tool to educate residents about professionalism. Vignettes may increase awareness about standards of professional behavior and facilitate discussion in the training program about appropriate standards of behavior and the importance of professionalism. Participants, including residents and faculty, may be asked to rate the severity of unprofessional behaviors that are described in the vignette.

Once attitudinal problems have been observed, careful documentation of deficiencies is an important first step in the process of remediation. Specific deficits, such as unmet professional responsibility, lack of effort toward self-improvement, poor adaptability, disrespect for others, dishonesty, or misconduct, must be documented carefully to begin the process. The use of 360° evaluations can be highly useful in assessing professionalism or behavior problems. The best approach is direct observation by multiple observers, including faculty members, peers, patients, and staff. Residents also may be asked to make self-assessments about attitudes and behaviors. Regularly scheduled faculty discussions also can help identify important resident performance issues that may not appear on written evaluations. It is important to elicit the faculty's and resident's perception of the issue and determine whether other contributing personal issues (eg, depression, anxiety, substance use, personal or family issues) are contributing to the resident's performance problems [21,27]. Occasionally, larger system issues within the residency program may be contributing. The development of an appropriate plan takes into consideration the potential impact of the problem on patient care, other residents, and faculty.

In some instances, the training director may be concerned about a single, discrete incident or behavior, such as disrespectful behavior toward a single individual or failure to prepare for a particular educational activity. In these cases, the training director can meet with the resident to discuss the situation and perceived problem to constructively enhance the resident's professional growth and prevent recurrence of this attitude or behavior.

The more challenging situations involve chronic, pervasive problems with inappropriate attitudes that result in a pattern of unacceptable behavior by a resident. This category may include the resident who is chronically late for appointments, seminars, or meetings or the resident who repeatedly fails to respond to pages while on call. Once the problem areas are identified with the resident, specific expected behaviors should be identified (eg, arrive on time for appointments, answer all pages within 5 minutes) and remediation goals established to address these behaviors. Residents with chronic, pervasive difficulties may become defensive or highly resistant to developing insight into the significance of their problematic behaviors, which may make remediation particularly difficult.

It is frequently useful to appoint a faculty mentor who can work with residents on attitudinal issues. The attitudinal mentor may be useful to monitor and provide feedback on the identified deficits. It is essential to involve residents in developing the intervention plan and selecting the mentor to enhance the likelihood that the intervention is perceived positively by residents rather than as a punitive situation that is met with opposition. The mentor should be non-authoritarian, direct, and clear [19]. The role of the mentor also must be specified clearly. The mentor is not an individual psychotherapist. Rather, the mentor is an advisor/advocate. The mentor serves the role of confidante and counselor—giving concrete advice, providing clear feedback, and closely monitoring resident progress toward professionalism goals. In cases in which personality disorder, chronic stress, or other personal issues are contributing to the problem, the addition of psychotherapy to the remediation recommendations should be considered.

The faculty in residency training programs in child and adolescent psychiatry are generally psychiatrists. This factor has the advantage of increasing awareness about the complexities of interpersonal and stress-related behaviors and issues of transference and countertransference in supervision. The risk of diagnosing psychiatric maladies in residents who have performance issues is ever-present, however. Residency training directors must be vigilant during residency review meetings that residents who are not performing up to expectations not be merely labeled with a psychiatric disorder—Axis I or II. It is the role of the training director to maintain a focus on performance and constructive plans to help the resident change inappropriate behavior while simultaneously considering the potential that a treatable disorder may be impairing the physician's functioning.

Problems with attitude and resident behavior may at times suggest serious underlying psychopathology or substance abuse. Residents whose ability to practice medicine is affected by substance abuse or medical or psychiatric illness pose a significant challenge to the residency training director. The duty to protect the public requires identification and early intervention with residents whose ability to practice medicine safely is impaired. The concern should be discussed directly with the resident and a plan of action determined. This plan may include a mandated evaluation and mandated treatment. Issues of monitoring compliance and effectiveness of treatment should be discussed with the graduate medical education and legal offices of the institution. Residents must be informed about the limits of confidentiality with the professional providing treatment and the nature of information required by the program. Most often, a written note about issues of impairment, compliance with treatment recommendations, and progress is required, as is a medical note indicating clearance to return to work. Residents require clear written criteria for returning to the program or ending treatment and may require ongoing monitoring and periodic follow-up with a professional to ensure continued competence to practice safely.

## When remediation becomes discipline: due process procedures

If a resident demonstrates deficiencies in competence that are severe, may pose a danger to the public, or have not been modified by a comprehensive remediation plan, the remediation process may enter the disciplinary phase. Each institution must have written due process procedures that outline the process clearly for the resident and training director. The graduate medical education and legal office for the institution should be involved whenever the remediation process enters this phase. The residency training director is responsible for ensuring competent graduating physicians, and faculty should not fear legal action because of a negative evaluation of a resident's performance. The courts have strongly supported the decision of academic faculty in dismissing residents unless evidence of discrimination or other wrongdoing by the faculty exists. Residents are viewed as clinicians/faculty rather than as students by the courts as far as disciplinary action is concerned. The court has supported disciplinary actions, including dismissal of residents, in the interest of public safety.

Steps in a remediation process include

- Providing performance evaluations
- Supplying written warnings
- Providing prescriptive/remedial procedures

One formal level of action is whether a resident's annual contract will be renewed. Graduate medical education offices have obligations that require timely notice of non-reappointment, typically 6 months in advance of the point of reappointment. In some instances, a decision to not renew a contract may be reconsidered upon successful addressing of areas of performance difficulty. This decision must be articulated in advance.

Other levels of the management of performance problems include the formal placement of a resident on probation. Terms of that probation must be articulated specifically. Typically, a resident is not placed on probation until lesser measures have been used and have not been successful. In the case of probation, grievance procedures are available to residents that they may pursue if they feel that placement on probation was an unfair judgment. Residents must be aware of these grievance procedures. When a resident is placed on probation, that finding is recorded in his or her permanent file.

In rare instances, a resident may be terminated for cause. In this case, informing grievance procedures is also absolutely essential. Types of disciplinary action include

- Probation, which involves strictly written expectations for which the trainee is closely monitored, with the explicit plan for termination if the expectations are not met
- Retention, extending the training time to remediate areas of deficiency
- Nonrenewal of appointment, which provides advanced warning and a planned nonrenewal of the training appointment before graduation
- Termination—dismissal from the program—usually for egregious or ongoing professional violations.
- Not certifying for board qualification. Some training directors have graduated residents but not attested to competency in the letter sent to the board for eligibility for specialty certification. Most programs and procedures for attestation of competency currently forbid this option.

**Special issues**

*Departmental resources*

In some instances residents with performance problems may not receive credit for portions of their training. Remediation may require extension of training. Mechanisms for funding extended training must be identified. Identification may be problematic because training budgets typically anticipate the numbers of residents to be funded. There often are problems securing additional stipends, particularly if the need is a result of unsatisfactory performance. The obligation of the training institution to remediate must be conveyed clearly to the division head and chair, so that a contingency plan may be made for this potential occurrence. Using rotations that provide stipend support and finding community agencies that may fund a resident stipend while faculty (regular and voluntary) provide intensive supervision and monitoring are potential funding sources of extended resident training. Engaging the graduate medical education office, chair of the department, and the division director early in the process of remediation is essential to their engagement in the serious and essential task of training competent physicians.

*The training environment*

Although remediation of competence assumes that the nature of the difficulty lies within the resident, several training variables may confound this assumption. A residency training program that is insensitive to issues of culture, gender, and level of stress in the program erodes morale and leaves residents at risk for poor performance. Playing favorites by faculty toward certain residents may encourage acting out or other noncollaborative behaviors in an effort to be recognized by persons in charge. Some suboptimal conditions violate training requirements (the 80-hour workweek and need to monitor resident stress), and others violate laws (discrimination or harassment based on race, culture, or gender). It is the training director's job to provide a training atmosphere that is respectful and professional and monitors for appropriate professional boundaries between faculty and residents.

Residents must be able to manage appropriate amounts of stress in the clinical environment, because the work with disturbed children and families can be stressful. Excessive stress within the program must be identified and remedied, however. Trends in resident performance should be monitored. If a single resident is displaying difficulties, the intervention targets assistance and remediation of the difficulty experienced by that resident. If several residents demonstrate suboptimal performance, however, training program variables may be contributing. The training director should take feedback about the program seriously, ensure that residents have a voice in curriculum assessment and modifications, and provide ongoing monitoring of the rotations, the curriculum, and the teaching and supervisory faculty to ensure that the program provides an environment that optimizes learning and skill acquisition.

Programs require remediation if competent training is not provided. "Beginning July, 2006, the accreditation focus will be on evidence that programs are making data-driven improvements, using not only resident performance data, but also external measures" [28]. Increasingly, residency training programs must demonstrate that residents are meeting quality criteria in terms of various measures (eg, psychiatry resident-in-training examination, PRITE and Child PRITE, National Board of Psychiatry and Neurology examination scores, in-training clinical assessments) to maintain accreditation. The success of residents in the program directly impacts accreditation status.

## Components of successful remediation: the next steps

Child and adolescent psychiatry educators strive to perfect the art and science of training competent to superior physicians who then become the next generation of clinicians, scientists, and educators. Training directors are, almost by definition, role models and mentors in addition to clinicians, educators, and sometimes researchers.

There has been a somewhat arbitrary delineation of clinician versus researcher. Most training directors fit in the "clinician educator" track of academic departments. This is appropriate, because the task of curriculum development and medical and postgraduate training is time consuming and a position that requires skill and substantial expertise in administration and teaching. Training directors tend to turn over rapidly (approximately two thirds are training directors for less than 5 years), whereas the career educator (approximately one third of child and adolescent psychiatry training directors) is an immensely satisfying academic niche for many [29].

The mission of medical educators in all fields is to perfect the science and the art of training competent physicians and the next generation of leaders. To do this, outcomes research regarding effective training and supervision techniques and curricula, the optimal educational environment, assessment, and remediation of competency is needed. The ACGME has provided the impetus, but it is incumbent upon training directors to continue to provide the primary leadership for the field of training. The areas that are ripe for research and development include effective curricula, effective evaluation and remediation of competency, and leadership skill development. As medicine becomes more complex, so does the task of training physicians. Joint monitoring and outcomes research of the training enterprise are the scholarly and academic missions of the present and the future.

## References

[1] Stubbe D, Beresin E. Education and training in child and adolescent psychiatry Martin A, Volkmar F, editors. Lewis textbook of child and adolescent psychiatry. 4th edition. New York: Lippincott Williams and Wilkins; 2007, in press.

[2] Kim WJ. Child and adolescent psychiatry workforce: a critical shortage and national challenge. Acad Psychiatry 2003;27:277–82.

[3] US Public Health Service. Report of the surgeon general's conference on children's mental health: a national action agenda. Washington, DC: Department of Health and Human Services; 2000.

[4] Accreditation Council for Graduate Medical Education. Outcome project: ACGME general competencies version 1.3. Chicago (IL): ACGME; 2000.

[5] Sargent J, Sexson S, Cuffe S, et al. Assessment of competency in child and adolescent psychiatry training. Acad Psychiatry 2004;28:18–26.

[6] Sexson S, Sargent J, Zima B, et al. Sample core competencies in child and adolescent psychiatry training: a starting point. Acad Psychiatry 2001;25:201–13.

[7] Dingle A, Beresin E. Competencies. Child Adolesc Psychiatr Clin N Am 2007;16(1): in press.

[8] Boiselle PM. A remedy for resident evaluation and remediation. Acad Radiol 2005;12:894–900.

[9] Doty CI, Lucchesi M. The value of a web-based testing system to identify residents who need early remediation: what are we waiting for? Acad Emerg Med 2004;11:324.

[10] Schwind CJ, Williams RG, Boehler ML, et al. Do individual attendings' post-rotation performance ratings detect residents' clinical performance deficiencies? Acad Med 2004;79:453–7.

[11] Turnbull J, Carbotte R, Hanna E, et al. Cognitive difficulties in physicians. Acad Med 2000;75:177–81.

[12] Hays RB, Jolly BC, Caldon LJ, et al. Is insight important? Measuring capacity to change performance. Med Educ 2002;36:965–71.

[13] Metro DG, Talarico JF. Your admission process can help you. American Council for Graduate Medical Education Bulletin 2006;7–9.

[14] Dawkins K, Ekstrom RD, Maltbie A, et al. The relationship between psychiatry residency application evaluations and subsequent residency performance. American Council for Graduate Medical Education Bulletin 2006;9–11.

[15] Larkin GL, McKay MP, Angelos P. Six core competencies and seven deadly sins: a virtues-based approach to the new guidelines for graduate medical education. Surgery 2005;138(3):490–7.

[16] Borus JF. Recognizing and managing resident's problems and problem residents. Acad Radiol 1997;4:527–33.

[17] Bernard JM, Goodyear RK. Fundamentals of clinical supervision. 3rd edition. New York: Allyn & Bacon; 2003.

[18] Falvey JE, Cohen C, Caldwell CF. Documentation in supervision: the Focused Risk Management Supervision System (Formss). New York: Wadsworth; 2001.

[19] Stubbe DE, Sexson S, Bartell A, et al. Competency remediation in child and adolescent psychiatry training. Acad Psychiatry, submitted for publication.

[20] Dudek NL, Marks MB, Regehr G. Failure to fail: the perspectives of clinical supervisors. Acad Med 2005;80(10):S84–7.

[21] Boiselle PM, Siewert B. A multi-faceted approach to resident evaluation and remediation. American Council for Graduate Medical Education Bulletin 2006;48–50.

[22] Friedman RS. A primer on stress for house staff, educators, administrators and risk managers. Risk Management Foundation of Harvard Medical Institute Forum 1993;14:10–1.

[23] Teherani A, Hodgson CS, Papadakis BM. Domains of unprofessional behavior during medical school associated with future disciplinary action by a state medical board. Acad Med 2005;80(10 Suppl):S17–20.

[24] Teherani A. How can we improve the assessment of professionalism behaviors in graduate medical education? American Council for Graduate Medical Education Bulletin 2006;5–7.

[25] Papadakis MA, Teherani A, Banach MA, et al. Disciplinary action by medical boards and prior behavior in medical school. N Engl J Med 2005;353:2673–82.

[26] Suchman AL, Williamson PR, Litzelman DK, et al. Toward an informal curriculum that teaches professionalism: transforming the social environment of a medical school. J Gen Intern Med 2004;19:501–4.

[27] Reamy BV, Harman JH. Residents in trouble: an in-depth assessment of the 25-year experience of a single family medicine residency. Fam Med 2006;38(4):252–7.

[28] Derstine P. Turning the challenge into opportunity. American Council for Graduate Medical Education Bulletin 2006;1–3.

[29] Beresin EV. The administration of residency training programs. Child Adolesc Psychiatr Clin N Am 2002;11:67–89.

**ELSEVIER
SAUNDERS**

Child Adolesc Psychiatric Clin N Am
16 (2007) 265–270

CHILD AND
ADOLESCENT
PSYCHIATRIC CLINICS
OF NORTH AMERICA

# Index

*Note:* Page numbers of article titles are in **boldface** type.

# Moving?

## Make sure your subscription moves with you!

To notify us of your new address, find your **Clinics Account Number** (located on your mailing label above your name), and contact customer service at:

E-mail: elspcs@elsevier.com

800-654-2452 (subscribers in the U.S. & Canada)
407-345-4000 (subscribers outside of the U.S. & Canada)

Fax number: 407-363-9661

**Elsevier Periodicals Customer Service**
6277 Sea Harbor Drive
Orlando, FL  32887-4800

*To ensure uninterrupted delivery of your subscription, please notify us at least 4 weeks in advance of move.